Antibacterial Therapy and Newer Agents

Guest Editors

KEITH S. KAYE, MD, MPH
DONALD KAYE, MD

MEDICAL CLINICS
OF NORTH AMERICA

www.medical.theclinics.com

July 2011 • Volume 95 • Number 4

SAUNDERS an imprint of ELSEVIER, Inc.

W.B. SAUNDERS COMPANY
A Division of Elsevier Inc.

1600 John F. Kennedy Boulevard • Suite 1800 • Philadelphia, Pennsylvania 19103-2899

http://www.theclinics.com

MEDICAL CLINICS OF NORTH AMERICA Volume 95, Number 4
July 2011 ISSN 0025-7125, ISBN-13: 978-1-4557-2291-4

Editor: Rachel Glover
Developmental Editor: Donald Mumford

Medical Clinics of North America (ISSN 0025-7125) is published bimonthly by Elsevier Inc., 360 Park Avenue South, New York, NY 10010-1710. Months of issue are January, March, May, July, September, and November. Periodicals postage paid at New York, NY, and additional mailing offices. Subscription prices are USD 218 per year for US individuals, USD 404 per year for US institutions, USD 110 per year for US students, USD 277 per year for Canadian individuals, USD 525 per year for Canadian institutions, USD 173 per year for Canadian students, USD 336 per year for international individuals, USD 525 per year for international institutions and USD 173 per year for international students. To receive student/resident rate, orders must be accompanied by name of affiliated institution, date of term, and the *signature* of program/residency coordinator on institution letterhead. Orders will be billed at individual rate until proof of status is received. Foreign air speed delivery is included in all *Clinics* subscription prices. All prices are subject to change without notice. **POSTMASTER:** Send address changes to *Medical Clinics of North America*, Elsevier Health Sciences Division, Subscription Customer Service, 3251 Riverport Lane, Maryland Heights, MO 63043. **Customer Service: Telephone: 1-800-654-2452** (U.S. and Canada); **1-314-447-8871** (outside U.S. and Canada). **Fax: 1-314-447-8029. E-mail: journalscustomerservice-usa@elsevier.com** (for print support); **journalsonlinesupport-usa@ elsevier.com** (for online support).

Reprints. For copies of 100 or more of articles in this publication, please contact the Commercial Reprints Department, Elsevier Inc., 360 Park Avenue South, New York, NY 10010-1710. Tel.: 212-633-3812; Fax: 212-462-1935; E-mail: reprints@elsevier.com.

Medical Clinics of North America is also published in Spanish by McGraw-Hill Interamericana Editores S. A., P.O. Box 5-237, 06500 Mexico, D.F., Mexico.

Medical Clinics of North America is covered in *MEDLINE/PubMed (Index Medicus), Current Contents, ASCA, Excerpta Medica, Science Citation Index*, and *ISI/BIOMED*.

Printed in the United States of America.

GOAL STATEMENT

The goal of *Medical Clinics of North America* is to keep practicing physicians up to date with current clinical practice by providing timely articles reviewing the state of the art in patient care.

ACCREDITATION

The *Medical Clinics of North America* is planned and implemented in accordance with the Essential Areas and Policies of the Accreditation Council for Continuing Medical Education (ACCME) through the joint sponsorship of the University of Virginia School of Medicine and Elsevier. The University of Virginia School of Medicine is accredited by the ACCME to provide continuing medical education for physicians.

The University of Virginia School of Medicine designates this educational activity for a maximum of 15 *AMA PRA Category 1 Credits*™ for each issue, 90 credits per year. Physicians should only claim credit commensurate with the extent of their participation in the activity.

The American Medical Association has determined that physicians not licensed in the US who participate in this CME activity are eligible for a maximum of 15 *AMA PRA Category 1 Credits*™ for each issue, 90 credits per year.

Credit can be earned by reading the text material, taking the CME examination online at http://www.theclinics.com/home/cme, and completing the evaluation. After taking the test, you will be required to review any and all incorrect answers. Following completion of the test and evaluation, your credit will be awarded and you may print your certificate.

FACULTY DISCLOSURE/CONFLICT OF INTEREST

The University of Virginia School of Medicine, as an ACCME accredited provider, endorses and strives to comply with the Accreditation Council for Continuing Medical Education (ACCME) Standards of Commercial Support, Commonwealth of Virginia statutes, University of Virginia policies and procedures, and associated federal and private regulations and guidelines on the need for disclosure and monitoring of proprietary and financial interests that may affect the scientific integrity and balance of content delivered in continuing medical education activities under our auspices.

The University of Virginia School of Medicine requires that all CME activities accredited through this institution be developed independently and be scientifically rigorous, balanced and objective in the presentation/discussion of its content, theories and practices.

All authors/editors participating in an accredited CME activity are expected to disclose to the readers relevant financial relationships with commercial entities occurring within the past 12 months (such as grants or research support, employee, consultant, stock holder, member of speakers bureau, etc.). The University of Virginia School of Medicine will employ appropriate mechanisms to resolve potential conflicts of interest to maintain the standards of fair and balanced education to the reader. Questions about specific strategies can be directed to the Office of Continuing Medical Education, University of Virginia School of Medicine, Charlottesville, Virginia.

The faculty and staff of the University of Virginia Office of Continuing Medical Education have no financial affiliations to disclose.

The authors/editors listed below have identified no professional or financial affiliations for themselves or their spouse/partner:
Jose A. Bazan, DO; Maureen K. Bolon, MD, MS; Barthomelow R. Bono, MD; Teena Chopra, MD; Rachel Glover (Acquisitions Editor); Donald Kaye, MD (Guest Editor); Lawrence L. Livornese Jr, MD, FIDSA; Stanley I. Martin, MD; Fozia Qamar, MD; Paul Robbins, DO; Andrew Wolf, MD (Test Author); and Jerry M. Zuckerman, MD.

The authors/editors listed below identified the following professional or financial affiliations for themselves or their spouse/partner:
Luke F. Chen, MBBS (Hons), MPH, CIC, FRACP is a consultant for Medscape, and is an industry funded research/investigator for Merck, Inc.
Brett Gilbert, DO is on the Speakers' Bureau for Pfizer and Merck.
Keith S. Kaye, MD, MPH (Guest Editor) is a consultant for Forest, Merck, and Pfizer, and is an industry funded research/investigator for Merck and Pfizer.
Elaine T. Kaye, MD owns stock in Merck, GlaxoSmithKline, Abbott, and Allergan.
Kenneth M. Kaye, MD owns stock in Merck, GlaxoSmithKline, Abbott, and Allergan.
Peter A. Lio, MD is on the Advisory Committee/Board of Galderma Laboratories, Modernizing Medicine, National Eczema Association, Onset Therapeutics; and owns stock with Modernizing Medicine.
Michael D. Nailor, PharmD is a consultant for Astellas Pharmaceuticals, and is on the Speakers' Bureau for Astellas Pharmaceuticals and Forest Pharmaceuticals.
Jack D. Sobel, MD is an industry funded research/investigator for Pfizer, Inc. and Merck, and is on the Speakers' Bureau for Merck and Astellas.

Disclosure of Discussion of Non-FDA Approved Uses for Pharmaceutical Products and/or Medical Devices.
The University of Virginia School of Medicine, as an ACCME provider, requires that all faculty presenters identify and disclose any off-label uses for pharmaceutical and medical device products. The University of Virginia School of Medicine recommends that each physician fully review all the available data on new products or procedures prior to clinical use.

TO ENROLL

To enroll in the Medical Clinics of North America Continuing Medical Education program, call customer service at 1-800-654-2452 or visit us online at http://www.theclinics.com/home/cme. The CME program is available to subscribers for an additional fee of USD 228.

RELATED INTEREST

Immunology and Allergy Clinics of North America,
November 2010 (Volume 30, Issue 4)
Infectious Diseases and Asthma
Shyam Mohapatra, PhD, and Gary Hellermann, PhD, *Guest Editors*

VISIT US ONLINE!
Access your subscription at:
www.theclinics.com

Contributors

GUEST EDITORS

KEITH S. KAYE, MD, MPH
Professor of Medicine, Corporate Director, Infection Prevention, Epidemiology and Antimicrobial Stewardship, Division of Infectious Diseases, Department of Medicine, Detroit Medical Center and Wayne State University, Detroit, Michigan

DONALD KAYE, MD
Professor of Medicine, Drexel University College of Medicine, Philadelphia, Pennsylvania

AUTHORS

JOSE A. BAZAN, DO
Clinical and Research Fellow, Division of Infectious Diseases, The Ohio State University Medical Center, Columbus, Ohio

MAUREEN K. BOLON, MD, MS
Assistant Professor of Medicine, Division of Infectious Diseases, Northwestern University Feinberg School of Medicine, Chicago, Illinois

BARTHOLOMEW R. BONO, MD
Assistant Professor of Medicine, Jefferson Medical College; Attending Physician, Division of Infectious Diseases, Department of Medicine, Albert Einstein Medical Center, Philadelphia, Pennsylvania

LUKE F. CHEN, MBBS (Hons), MPH, CIC, FRACP
Assistant Professor of Medicine, Division of Infectious Diseases and International Health, Department of Medicine, Duke University Medical Center, Durham, North Carolina

TEENA CHOPRA, MD
Fellow, Division of Infectious Diseases, Department of Medicine, Harper Hospital, Detroit Medical Center and Wayne State University, Detroit, Michigan

BRETT GILBERT, DO, FACOI
Clinical Instructor of Medicine, Thomas Jefferson University Hospital, Philadelphia; Division of Infectious Diseases, Lankenau Hospital, Wynnewood, Pennsylvania

DONALD KAYE, MD
Professor of Medicine, Drexel University College of Medicine, Philadelphia, Pennsylvania

ELAINE T. KAYE, MD
Clinical Assistant Professor in Dermatology, Department of Dermatology, Harvard Medical School, Children's Hospital Medical Center, Boston, Massachusetts

KEITH S. KAYE, MD, MPH
Professor of Medicine, Corporate Director, Infection Prevention, Epidemiology and Antimicrobial Stewardship, Division of Infectious Diseases, Department of Medicine, Detroit Medical Center and Wayne State University, Detroit, Michigan

KENNETH M. KAYE, MD
Associate Professor, Division of Infectious Diseases, Harvard Medical School, Channing Laboratory, Brigham and Women's Hospital, Boston, Massachusetts

PETER A. LIO, MD
Assistant Professor in Pediatrics and Dermatology, Department of Dermatology, Northwestern University Feinberg School of Medicine, Chicago, Illinois

LAWRENCE L. LIVORNESE Jr, MD, FACP, FIDSA
Clinical Assistant Professor of Medicine, Drexel University College of Medicine, Philadelphia; Chief, Division of Infectious Diseases, Lankenau Hospital, Wynnewood, Pennsylvania

STANLEY I. MARTIN, MD
Assistant Professor of Clinical Internal Medicine, Division of Infectious Diseases, The Ohio State University Medical Center, Columbus, Ohio

MICHAEL D. NAILOR, PharmD
Clinical Assistant Professor, University of Connecticut School of Pharmacy, Storrs, Connecticut; Formerly Clinical Assistant Professor, Division of Infectious Diseases, Department of Internal Medicine, Wayne State University School of Medicine, Detroit, Michigan

FOZIA QAMAR, MD
University of Massachusetts Medical School; Department of Medicine, UMass Medical Memorial Center, Worcester, Massachusetts

PAUL ROBBINS, DO
Division of Nephrology, Department of Medicine, Lankenau Hospital, Wynnewood, Pennsylvania

JACK D. SOBEL, MD
Chief, Division of Infectious Diseases, Department of Internal Medicine, Wayne State University, Detroit, Michigan

JERRY M. ZUCKERMAN, MD
Assistant Professor of Medicine, Jefferson Medical College; Attending Physician, Division of Infectious Diseases, Department of Medicine, Albert Einstein Medical Center, Philadelphia, Pennsylvania

Contents

Rifaximin is a new rifamycin that is a strict enteric antibiotic approved for treatment of traveler's diarrhea and is showing promise as a possible agent for refractory *Clostridium difficile* infections. The aminoglycosides are used mainly as companion drugs for the treatment of resistant gram-negative bacillary infections and for gram-positive coccal endocarditis.

Preface

Antibacterial Therapy and Newer Agents

Keith S. Kaye, MD, MPH   Donald Kaye, MD
Guest Editors

The discipline of infectious diseases is one of the most rapidly changing fields in medicine. In most specialties of medicine, diseases remain relatively stable, and diagnostic and therapeutic approaches change slowly. In infectious diseases, the syndromes change with the emergence of new organisms, development of resistant pathogens, and resurgence of infections that have virtually disappeared. Clearly, the diagnostic and therapeutic approaches must change rapidly to keep pace with the changing epidemiology of infections. In no area of medicine does the knowledge and art of clinical practice change as rapidly as in the use of antimicrobial agents.

In this issue of *Medical Clinics of North America*, we deal with antibacterial agents and their use, with concentration on newer agents and recent changes in the use of some older antibacterial agents. Pneumococci, enterococci, and gram-negative bacilli have continued to become increasingly resistant to existing antimicrobial agents, and in addition, community-acquired methicillin-resistant *Staphylococcus aureus* has spread dramatically. Criteria for susceptibility of pneumococci and enterococci to various antibacterial agents have recently changed. New β-lactam, antistaphylococcal, and glycylcycline antibiotics have been developed or are in development.

This issue reviews various aspects of the clinical use and management of certain antibacterial agents. Problems with resistant bacteria as well as specific use of antibacterial agents in renal insufficiency are covered. The current status of important older antibiotics is summarized. Newer antibiotics are described, as is the use of topical agents.

In choosing authors to address the different topics, an effort was made to select individuals who are experts in the areas assigned. The end result of their efforts is

A version of this article appeared in the 23:4 issue of the *Infectious Disease Clinics of North America*.

Med Clin N Am 95 (2011) xi–xii
doi:10.1016/j.mcna.2011.05.001
0025-7125/11/$ – see front matter © 2011 Elsevier Inc. All rights reserved.

medical.theclinics.com

a state-of-the-art review on the subject of the use of antibacterial agents and their interactions with bacteria.

Keith S. Kaye, MD, MPH
Division of Infectious Diseases
Department of Medicine
Detroit Medical Center and Wayne State University
4201 Saint Antoine, Suite 2B, Box 331
Detroit, MI 48201, USA

Donald Kaye, MD
Department of Medicine
Drexel University
College of Medicine
Philadelphia, PA 19102, USA
1535 Sweet Briar Road
Gladwyne, PA 19035, USA

E-mail addresses:
KKaye@dmc.org (K.S. Kaye)
donjank@aol.com (D. Kaye)

Pathogens Resistant to Antibacterial Agents

Luke F. Chen, MBBS (Hons), MPH, CIC, FRACP[a],*, Teena Chopra, MD[b],
Keith S. Kaye, MD, MPH[c]

KEYWORDS

- Drug resistance • Methicillin-resistant *Staphylococcus aureus*
- Vancomycin-resistant *Enterococcus*
- Vancomycin intermediate-susceptible *Staphylococcus aureus*
- Extended-spectrum β-lactamase
- Penicillin-resistant *Streptococcus pneumoniae*
- *Klebsiella pneumoniae* carbapenemase
- *Acinetobacter baumanii*

Multidrug-resistant pathogens historically were limited to the hospital setting. In the 1990s, multidrug-resistant pathogens were described to be affecting outpatients in health care–associated settings (nursing homes, dialysis centers, infusion centers, among patients recently hospitalized). More recently, multidrug-resistant pathogens have become major issues in the community, affecting persons with limited or in many cases no contact with health care. This article reviews the molecular mechanisms by which resistance traits are conferred and disseminated and the epidemiology of such bacterial resistance.

MECHANISMS OF RESISTANCE

It is important to distinguish the many ways by which an organism may demonstrate resistance. Intrinsic resistance to an antimicrobial agent characterizes resistance that is an inherent attribute of a particular species; all organisms of the species may lack the appropriate drug-susceptible target or possess natural barriers that prevent an

A version of this article appeared in the 23:4 issue of the *Infectious Disease Clinics of North America*.

[a] Division of Infectious Diseases and International Health, Department of Medicine, Duke University Medical Center, Box 102359, Hanes House, Durham, NC 27710, USA
[b] Division of Infectious Diseases, Department of Medicine, Harper Hospital, Detroit Medical Center and Wayne State University, 3990 John R. Street, 5 Hudson, Detroit, MI 48201, USA
[c] Division of Infectious Diseases, Department of Medicine, Detroit Medical Center and Wayne State University, 4201 Saint Antoine, Suite 2B, Box 331, Detroit, MI 48201, USA
* Corresponding author.
E-mail address: luke.chen@duke.edu

Med Clin N Am 95 (2011) 647–676
doi:10.1016/j.mcna.2011.03.005
0025-7125/11/$ – see front matter © 2011 Elsevier Inc. All rights reserved.

medical.theclinics.com

antimicrobial agent from reaching its target. Some examples are the natural resistance of gram-negative bacteria to vancomycin because the drug cannot penetrate the gram-negative outer membrane, or the intrinsic resistance of the penicillin-binding proteins (PBPs) of enterococci to the effects of the cephalosporins.

Acquired resistance, the primary focus of this article, reflects a change in the genetic composition of a bacterium so that a drug that once was effective is no longer active, resulting in clinical resistance. Sometimes genetic change results in diminished antimicrobial activity, but not complete loss of drug effectiveness.

The major strategies used by bacteria to avoid the actions of antimicrobial agents are outlined in **Table 1**. These include limiting the intracellular concentration of an antimicrobial agent by decreased influx or increased efflux, neutralization of the antimicrobial agent by enzymes, alteration of the target so that the agent no longer interferes with it, and elimination of the target altogether by the creation of new metabolic pathways.[1] Bacteria may use one or multiple mechanisms against a single agent or class of agents or a single change may result in resistance to several different agents or even multiple unrelated drug classes.

Gram-positive and gram-negative bacteria possess different structural characteristics and these differences determine the mechanisms for primary resistance. The targets of most antimicrobial agents are located either in the cell wall, cytoplasmic membrane, or within the cytoplasm. In gram-negative bacteria, the outer membrane may provide an additional intrinsic barrier that prevents drugs from reaching these targets. Additionally, modifications in outer membrane permeability by both alterations in porin channels and by upregulation of multidrug efflux pumps may contribute to resistance in many gram-negative organisms. Moreover, inactivating enzymes

Table 1
General mechanisms of resistance to antimicrobial agents

Resistance Mechanism	Specific Examples	References
Diminished intracellular drug concentration		
Decreased outer membrane permeability	β-Lactams (eg, OmpF, OprD)	4
Decreased cytoplasmic membrane transport	Quinolones (eg, OmpF)	2
	Aminoglycosides (decreased energy)	6
Increased efflux	Tetracyclines (eg, tetA)	208
	Quinolones (eg, norA)	209
	Macrolides (eg, mefA)	209
	Multiple drugs (eg, mexAB-OprF)	3
Drug inactivation (reversible or irreversible)	β-Lactams (β-lactamases)	104
	Carbapenemases (carbapenems)	115,105
	Aminoglycosides (modifying enzymes)	6
	Chloramphenicol (inactivating enzymes)	1
Target modification	Quinolones (gyrase modifications)	9
	Rifampin (DNA polymerase binding)	9
	β-Lactams (PBP changes)	9
	Macrolides (rRNA methylation)	8
	Linezolid (23s rRNA modifications)	58
Target bypass	Glycopeptides (vanA, vanB)	10
	Trimethoprim (thymidine-deficient strains)	—

released across the cytoplasmic membrane can function more efficiently within the confines of the periplasmic space.

The mechanisms by which intracellular concentrations of drugs are limited include decreased outer membrane permeability, decreased uptake through the cytoplasmic membrane, and active efflux out of both the cytoplasmic membrane and the outer membrane. Acquired outer membrane permeability changes in gram-negative organisms previously attributed solely to alterations in outer membrane porin proteins are now also understood to be related to the upregulation of complex multidrug efflux pumps whose expression is linked to that of outer membrane proteins, such as the *MexAB-OprM* system of *Pseudomonas aeruginosa*.[5] These efflux systems are widely distributed among gram-negative pathogens, such as *P aeruginosa* and Enterobacteriaceae, and may be an important component of resistance to β-lactams, but usually result in high-level resistance only when associated with β-lactamase production.[2] Imipenem resistance in *P aeruginosa* can be mediated by alteration of a specific porin OprD that is used preferentially by this agent.[2] Decreased outer membrane permeability through porin changes and efflux may also play a role in resistance to fluoroquinolones and aminoglycosides. Resistance mediated by decreased uptake across the metabolically active cytoplasmic membrane is best demonstrated by small-colony aminoglycoside-resistant mutants of staphylococci, but this mechanism is less important than other mechanisms of aminoglycoside resistance.[6] Active antimicrobial efflux systems play a role in resistance to many different agents, including macrolides, tetracyclines, quinolones, chloramphenicol, and β-lactams.

Inactivating enzymes remain the predominant mechanism of resistance to several major classes of antimicrobial agents. Resistance to β-lactams is mediated by a wide variety of β-lactamases that hydrolytically inactivate these drugs. β-lactamases can be either plasmid or chromosomally-mediated, and their expression can be constitutive or induced. Unlike those of gram-positive organisms, β-lactamases of gram-negative organisms are confined to the periplasmic space, which may explain some of the differences in their phenotypic expression and ease of laboratory detection. Of particular importance in the hospital setting are the class I chromosomal β-lactamases in organisms, such as *Enterobacter cloacae*, which are produced in high levels after exposure to an inducing β-lactam agent (particularly to third-generation cephalosporins), and the extended-spectrum β-lactamases (ESBLs), mediating resistance to third-generation cephalosporins and aztreonam.[7] Carbapenemases are an emerging, and important class of inactivating enzymes that mediate resistance to carbapenem antibiotics in gram-negative organisms. Another major class of inactivating enzymes is the family of aminoglycoside-modifying enzymes. These enzymes are widely distributed in gram-positive and gram-negative bacteria, and usually are plasmid-mediated.[6] Resistance to chloramphenicol and macrolides also can be mediated by modifying or inactivating enzymes.[8]

Target modifications are used by bacteria to mediate resistance to a wide variety of antimicrobial agents.[9] Some of these alterations may require as little as a single mutational event at a critical gene sequence in the primary target to create a new, functional target with reduced affinity for the antimicrobial agent. Such changes account for the relative ease of selection of rifampin-resistant mutants of staphylococci and streptococci by changes in DNA polymerase or the selection of high-level streptomycin-resistant mutants with altered ribosomes. Although some resistance secondary to target modifications can be directly selected, others, such as development of resistance to semisynthetic penicillins in staphylococci, require acquisition of novel exogenous DNA. Modification of PBPs is the primary mode of penicillin resistance in *Streptococcus pneumoniae*, *Neisseria meningitidis*, and *Enterococcus faecium*. Modification of genes encoding DNA gyrases and topoisomerases is the main mechanism of resistance to quinolones, while target modification is important in resistance to macrolides, tetracyclines, rifampin, and mupirocin.[9]

Some bacteria have gone beyond simple target modification and have acquired novel systems in which the antimicrobial target is no longer necessary for survival of the organism. This is achieved by creation of new metabolic pathways to bypass the primary target. Perhaps the most elaborate examples of this are the *vanA* and *vanB* clusters that mediate resistance to glycopeptides in enterococci.[10] Target bypass also is the major mechanism of acquired resistance to folate antagonists.

MECHANISMS OF DISSEMINATION OF RESISTANCE GENES

In addition to the complex strategies used to express resistance to antimicrobial agents, bacteria also can avail themselves of a variety of efficient mechanisms for the transfer of resistance genes to other organisms and to other species.[11] The bacterial genome consists of chromosomal DNA, and encodes the following cellular characteristics: metabolic and repair pathways, smaller circular DNA elements or plasmids that encode for supplemental bacterial activities, such as virulence factors and resistance genes, and genes essential to the independent mobilization and transmission of the plasmid elements. Most resistance genes are plasmid-mediated, but plasmid-mediated traits can interchange with chromosomal elements. Transfer of genetic material from a plasmid to the chromosome can occur by simple recombination events, but the process is greatly facilitated by transposons. Transposons are small, mobile DNA elements capable of mediating transfer of DNA by removing and inserting themselves into host chromosomal and plasmid DNA. Many resistance genes, such as plasmid-mediated β-lactamases, tetracycline-resistance genes, and aminoglycoside-modifying enzymes, are organized on transposons, which may have a broader host range than their parent plasmids. Multiple resistance transposons can then be clustered together on even larger composite transposable elements capable of simultaneously transferring multiple unrelated resistance genes.[11]

Resistance determinants carried on the chromosome are vertically transmitted by clonal dissemination. Resistance determinants on plasmids can also be vertically transferred, although plasmids may be lost from the bacterial population if they no longer confer a particular selective advantage. Plasmids also are capable of horizontal transfer by conjugation, although the efficiency of plasmid transfer both within and between species can vary tremendously. Plasmid transfer between gram-positive and gram-negative bacteria, once thought to be an unlikely event, can occur both in the laboratory and in the gastrointestinal tract of gnotobiotic mice, suggesting that such transfer events between even remotely related organisms may be important in nature.[12]

Conjugative transposons of gram-positive bacteria are capable of directly mediating gene transfer without plasmids. Transformation, direct incorporation of free DNA by bacterial cells, may also be important for the evolution of resistance in *Neisseria* and streptococcal species.[9,11]

Resistant Gram-Positive Cocci

Multidrug-resistant enterococci
Epidemiology and characteristics of resistance Enterococci are naturally tolerant of penicillins, and are resistant to cephalosporins, clindamycin, and achievable serum levels of aminoglycosides. Cephalosporin resistance is caused by poor affinity of cephalosporins for enterococcal PBPs. Natural low-level aminoglycoside resistance

is attributed to the inability of aminoglycosides to penetrate the enterococcal cell wall, but activity is enhanced in the presence of cell wall–active drugs, such as ampicillin or vancomycin.[13] Enterococci are usually intrinsically tolerant, or lysis resistant, to the effects of penicillins and glycopeptides alone. Until the emergence of drug-resistant isolates, bactericidal therapy was reliably achieved with synergistic combinations of cell wall–active drugs plus aminoglycosides.

Enterococci demonstrate several types of penicillin resistance Penicillin resistance in *E faecalis* is mediated by β-lactamase production and has been reported from a few nosocomial outbreaks both within and outside of the United States,[14] but infections with such strains are still very uncommon. Chromosomal high-level penicillin resistance is a species-specific characteristic of *E faecium*, but is occasionally found in other species.[15] *E faecium* with low-level penicillin-resistance are found in normal fecal flora, but high-level resistant strains are likely to be nosocomially acquired.[16] Intermediate level of ampicillin resistance (minimum inhibitory concentrations [MICs] of 16–64 μg/mL) is attributable to alterations in PBPs and in most cases, is associated with the overexpression of PBP5, a PBP with low affinity for penicillins.[17] High-level penicillin-resistant *E faecium* are also resistant to imipenem and β-lactam–β-lactamase inhibitors and are often also glycopeptide-resistant.[18]

High-level gentamicin resistance, mediated by a bifunctional inactivating enzyme, first appeared in 1978 and rapidly spread worldwide. As many as 60% of enterococci from some hospitals are high-level gentamicin resistant, but resistance remains strongly associated with nosocomial acquisition.[19] High-level gentamicin resistant enterococci are highly resistant to all other aminoglycosides in clinical use in the United States, with the possible exception of streptomycin. Importantly, highly resistant strains do not demonstrate synergistic killing of enterococci when aminoglycosides are combined with penicillin or vancomycin.[20] Most high-level gentamicin resistance is carried on transposons and is plasmid mediated.[20] Detection of high-level gentamicin resistance requires either special susceptibility wells or screening plates with high concentrations of gentamicin or streptomycin (eg, $\geq$500 μg/mL for gentamicin and $\geq$1,000 μg/mL for streptomycin).

Vancomycin-resistant enterococci (VRE) were first isolated in Europe in 1988 and in the United States in 1989. Since then, VRE have spread rapidly throughout the United States and the world and have become a significant infection control problem for many hospitals.[21] VRE are established throughout the United States and Europe, but are less frequently isolated in Asia and Latin America.[22] The prevalence of VRE remains low in true community-acquired isolates in the United States.

The increase in glycopeptide resistance in the United States followed the marked increase in vancomycin usage in many hospitals, just as methicillin-resistant *Staphylococcus aureus* (MRSA) strains became established in the 1980s. Most VRE seem to have been acquired nosocomially or institutionally, and spread of epidemic strains both within and between institutions is well documented.[23] From 1989 to 2002, the proportion of enterococcal isolates from ICUs that were resistant to vancomycin increased from 0.3% in 1989 to 23.9% in 1998, and further increased to 33.3% in 2008.[21] As of October 2008, the National Nosocomial Infections Surveillance system reported that more than one third of healthcare–associated enterococcal infections were associated with organisms resistant to vancomycin.[21] Some risk factors for VRE colonization or infection include exposure to antibiotics, such as broad-spectrum cephalosporins, fluoroquinolones, vancomycin, and antianaerobic drugs, prolonged hospital and ICU stays, intrahospital transfer between patient floors, use of enteral tube feedings, or sucralfate and liver transplant requiring surgical re-exploration.[24]

Glycopeptides are large, complex molecules that do not enter the bacterial cell. They interfere with cell wall synthesis by tightly binding to the D-alanine-D-alanine terminal dipeptide on the peptidoglycan precursor, sterically blocking the subsequent transglycosylation and transpeptidation reactions. The vancomycin-resistance mechanism involves a complex series of reactions that ultimately result in the building of the cell wall by bypassing the D-alanine-D-alanine–containing pentapeptide intermediate structure, thereby eliminating the glycopeptide target.[25]

VRE initially were characterized phenotypically as *vanA*, *vanB*, and *vanC* strains based on levels of resistance to vancomycin, cross-resistance to teicoplanin, and the inducible or constitutive nature of resistance.[26] The genotype and molecular basis for each resistance type have now been characterized (**Table 2**). The *vanA* cluster has been identified predominantly in *E faecium* and *E faecalis* but has also been found in other enterococci, streptococci, *Oerskovia*, *Bacillus*, and has been found in *S aureus*.[27–31] Furthermore, there is evidence for in vivo transfer of *vanA* resistance on plasmids.[32]

vanB is found almost exclusively in *E faecium* and *E faecalis*. *vanC1*, *C2*, *C3*, *D*, *E*, and *G* are rarely found in enterococci causing human infections.[33–35]

Resistance to linezolid in enterococci is mediated by the G2576U mutation or similar mutations of the 23S ribosome.[36] Recent studies have shown high rates of linezolid resistance among enterococcal isolates; 11% to 20% of VRE colonizing or infecting isolates were resistant to linezolid.[37,38] Risk factors associated with isolation of linezolid-resistant VRE were receipt of a solid organ transplant; receipt of parenteral nutrition; peripheral vascular disease; and prior receipt of linezolid, piperacillin-tazobactam, or cefepime.[38]

Enterococcal resistance to daptomycin rarely occurs and is associated with previous treatment with daptomycin. The mechanism of resistance is not well understood.[39]

Multidrug-Resistant Staphylococcus Aureus

The first strain of penicillinase-producing *S aureus* was reported in 1941[40] and 90% of *S aureus* isolates in the world are now penicillin-resistant as a result of β-lactamase

Table 2
Glycopeptide-resistant enterococci

Genotype	Vancomycin MIC (μg/mL)	Teicoplanin MIC (μg/mL)	Expression	Typical Location
vanA	64–1024	≥16	Inducible	Plasmid[a]
vanB	4–1024	≤1[b]	Inducible[c]	Chromosome[d]
vanC[f]	2–32	≤1	Constitutive and inducible	Chromosome
vanD	64–256	4–32	Constitutive and inducible[e]	Chromosome
vanE	16	0.5	Inducible	Chromosome
vanG	16	0.5	Inducible	Chromosome

[a] Strains with *vanA* on the chromosome have been described.
[b] Teicoplanin-resistant strains have emerged with MIC ≥16.
[c] Constitutively expressing strains have been described.
[d] Plasmids containing *vanB* have been described.
[e] Both have been described.
[f] Species-specific variants *vanC-1*, *vanC-2*, and *vanC-3* have been described.

production. Over the ensuing decades, S aureus continued to predominate as a major human pathogen and it became increasingly resistant to drugs in the face of antimicrobial selection pressure. For example, since 1996, there have been several reports of infections caused by MRSA with intermediate susceptibility to vancomycin (vancomycin-intermediate S aureus [VISA]; MIC 4–8 µg/mL).[41] Furthermore, there are now several strains of S aureus in the United States that are fully resistant to vancomycin (vancomycin-resistant S aureus [VRSA]; MIC $\geq$16 µg/mL)[42] and to other recently approved antibiotics specifically developed to treat MRSA, such as linezolid[43] and daptomycin. The Infectious Diseases Society of America addressed many management implications of these resistant S aureus isolates in its recently published Clinical Practice Guidelines for the Treatment of MRSA infections in adults and children.[44,45]

Mechanism of resistance in MRSA

Resistance to methicillin and other β-lactam antibiotics is mediated by the mecA gene, which encodes for a specific PBP (PBP2a), which has low affinity for β-lactams. Strains with mecA-mediated methicillin resistance are classically referred to as MRSA. These mecA genes are situated on a mobile genetic element, known as the Staphylococcal Cassette Chromosome mec (SCCmec). To date, eight types of SCCmec (I–VIII) have been reported, and these are widely distributed in both coagulase-positive and coagulase-negative staphylococci.[46–48] The SCCmec element also includes two regulatory loci, the repressor MecI and the trans-membrane β-lactam–sensing signal-transducer MecRI.[49] Some SCCmec components may contain additional genes encoding for resistance against non–β-lactam antibiotics.

The expression of mecA can be either constitutive or inducible. Additionally, expression of the resistance phenotype also depends, in part, on other chromosomal genes, which are part of cellular peptidoglycan metabolism and can regulate the degree of resistance without altering levels of PBP2a.

Community-acquired MRSA Community-acquired MRSA is both phenotypically and genotypically distinct from healthcare–associated MRSA. Frequently, community-acquired MRSA isolates produce toxins including Panton-Valentine leukocidin, which is an exotoxin encoded by two cotranscribed genes: lukF-PV and lukS-PV. Although the actual virulence of the Panton-Valentine leukocidin gene remains uncertain, presence of the Panton-Valentine leukocidin protein has been associated with skin and soft tissue infections and severe necrotizing pneumonia.[50] Furthermore, community-acquired MRSA strains are susceptible to non–β-lactam antibiotics[51] and this is explained by the fact that resistance genes to non–β-lactam antibiotics are not usually included in the smaller type IV SCCmec elements that are common in community-acquired MRSA isolates. In contrast to nosocomial MRSA isolates, most community-acquired MRSA strains are susceptible to multiple classes of antibiotics other than β-lactams, including trimethoprim-sulfamethoxazole (TMP-SMX), clindamycin, aminoglycosides, tetracyclines, and fluoroquinolones. Recently, isolates of community-acquired MRSA with resistance to clindamycin, tetracyclines and macrolides were reported among men who have sex with men.[52]

Reduced susceptibility to vancomycin Vancomycin is the mainstay of treatment of MRSA infections. Failure of vancomycin therapy, however, is not uncommon and is increasing. Reduced susceptibility of MRSA to vancomycin, which occurs predominantly among strains of healthcare–associated MRSA, is being studied in the following three contexts: (1) VRSA; (2) VISA; and (3) the trend of MRSA isolates with increased vancomycin MICs (MIC creep).

VRSA, fortunately, continues to be rare. There have only been eleven reports of clinical isolates of VRSA in the United States as of this writing; eight of the eleven occurred within the greater Michigan area.[53] MICs of VRSA isolates to vancomycin are generally greater than 128 μg/mL. In these isolates, vancomycin resistance has been conferred by the *vanA* resistance cluster, which also mediates glycopeptide resistance in some enterococcal species. In these patients from whom VRSA was isolated, prior dual infection with MRSA and VRE was documented in most patients. The transfer of the *vanA* gene has been demonstrated in vitro from enterococcus to *S aureus*.[54] More recently, investigators found that *Enterococcus* spp that harbored the Inc 18-like vanA plasmids were probably more likely than other vanA plasmids to transfer to *S aureus* and produce VRSA.[55] Vancomycin acts by binding the D-Ala-D-Ala terminus of peptidoglycan precursors and the resistance to vancomycin in VRSA is mediated by the presence of enzymes that produce low-affinity precursors, such as D-Ala-D-lactate or D-Ala-D-Ser, or the presence of enzymes that eliminate the high-affinity peptidoglycan precursors that are normally produced in susceptible *S aureus*.[56]

Among VISA isolates, the MIC to vancomycin is 4 to 8 μg/mL. The mechanism conferring glycopeptide resistance in VISA is not well understood at the genetic level but seems to involve cell wall thickening with reduced levels of peptidoglycan cross-linking and does not seem to require the acquisition of new DNA. It is postulated that reduced levels of peptidoglycan cross-linking leads to more D-alanyl-D-alanine side chains. These side chains can bind vancomycin outside the cell membrane and prevent vancomycin from reaching its cell membrane targets.

Independent risk factors for infections caused by VISA include prior infection caused by MRSA and antecedent vancomycin use within 3 months before VISA infection. Most patients in the United States with VISA infections received repeated, prolonged exposures to vancomycin and received dialysis at the time of infection.

Several investigators have observed increased rates of vancomycin treatment failures in patients with MRSA infections where the isolates have increased vancomycin MICs but are still classified as susceptible by Clinical and Laboratory Standards Institute (CLSI) definitions.[57] One study showed less than 10% treatment success when vancomycin was used to treat bacteremia caused by MRSA strains with vancomycin MICs of 1 to 2 μg/mL, compared with 56% success when the vancomycin MIC was less than or equal to 0.5 μg/mL.[58] Partly in response to this study and others, in 2007, the susceptibility breakpoints for *S aureus* to vancomycin were lowered from 8 to 16 μg/mL to 4 to 8 μg/mL for intermediate and from less than or equal to 4 μg/mL to less than or equal to 2 μg/mL for susceptible.[57]

Several investigators from different geographic locales have reported that the MICs of *S aureus* isolates to vancomycin have increased over time. This phenomenon has been described as "MIC creep."[59] Debate is ongoing with respect to the significance of the MIC creep and the degree to which it is actually occurring.[60] For example, a study of more than 35,000 *S aureus* isolates from the SENTRY database collected from sites around the world between 1997 and 2003 showed no evidence of increasing vancomycin MICs over time.[61] Another study of more than 6000 *S aureus* isolates collected over 5 years in southern California found a clear and statistically significant drift of vancomycin MICs toward reduced susceptibility, with an increase in the proportion of isolates with a MIC equal to 1 μg/mL from 19.9% in 2000 to 70.4% in 2004.[62] Despite these conflicting results, reports of vancomycin treatment failures for susceptible MRSA strains and reports of MIC creep from some geographic locales raise concerns about the future of vancomycin as an effective agent for treatment of invasive MRSA infections. Recently, guidelines were published regarding optimal dosing of vancomycin for the treatment of infections caused by *S aureus*.[63]

Resistance to alternative agents for treatment of MRSA

Linezolid is bacteriostatic against *S aureus* and binds to the 50S subunit of the bacterial ribosome, resulting in the inhibition of bacterial protein synthesis.[64] In vitro resistance to linezolid have been reported in *S aureus*.[65] Fortunately, such resistant isolates remain a rare phenomenon. Linezolid may fail to bind its bacterial target site in the presence of single point mutations in the bacterial 23S rRNA of the 50S subunit.[66] Notably, 23S rRNA mutations that confer resistance to linezolid can produce cross-resistance to chloramphenicol and quinupristin-dalfopristin, which also bind to the same 23S rRNA domain.[66] Prior therapy with linezolid seems to be an important risk factor for subsequent isolation of linezolid-resistant *S aureus*.[67]

Daptomycin is rapidly bactericidal against *S aureus* and its primary mechanism of action is a calcium-dependent depolarization of bacterial cell wall.[68] Daptomycin is inactivated by alveolar surfactants, and should not be used for pulmonary infections.[69] Clinical failures caused by emergence of resistance have been reported during daptomycin for chronic infections.[70] The exact mechanisms of resistance to daptomycin have not been completely elucidated. Studies have shown that daptomycin resistance gradually emerges by a multistep process[71] and generally results in a heteroresistant bacterial subpopulation with higher MICs to daptomycin. Current evidence suggests that resistance is caused by impairment of daptomycin binding by a change in cell membrane potential leading to (1) reduced daptomycin binding to the cell membrane, (2) changes in cell membrane surface charge, and (3) reduced susceptibility to daptomycin-induced depolarization.[72] Furthermore, there is a correlation between daptomycin-resistance and vancomycin nonsusceptibility in isolates of VISA.[73] The cross-resistance between vancomycin and daptomycin in VISA is thought to be caused by the thickened cell wall, which acts as a common obstacle to daptomycin and vancomycin cellular penetration.

Quinupristin-dalfopristin is a concentration-dependent antibiotic that is bactericidal against staphylococci. Staphylococcal isolates constitutively expressing macrolide-lincosamide-streptogramin B resistance (eg, erm A or erm C) may be resistant to the quinupristin component of quinupristin-dalfopristin. In such cases, the activity of quinupristin-dalfopristin may be significantly altered.[74]

Clinical failures associated with resistance to quinupristin-dalfopristin have already been described in some isolates of MRSA even in the relatively short timeframe that the drug has been available.[75] Isolates of staphylococci that are resistant to quinupristin-dalfopristin are more likely to have resistances to the dalfopristin component, which is caused by genes encoding acetyltransferases (*vatA*, *vatB*, and *vatC*) or efflux pumps (*vgaA* and *vgaB*).[76] Resistance to quinupristin-dalfopristin can also be mediated by resistance to the quinupristin component, caused by production of ribosomal methylases encoded by *erm* genes; and the macrolide-lincosamide-streptogramin B phenotype, which also confers cross-resistance to macrolides and lincosamides.

Resistance of MRSA to other classes of antibiotics

MRSA isolates containing *mecA* are resistant to all β-lactam antibiotics. Most nosocomial and health care–associated isolates frequently carry multiple other resistance determinants. Many of these resistance determinants can be found on transferable genetic elements or plasmids, whereas others are chromosomal in origin. The plasmid-mediated determinants include aminoglycoside-modifying enzymes, tetracycline efflux genes, and macrolide-methylating enzymes, and resistance determinants for TMP-SMX. Quinolone resistance is mediated primarily by alterations in DNA topoisomerases, but also by the staphylococcal *norA* gene by active efflux. Resistance to macrolide, lincosamide, and streptogramin antibiotics may be conferred by modifications of target sites, active efflux, and by inactivating enzymes. Gentamicin resistance also can occur by selection of small-colony, membrane energy-deficient mutants.

Penicillin and Multidrug-Resistant Pneumococci

Mechanisms of resistance

Beta-lactam-resistance in *S pneumoniae* is caused by reduced affinity between the PBPs and β-lactam antibiotics. Such resistance is mediated through changes in genes that encode one of the six high-molecular-weight PBPs of the organism.[77] There are two notable features of PBP-mediated resistance in pneumococci. First, highly resistant strains generally show more PBP alterations than do those of low-level resistant strains.[78] Second, pneumococcal resistance can occur by homologous recombination of PBP genes of different strains, in addition to direct clonal dissemination of resistant strains.[79] Such events can occur both between different pneumococcal species and between pneumococci and the closely related viridans streptococcal species. Oral streptococci have been postulated to be the major reservoir for the novel DNA required to create the genetic sequences demonstrated by some of the altered pneumococcal PBP genes.[9]

Tolerance to penicillins in pneumococci can also be mediated by altered peptidoglycan structures. Additionally, penicillin tolerance has been found in strains with reduced penicillin susceptibility that fails to lyse at penicillin concentrations far above the MIC; however, the clinical significance of this observation remains unclear.

Changes in PBP of penicillin-resistant strains also result in diminished susceptibility to other β-lactam agents.[80] The levels of resistance to different agents vary greatly. Penicillin-resistant strains are uniformly resistant to penicillin derivatives, such as ampicillin and the ureidopenicillins (eg, piperacillin), and generally are resistant to first- and second-generation cephalosporins. Certain third-generation agents, particularly cefotaxime and ceftriaxone, are often effective, in part because of their high level of activity and in part because of the high tissue levels attained by these agents. Many strains of pneumococci also harbor high-level resistance to cefotaxime and ceftriaxone (MIC ≥ 2 μg/mL) (3.3% of all strains reported in a recent United States study were ceftriaxone-resistant and 5% of all isolates in a recent Taiwanese study were ceftriaxone-resistant).[81,82] Interestingly, several studies also show that isolates of penicillin-resistant pneumococci may be disproportionately more susceptible to ceftriaxone than to cefotaxime.[83] Regardless of the pattern of β-lactam nonsusceptibility, debate is still ongoing as to infections caused by these resistant strains are associated with poorer outcomes than infections caused by susceptible strains.[84]

Resistance of pneumococci to non–β-lactam antimicrobial agents

Penicillin-resistant strains are frequently resistant to non–β-lactam antimicrobial agents and are often multidrug resistant. Resistance to erythromycin, tetracycline, TMP-SMX, and chloramphenicol are the most common.

A recent surveillance study in the United States shows that prevalence of macrolide resistance in *S pneumoniae* is approximately 26.2%.[85] The most common mechanism of macrolide resistance in *S pneumoniae* is caused by target-site modification encoded by erythromycin ribosome methylation (erm) genes that provide inducible cross-resistance to all macrolides, lincosamides, and streptogramin B. Two other mechanisms of resistance to macrolides include active efflux pump encoded by macrolide efflux genes (*mefA*, *mefE*) that result in resistance to macrolides alone (M phenotype); and ribosomal mutations in the 23S rRNA gene for ribosomal protein L4 or L22.

Although vancomycin-tolerant pneumococcal isolates have recently been isolated, no strains fully resistant to vancomycin have been reported.[86]

Fluoroquinolone resistance has been described during therapy, especially in patients with prior fluoroquinolone exposures, leading to clinical failure.[87] The older fluoroquinolones (eg, ciprofloxacin) lack reliable activity against pneumococci (18.6% of pneumococcal isolates in a 2008 study were nonsusceptible to ciprofloxacin).[85] Newer fluoroquinolones, such as levofloxacin, moxifloxacin, and gemifloxacin, inhibit most strains at achievable levels (only 1.3% of the isolates were nonsusceptible to levofloxacin in a study by Sahm and colleagues[85]). The mechanism of decreased susceptibility to the newer fluoroquinolones is primarily caused by mutations in the *parC* gene of topoisomerase IV and the *gyrA* gene of DNA gyrase.

RESISTANT GRAM-NEGATIVE MICROORGANISMS
Escherichia Coli and Klebsiella spp Resistant to Broad-Spectrum Cephalosporins

Resistance of *Escherichia coli* and *Klebsiella* spp to broad-spectrum cephalosporins is largely mediated by ESBLs, designated as Bush-Jacoby-Medeiros Group 2be.[88] These enzymes confer resistance to oxyimino-β-lactam antibiotics. Most ESBLs are derivatives of TEM and SHV, which have undergone amino acid substitutions at the active site of the enzyme. Such ESBL enzymes are often plasmid-borne. Depending on the location of the substitution, the resultant β-lactamase can cause variably diminished susceptibility to cefotaxime, ceftazidime, and aztreonam. ESBLs are most commonly expressed in *Klebsiella pneumoniae*, *Klebsiella oxytoca*, and *E coli*, although they have been detected in other organisms including *Salmonella* spp, *Pseudomonas aeruginosa*, *Proteus mirabilis*, and other Enterobacteriaceae. Plasmids that encode ESBLs often carry resistance to other antibiotics. The effective control and treatment of ESBLs are a growing challenge because of the role of ESBLs in outbreaks in hospitals and nursing homes, and because of the ability of ESBLs to be transferred to other bacterial species by plasmids.

Epidemiology and mechanisms of resistance

ESBLs were first discovered in Europe in 1983 and soon after in the United States. Since then their prevalence has increased. By 1990, 14% of all *K pneumoniae* isolated from French hospitals were ESBL producers, with rates approaching 50% in some hospitals.[89] In some United States hospitals, the prevalence of ESBLs in *K pneumoniae* has been reported to be as high as 40%.[90] The Centers for Disease Control and Prevention reported, in 2006 to 2007, the rate of ceftazidime-resistant *K pneumoniae* strains associated with device-related infection exceeded 20%, and the rate of ceftazidime-resistant *E coli* ranged between 5% and 11%.[91] Teaching hospitals have a higher prevalence of ESBL resistance.[92]

ESBL-producing organisms are generally found in hospitals, although nursing home outbreaks have been reported.[93] Outbreaks can occur through either clonal spread of a specific plasmid-carrying strain or through transfer of a particular plasmid to other bacterial strains, or even to different bacterial genera.[93] Resistant organisms can pass from patient to patient on the hands of healthcare providers.[94] Risk factors for acquisition of ESBLs are similar to those reported for other hospital-acquired organisms and include emergency abdominal surgery, mechanical ventilation, presence of percutaneous devices, tracheostomy, prolonged hospital stay, and increased patient morbidity.[92,93,95] Risk factors associated with antibiotics are of increasing interest to researchers. Exposure to antibiotics, particularly to ceftazidime and aztreonam, has been associated with an increased prevalence of ESBL-producing organisms.[96,97] Other studies, however, have found no association between use of third-generation cephalosporins and emergence of ESBL resistance.[93,98] Exposure to TMP-SMX has also been associated with acquisition of ESBLs.[93] Restriction of cephalosporin use has been associated with control of hospital outbreaks.[99,100] Recently, a study showed use of piperacillin-tazobactam and vancomycin was an independent risk factor for colonization with ESBL organisms.[101]

Many different types of ESBLS have been described, including greater than 160 in the TEM class, over 100 in the SHV family, over 80 in the CTX-M class, and more than 140 in the OXA family. A Web site maintains an up-to-date, complete listing of all identified ESBLs: http://www.lahey.org/studies/.[102]

Each ESBL has unique amino acid substitutions at active sites of the enzyme, affecting its isoelectric point and affecting the enzyme's affinity for and hydrolytic activity of oxyimino-β-lactams.[92] Most ESBLs have higher hydrolytic activity against ceftazidime and aztreonam and less activity against cefotaxime, although the opposite may be true in some cases. For example, in SHV and TEM β-lactamases a serine substitution for glycine at amino acid 238 causes decreased hydrolytic activity against ceftazidime but increases activity against cefotaxime.[92] CTX-M–type ESBLs, however, generally have higher hydrolytic activity against cefotaxime than ceftazidime.[103] Multiple β-lactamases conferring resistance to different classes of β-lactam antibiotics can be found within a single bacterial strain. The diversity of cephalosporin susceptibility profiles manifested by different ESBL enzymes makes detection of some ESBL-producing strains a major challenge for the clinical laboratory. These enzymes are not capable of hydrolyzing cephamycins and carbapenems.[104]

Carbapenemase-producing gram-negative organisms can hydrolyze all penicillins, cephalosporins, and carbapenems and they have been reported in several large outbreaks in hospitalized patients since 2001.[105] KPC,[106] a class A plasmid-mediated β-lactamase, has been associated with outbreaks in hospitals in the northeastern regions of the United States,[107–109] and in other countries, such as China, Brazil, and Israel. KPCs are classically associated with *K pneumoniae*; however, outbreaks of KPCs have been reported with *E coli*, *K oxytoca*, *Enterobacter* spp, *Salmonella*,[102,110] and *Pseudomonas*.[111] Some preliminary evidence demonstrates propagation of KPC-producing organisms in diverse geographic regions in the United States; inside and outside of hospitals; and in community-based health care services, such as nursing homes.[112]

Metallo-β-lactamases are class B β-lactam hydrolyzing enzymes that contain a zinc moiety and have caused several extended outbreaks of nosocomial infections in patients in ICUs and burns units in Europe and Australia.[113] VIM and IMP metallo-β-lactamases are more commonly found in *Pseudomonas* and *Acinetobacter* species. These metallo-β-lactamases can also rapidly hydrolyze cephalosporins and penicillins (but not aztreonam), and can be encoded by integrins, raising concerns regarding horizontal spread of this resistance mechanism. OXA-type carbapenemases are class D β-lactamases that have caused limited outbreaks in the United States.[114] Metallo-β-lactamases are a diverse group of β-lactamases that are active not only against the oxyimino-cephalosporins and cephamycins but also against carbapenems.[115] There are two major groups of metalloid-β-lactamases: the IMP-type carbapenemases and the Verona integron-encoded metallo-β-lactamase (VIM) carbapenemases.[116] In 2010, a new metallo-β-lactamase was described. This new carbapenemase, known as New Delhi metallo-β-lactamase (NDM-1), was reported in patients in the UK, USA, Canada, Belgium, Taiwan and Australia. Although some patients infected with NDM-1-producing organisms had a travel history through the Indian subcontinent, the origin and the extent of NDM-1 remains uncertain. The fact that NDM-1 was detectable in patients who did not travel to the Indian subcontinent led many experts to believe that NDM-1 may already be widely disseminated globally and was posing a problem possibly bigger than even resistance mediated by KPC production.[117]

Another mechanism facilitating β-lactamase activity involves loss of porin channels in the outer cellular membrane and upregulation of efflux pumps, decreasing antibiotic concentrations in the periplasmic space and facilitating hydrolysis by β-lactamases. This mechanism often results in increased resistance to cephalosporins, cephamycins, and β-lactamase inhibitors.[92,118,119] Plasmids producing ESBLs often carry resistance to other antibiotics, including aminoglycosides, tetracyclines, chloramphenicol, TMP, and sulfonamides.[92]

Escherichia coli and *Klebsiella* possess other mechanisms of β-lactam antibiotic resistance unrelated to ESBL production. Resistance to extended-spectrum cephalosporins, cephamycins, oxyimino-β-lactams, and β-lactamase inhibitors in *E coli* and *K pneumoniae* can be mediated by plasmid-mediated β-lactamases similar to those chromosomal AmpC enzymes produced in species such as *E cloacae* and *Serratia marcescens*.[120,121] Additional porin mutations can result in carbapenem resistance.[92] Resistance to β-lactam–β-lactamase inhibitor combinations can occur by alterations in porin channels, TEM and SHV hyperproduction, by the production of inhibitor-resistant TEM enzymes (Bush-Jacoby-Medeiros Group 2br) and in *E coli*, by chromosomal cephalosporinase AmpC production.[92,104,120]

β-lactam–resistant *Klebsiella* and *E coli* strains are often resistant to quinolones and aminoglycosides, leaving few alternatives for treatment.[122] Alterations in DNA gyrase (topoisomerase II and to a lesser extent topoisomerase IV), porin channel mutations, and efflux mechanisms can confer quinolone resistance.[123] Enzymatic modifications can lead to aminoglycoside resistance.[124]

Tigecycline has potent in vitro activity against multidrug-resistant gram-negative bacilli including ESBL-producing organisms.[125] Unfortunately, there are few data from the clinical setting to support the use of tigecycline as a single agent for the treatment of invasive infections caused by multidrug-resistant gram-negative bacilli. A recent study reported failure of tigecycline among patients with serious infections caused by gram-negative bacilli. Of note, these treatment failures occurred among isolates considered to be susceptible to tigecycline.[126]

Pseudomonas and Other Gram-Negative Rods Producing AmpC

AmpC β-lactamase production is another important mechanism of antimicrobial resistance in gram-negative organisms.[127] These hydrolyzing enzymes were discovered in the 1980s and were extensively studied. AmpC enzymes were initially identified only as inducible, chromosome-encoded β-lactamases found in certain species of *Enterobacter*, *Serratia*, *Pseudomonas*, *Providencia*, *Citrobacter*, and indole-positive *Proteus*.[128] Further research into gram-negative resistance also detected AmpC genes on transferrable plasmids in gram-negative bacilli, which do not chromosomally express these types of β-lactamases, including *Klebsiella* spp, *E coli*, or *Salmonella* spp.[129] Plasmid-mediated AmpC hyperproduction and antimicrobial resistance caused by chromosome-encoded AmpC enzymes can substantially complicate the management of gram-negative infections and adversely impact the clinical outcomes of patients.[130]

β-Lactam resistance among gram-negative organisms can also be mediated by two other classes of plasmid-mediated β-lactamases: hydrolyzing carbapenemases and

ESBL. The former is briefly discussed in this section, whereas ESBL resistance was covered previously in the section on multidrug-resistant Enterobacteriaceae.

Epidemiology and mechanisms of resistance

The production of AmpC is regulated through a series of complex interactions among chromosomal bacterial genes. Such interactions are influenced by changes in the cytoplasmic concentrations of intermediates of murein peptidoglycan synthesis and degradation.[131] AmpC is usually not produced at high levels initially, but exposure to particular β-lactam antibiotics, including cephalosporins, cephamycins, monobactams, and extended-spectrum penicillins, can "induce" or "derepress" the production of AmpC enzymes.[132] Additionally, certain genetic mutations lead to constitutive cephalosporinase production.[133] In both of these cases, the increase in AmpC production is regulated by changes in the homeostatic levels of intermediate products of murein synthesis.[131] There is a 20% to 30% risk of clinical failure when a third-generation cephalosporin is used to treat bacteremia secondary to AmpC-producing Enterobacter. The risk of such failure is much lower in urinary tract infections because of the high local cephalosporin concentrations.[134] AmpC-mediated resistance can be partially overcome by fourth-generation cephalosporins cefepime and cefpirome, which are more stable against AmpC-derepressed strains.[135]

Although AmpC production mediates much of the antibiotic resistance in certain gram-negative organisms, the impermeability of the outer cellular membrane and alterations in the outer membrane often also contribute to β-lactam resistance.[136] Cefepime, a fourth-generation cephalosporin, has neutral charge and a lower affinity for β-lactamases than third-generation cephalosporins, penetrates the outer membrane more effectively, and exhibits increased affinity for some essential PBP.[137] Cefepime often exhibits greater activity against AmpC-producing organisms than other cephalosporins.[138]

Acinetobacter spp

Resistance mechanisms to β-lactam antibiotics in Acinetobacter are not clearly understood, but resistance is common. Resistance frequently seems to be related to β-lactamase production, but other mechanisms have been identified. TEM-I and CARB enzymes seem to confer resistance to penicillins and some narrow-spectrum cephalosporins, whereas chromosomally produced cephalosporinases and plasmid-mediated ESBLs are thought to modulate resistance to broader-spectrum cephalosporins.[104,139] Carbapenem resistance is conferred by multiple different mechanisms including carbapenemase production of the IMP- and VIM-type, production of OXA-type β-lactamases, reduced cellular uptake, target mutations, and alterations in the PBP.[140–143] IMP metallo-β-lactamases were first described in a strain of P aeruginosa in Japan in 1988. In Acinetobacter baumannii IMP metallo-β-lactamases are usually present as part of a class 1 integron. Although metallo-β-lactamases are not the predominant carbapenemases in A baumannii, several have been described including IMP-1, IMP-2, IMP-4, IMP-5, IMP-6, and IMP-11.[144] Aminoglycoside resistance is mediated by aminoglycoside-modifying enzymes, and quinolone resistance by mutational changes of topoisomerase IV.[145,146]

Carbapenems are the most reliable therapeutic agents for infections caused by Acinetobacter, but resistance has begun to emerge in multiple geographic areas. Recent studies have reported rates of carbapenem resistance in A baumannii, the more resistant Acinetobacter species, as high as 11%.[147] A recent Centers for Disease Control and Prevention report noted that greater than 25% of Acinetobacter strains associated with device-related infections were carbapenem-resistant.

Additionally, the study by Reddy and colleagues revealed a increase of incidence of *A baumannii* from 1.7 to 3.7/1000 patient days from 2003 to 2008 along with a decrease in susceptibility to ampicillin-sulbactum and imipenem from 90% to 40% over the same time period.[148] A 1999 study reported meropenem resistance at greater than 50% in all isolates of *A baumannii* recovered from 15 hospitals in Brooklyn, New York.[149] A more recent study from the same area reported that rates of carbapenem resistance have exceeded 60% in some hospitals.[150] β-lactam–β-lactamase inhibitor combination antibiotics have good in vitro activity against *Acinetobacter lwoffi* (approximately 15% are resistant) but are less effective against *A baumannii* (20%–30% are resistant to piperacillin-tazobactam).[147] Ampicillin-sulbactam may be active against strains of *Acinetobacter* resistant to all other β-lactam agents, perhaps because of the unique antimicrobial activity of the sulbactam component against some acinetobacters. Ceftazidime and cefepime have modest activity, but approximately 35% of *A lwoffi* and *A baumannii* strains are resistant.[147] Aminoglycoside resistance occurs in approximately 20% to 30% of *A baumannii* isolates.[151] Resistance to quinolones is variable–precluding use of these drugs empirically before the results of susceptibility tests are known. In one study, approximately 80% of isolates tested were found to be ciprofloxacin-resistant.[152] Tigecycline, a relatively new glycylcycline agent, has bacteriostatic activity against multidrug-resistant *Acinetobacter* species. High-level resistance to tigecycline has been detected among some multidrug-resistant *Acinetobacter* isolates, and there is concern that the organism can rapidly evade this antimicrobial agent by upregulating chromosomally mediated efflux pumps. Given these findings and concern about whether adequate peak serum concentrations can be achieved, currently tigecycline is best reserved for salvage therapy.[153]

Stenotrophomonas Maltophilia

Stenotrophomonas maltophilia (formerly *Xanthomonas maltophilia*) is an aerobic gram-negative rod that causes bacteremia, respiratory tract infection, skin and soft tissue infection, and endocarditis. The virulence factors associated with *S maltophilia* include the production of proteases and elastases and the ability to adhere to synthetic materials. Nosocomial *S maltophilia* pneumonia is associated with adverse outcomes, particularly when the pneumonia is postobstructive or associated with bacteremia. In uncontrolled clinical trials, mortality rates associated with *S maltophilia* bacteremia range from 21% to 69%.[154]

The inducible, chromosomal enzymes *L1* and *L2* in *S maltophilia* confer resistance to β-lactam antibiotics. *L1* is a Bush-Jacoby-Medeiros class 3 enzyme (or metallo-β-lactamase) with broad activity against penicillins, carbapenems, cephalosporins, and β-lactamase inhibitors.[116,155] *L2* is a cephalosporinase (Bush-Jacoby-Medeiros class 2e) active against cephalosporins and monobactams. A TEM-2 β-lactamase encoded on a Tn-1 like transposon was also recently cloned from an *S maltophilia* isolate.[156] Decreased membrane permeability secondary to porin mutations often leads to quinolone resistance.[157] Aminoglycosides generally are not active against *S maltophilia*, probably caused by inactivating enzymes and alterations in the cell surface.[155] Overexpression of the multidrug efflux pump *SmeDEF* in *S maltophilia* may contribute to decreased susceptibility to tetracyclines, erythromycin, quinolones, and chloramphenicol.[158] Recent studies have reported that TMP-SMX resistance is mediated by the sul2 gene, which is associated with production by plasmids and class 1 integrons.[159,160]

TMP-SMX, a bacteriostatic agent, is the treatment of choice for infections caused by *S maltophilia*. Ticarcillin-clavulanate is the only β-lactam–β-lactamase inhibitor combination antibiotic that is reliably effective and may be used in patients who are intolerant of or infected with an isolate resistant to TMP-SMX.[155] Resistance to both of these agents is increasing; studies have reported that 5% of S maltophilia in the United States and 10% of isolates in Europe were resistant to TMP-SMX.[161] Ceftazidime does not possess reliable activity and should not be used empirically.[161] Cefepime has greater activity than ceftazidime (susceptibility was 88.7% vs 35.3% of United States bloodstream isolates in one study).[162] Resistance to imipenem approaches 100%.[162] Among the available fluoroquinolones, levofloxacin and moxifloxacin have better in vitro activity than ciprofloxacin. Minocycline has good in vitro activity,[163] but clinical experience is limited.

Tigecycline, a glycylcycline derived from minocycline, is a compound that has demonstrated good in vitro activity against S maltophilia strains including TMP-SMX–resistant S maltophilia, so it may be considered as a promising therapeutic option for the treatment of nosocomial infections caused by S maltophilia.[164] Use of antibiotic combinations, including TMP-SMX plus ticarcillin-clavulanate or a third-generation cephalosporin, and TMP-SMX plus minocycline plus ticarcillin-clavulanate, is being explored for the treatment of serious S maltophilia infections.[165] Although aztreonam is usually inactive against S maltophilia, one study demonstrated synergistic activity in vitro when combined with ticarcillin-clavulanate.[165] Although data are limited, resistance to TMP-SMX seems to be emerging, and recent in vitro modeling studies suggest that combination therapies of TMP-SMX plus ciprofloxacin and TMP-SMX plus tobramycin exhibit a greater killing capacity than TMP-SMX alone.[166]

The choice of monotherapy or combination therapy remains controversial. Use of multidrug therapy should be considered in cases of severe infection, particularly if local rates of resistance to TMP-SMX are high.[154]

Salmonella spp

Nontyphoidal species of Salmonella, such as S enteritidis and S enterica, are foodborne pathogens that can asymptomatically colonize the human intestine or cause clinical illnesses, such as gastroenteritis and bacteremia. Resistance to antimicrobial agents used to treat typhoidal and nontyphoidal species has rapidly emerged and disseminated around the world.[167]

Resistance to chloramphenicol in Salmonella typhi emerged in the 1970s, and several major outbreaks have been caused by chloramphenicol-resistant strains.[168] Resistance to chloramphenicol is often mediated by a self-transferable plasmid (IncHI) that also mediates resistance to sulfonamides, tetracycline, amoxicillin, TMP-SMX, and streptomycin.[167,169,170]

Resistance to the fluoroquinolones is an emerging problem, particularly in Asia,[171,172] and is usually mediated by chromosomal point mutations in the gyrA gene.[173] These quinolone-resistant strains are usually sensitive to ceftriaxone, cefixime, and azithromycin but the clinical response to treatment is usually slower and, with clearance of fever, sometimes exceeding taking 7 days or more. Failure rates are higher (>20%) when infection is caused by quinolone-resistant strains.[174] Resistance to nalidixic acid may predict clinical failure of quinolone therapy, even among isolates with in vitro quinolone susceptibility.[175] Such resistance to nalidixic acid was detected among 23% of S typhi isolates identified through the National Antimicrobial Resistance Monitoring System in 2000.[176] Resistance to third-generation cephalosporins (eg, ceftriaxone and cefotaxime) has occurred sporadically.[177]

The quinolones, such as ciprofloxacin, are considered the drugs of choice for empiric treatment of typhoid fever, except in areas of the world where quinolone resistance is common (eg, Asia).[178] So far, resistance to ciprofloxacin is infrequent in the

United States, but was found in up to 23% of *S typhi* isolates in the United Kingdom in 1999.[179] In that study, multidrug resistance to chloramphenicol, ampicillin, and TMP was reported in 26% of all *S typhi* isolates.[179] Other potential oral alternatives for treatment of *S typhi* infections include amoxicillin, TMP-SMX, cefixime, azithromycin, and chloramphenicol, as long as these agents possess in vitro activity against a given strain.[167] Third-generation cephalosporins, such as ceftriaxone and cefotaxime, remain active but require intravenous administration.[180]

Resistance among nontyphoidal strains of salmonellae emerged in the 1990s and spread rapidly.[167] Emergence of multiresistance to ampicillin, chloramphenicol, and TMP-SMX is caused in part by the widespread dissemination of *Salmonella typhimurium* definitive phage type 104 (DT 104).[181] This strain contains chromosomal determinants that mediate resistance to ampicillin, chloramphenicol, TMP-SMX, streptomycin, and tetracycline.[182] Resistance to fluoroquinolones has also emerged among nontyphoidal salmonellae in the United Kingdom (including DT104) and in the United States. Resistance to the fluoroquinolones is often mediated by *gyrA* mutations and fortunately this remains uncommon in isolates in the United States.[183] Resistance to broad-spectrum cephalosporins is conferred by plasmid-mediated AmpC-type cephalosporinase production[184] and sometimes by ESBL production.[185] Resistance to the carbapenems has been reported and is mediated by porin loss; cephalosporinase production; and carbapenemase production (including KPCs).[110,186]

Campylobacter Jejuni

Campylobacter spp are fastidious, curved, seagull-shaped, motile gram-negative bacilli and are the leading cause of foodborne diarrhea and a common cause of travelers' diarrhea.[187] Fluoroquinolone resistance in *Campylobacter* spp has been present since the early 1990s in Asia and Europe, which coincided with the addition of enrofloxacin to animal feed. In Spain, quinolone resistance is well above 50%. Elsewhere in Europe, resistance rates are approximately 10% to 20% and many of the resistant strains are acquired outside the reporting country.[188,189] Thailand experienced a similar increase in the rates of fluoroquinolone resistance in campylobacter during the 1990s (0% in 1990 to 84% in 1995).[190] Rates of fluoroquinolone resistance among *Campylobacter* are lower in the United States, but agricultural use of fluoroquinolones again coincided with increased resistance. In one United States study, resistance increased from 1.3% in 1992 to 10.2% in 1998.[191] Imported isolates can contribute significantly to local resistance patterns.

Resistance to the macrolides is low (<5% in most regions).[192] Most isolates are still susceptible to aminoglycosides, chloramphenicol, clindamycin, nitrofurantoin, and imipenem.[193] A point mutation at codon 86 in the *gyrA* DNA gyrase gene is the most common mutation conferring quinolone resistance.[192] Mutations in the *parC* gene occur less frequently,[194] but the presence of mutations in both regions confers high-level quinolone resistance.[194] Multidrug efflux pumps may also have a role in the development of quinolone resistance.[195] Erythromycin resistance in *Campylobacter* is caused by ribosomal alterations.[192]

Neisseria Gonorrhoeae

Antimicrobial resistance has been a concern with *Neisseria gonorrhoeae* since the 1940s when resistance to sulfonamides was first noted; this was followed by penicillin resistance in the 1950s, tetracycline resistance in the 1980s, and fluoroquinolone resistance in the 1990s.[196,197]

High-level penicillin resistance (MIC $\geq$16 μg/mL) in *N gonorrhoeae* is most often mediated by penicillinase production.[198] Penicillin resistance caused by production of a plasmid-encoded TEM-1 type β-lactamase was first detected in *N gonorrhoeae* in 1976 and has now disseminated worldwide.[199] In the United States, the percentage of penicillinase-producing *N gonorrhoeae* peaked in 1991 at 11% but declined to 0.4% in 2006.[200]

Multiple chromosomal mutations can mediate lower-level penicillin (MIC >2 μg/mL) resistance. Resistance genes typically accumulate in a stepwise fashion, leading to gradually increasing penicillin MICs.[198] These resistance genes include *penA*, which encodes an altered PBP 2; *mtr*, which increases expression of an efflux pump; and *penB*, which decreases antibiotic permeability across the cell membrane through a porin gene mutation.[198,201] Chromosomally mediated resistance to penicillin was present in 1.2% of isolates in a recent United States survey.[200]

Resistance to tetracycline occurs through chromosomally mediated changes in cell membrane porins or by ribosomal protection by the plasmid mediated tetM resistance gene. Additional chromosomal mutations led to resistance to spectinomycin.[202] Macrolide resistance can occur through efflux pumps, *erm* methylases, and changes in the 23S ribosome.[203]

Fluoroquinolone-resistant *N gonorrhoeae* (MIC ≥1 μg/mL) has disseminated to many countries,[204] and is widespread in certain parts of Asia. In a recent study, greater than 35% of *N gonorrhoeae* isolates in the Philippines and Vietnam were quinolone resistant.[205] There have also been alarming increases in quinolone resistance reported recently in England and Wales.[204] The overall prevalence of quinolone-resistant gonococci in the United States was 2.2% in 2002, but this increased to greater than 13% by 2005.[196] The rate of quinolone resistance is particularly high among men who have sex with men (29%). Decreased susceptibility to fluoroquinolones is caused by mutations in the *parC* gene of topoisomerase IV and *gyrA* of DNA gyrase.[206,207]

SUMMARY

The emergence of resistance to antimicrobial agents continues to evolve substantially, influencing the evaluation and treatment of infections in nosocomial and health care–associated settings and in the community. Bacteria use several strategies to avoid the effects of antimicrobial agents, and have evolved highly efficient means for clonal spread and for the dissemination of resistance traits. Control of antibiotic-resistant pathogens provides a major challenge for the medical and public health communities and for society. Control of the emergence of resistant pathogens requires adherence to infection control guidelines, such as those issued by the Centers for Disease Control and Prevention (http://www.cdc.gov/ncidod/dhqp/guidelines.html), and physicians, patients, and health care consumers must all understand the need for judicious use of antibiotics (http://www.cdc.gov/drugresistance/healthcare/default.htm).

REFERENCES

1. Neu HC. The crisis in antibiotic resistance [see comments]. Science 1992; 257(5073):1064–73.
2. Kishii R, Takei M. Relationship between the expression of ompf and quinolone resistance in escherichia coli. J Infect Chemother 2009;15(6):361–6.
3. Nikaido H. Preventing drug access to targets: cell surface permeability barriers and active efflux in bacteria. Semin Cell Dev Biol 2001;12(3):215–23.
4. Hu WS, Lin JF, Lin YH, et al. Outer membrane protein stm3031 (ail/ompx-like protein) plays a key role in the ceftriaxone resistance of salmonella enterica serovar typhimurium. Antimicrob Agents Chemother 2009;53(8):3248–55.

5. Ivaneson M, Mikkelsen H, Ventre I, et al. Two-component regulatory systems in pseudomonas aeruginosa: an intricate network mediating fimbrial and efflux pump gene expression. Molecular Microbiology 2011;79(5):1353–66.
6. Smith CA, Baker EN. Aminoglycoside antibiotic resistance by enzymatic deactivation. Curr Drug Targets Infect Disord 2002;2(2):143–60.
7. Bush K. Bench-to-bedside review: The role of beta-lactamases in antibiotic-resistant gram-negative infections. Crit Care 2010;14(3):224.
8. Davies J. Inactivation of antibiotics and the dissemination of resistance genes. Science 1994;264(5157):375–82.
9. Spratt BG. Resistance to antibiotics mediated by target alterations. Science 1994;264(5157):388–93.
10. Courvalin P. Vancomycin resistance in gram-positive cocci. Clin Infect Dis 2006; 42(Suppl 1):S25–34.
11. Normark BH, Normark S. Evolution and spread of antibiotic resistance. J Intern Med 2002;252(2):91–106.
12. Courvalin P. Transfer of antibiotic resistance genes between gram-positive and gram-negative bacteria. Antimicrob Agents Chemother 1994;38(7):1447–51.
13. Adhikari L. High-level aminoglycoside resistance and reduced susceptibility to vancomycin in nosocomial enterococci. J Glob Infect Dis 2010;2(3):231–5.
14. Murray BE, Singh KV, Markowitz SM, et al. Evidence for clonal spread of a single strain of beta-lactamase-producing *Enterococcus (Streptococcus) faecalis* to six hospitals in five states. J Infect Dis 1991;163(4):780–5.
15. Grayson ML, Eliopoulos GM, Wennersten CB, et al. Increasing resistance to beta-lactam antibiotics among clinical isolates of *Enterococcus faecium*: a 22-year review at one institution. Antimicrob Agents Chemother 1991;35(11):2180–4.
16. Boyce JM, Opal SM, Potter-Bynoe G, et al. Emergence and nosocomial transmission of ampicillin-resistant enterococci. Antimicrob Agents Chemother 1992;36(5):1032–9.
17. Williamson R, le Bouguenec C, Gutmann L, et al. One or two low affinity penicillin-binding proteins may be responsible for the range of susceptibility of *Enterococcus faecium* to benzylpenicillin. J Gen Microbiol 1985;131(8):1933–40.
18. Rupp ME, Marion N, Fey PD, et al. Outbreak of vancomycin-resistant *Enterococcus faecium* in a neonatal intensive care unit. Infect Control Hosp Epidemiol 2001;22(5):301–3.
19. Patterson JE, Zervos MJ. High-level gentamicin resistance in *Enterococcus*: microbiology, genetic basis, and epidemiology. Rev Infect Dis 1990;12(4):644–52.
20. Krogstad DJ, Korfhagen TR, Moellering RC Jr, et al. Aminoglycoside-inactivating enzymes in clinical isolates of *Streptococcus faecalis*: an explanation for resistance to antibiotic synergism. J Clin Invest 1978;62(2):480–6.
21. Hidron AI, Edwards JR, Patel J, et al. NHSN annual update: antimicrobial-resistant pathogens associated with healthcare-associated infections: annual summary of data reported to the National Healthcare Safety Network at the Centers for Disease Control and Prevention, 2006–2007. Infect Control Hosp Epidemiol 2008;29(11):996–1011.
22. Mutnick AH, Biedenbach DJ, Jones RN. Geographic variations and trends in antimicrobial resistance among *Enterococcus faecalis* and *Enterococcus faecium* in the SENTRY Antimicrobial Surveillance Program (1997–2000). Diagn Microbiol Infect Dis 2003;46(1):63–8.
23. Livornese LL Jr, Dias S, Samel C, et al. Hospital-acquired infection with vancomycin-resistant *Enterococcus faecium* transmitted by electronic thermometers. Ann Intern Med 1992;117(2):112–6.

24. Carmeli Y, Eliopoulos GM, Samore MH. Antecedent treatment with different antibiotic agents as a risk factor for vancomycin-resistant *Enterococcus*. Emerg Infect Dis 2002;8(8):802–7.
25. Arthur M, Courvalin P. Genetics and mechanisms of glycopeptide resistance in enterococci. Antimicrob Agents Chemother 1993;37(8):1563–71.
26. Shlaes DM, Etter L, Gutmann L. Synergistic killing of vancomycin-resistant enterococci of classes A, B, and C by combinations of vancomycin, penicillin, and gentamicin. Antimicrob Agents Chemother 1991;35(4):776–9.
27. Power EG, Abdulla YH, Talsania HG, et al. vanA genes in vancomycin-resistant clinical isolates of *Oerskovia turbata* and *Arcanobacterium (Corynebacterium) haemolyticum*. J Antimicrob Chemother 1995;36(4):595–606.
28. Ligozzi M, Lo Cascio G, Fontana R. vanA gene cluster in a vancomycin-resistant clinical isolate of *Bacillus circulans*. Antimicrob Agents Chemother 1998;42(8):2055–9.
29. Mevius D, Devriese L, Butaye P, et al. Isolation of glycopeptide resistant *Streptococcus gallolyticus* strains with vanA, vanB, and both vanA and vanB genotypes from faecal samples of veal calves in The Netherlands. J Antimicrob Chemother 1998;42(2):275–6.
30. Dutka-Malen S, Blaimont B, Wauters G, et al. Emergence of high-level resistance to glycopeptides in *Enterococcus gallinarum* and *Enterococcus casseliflavus*. Antimicrob Agents Chemother 1994;38(7):1675–7.
31. Centers for Disease Control and Prevention (CDC) *Staphylococcus aureus* resistant to vancomycin—United States, 2002. MMWR Morb Mortal Wkly Rep 2002;51(26):565–7.
32. Noble WC, Virani Z, Cree RG. Co-transfer of vancomycin and other resistance genes from *Enterococcus faecalis* NCTC 12201 to *Staphylococcus aureus*. FEMS Microbiol Lett 1992;72(2):195–8.
33. Perichon B, Reynolds P, Courvalin P. VanD-type glycopeptide-resistant *Enterococcus faecium* BM4339. Antimicrob Agents Chemother 1997;41(9):2016–8.
34. McKessar SJ, Berry AM, Bell JM, et al. Genetic characterization of vanG, a novel vancomycin resistance locus of *Enterococcus faecalis*. Antimicrob Agents Chemother 2000;44(11):3224–8.
35. Fines M, Perichon B, Reynolds P, et al. VanE, a new type of acquired glycopeptide resistance in *Enterococcus faecalis* BM4405. Antimicrob Agents Chemother 1999;43(9):2161–4.
36. Prystowsky J, Siddiqui F, Chosay J, et al. Resistance to linezolid: characterization of mutations in rRNA and comparison of their occurrences in vancomycin-resistant enterococci. Antimicrob Agents Chemother 2001;45:2154–6.
37. Bonora MG, Solbiati M, Stepan E, et al. Emergence of linezolid resistance in the vancomycin-resistant *Enterococcus faecium* multilocus sequence typing C1 epidemic lineage. J Clin Microbiol 2006;44(3):1153–5.
38. Pogue JM, Paterson DL, Pasculle AW, et al. Determination of risk factors associated with isolation of linezolid-resistant strains of vancomycin-resistant *Enterococcus*. Infect Control Hosp Epidemiol 2007;28(12):1382–8.
39. Kelesidis T, Humphries R, Uslan DZ, et al. Daptomycin nonsusceptible enterococci: An emerging challenge for clinicians. Clin Infect Dis 2011;52(2):228–34.
40. Kirby WM. Extraction of a highly potent penicillin inactivator from penicillin resistant staphylococci. Science 1944;99(2579):452–3.
41. Clinical and Laboratory Standards Institute (CLSI) Performance standards for antimicrobial susceptibility testing. Wayne (PA): Clinical and Laboratory Standards Institute (CLSI); 2008.

42. Zhu W, Murray PR, Huskins WC, et al. Dissemination of an enterococcus inc18-like vana plasmid associated with vancomycin-resistant *Staphylococcus aureus*. Antimicrob Agents Chemother 2010;54(10):4314–20.
43. Ikeda-Dantsuji Y, Hanaki H, Nakae T, et al. Emergence of linezolid-resistant mutants in the susceptible cell population of methicillin-resistant *Staphylococcus aureus*. Antimicrob Agents Chemother 2011;55(5):2466–8.
44. van Hal SJ, Paterson DL, Gosbell IB. Emergence of daptomycin resistance following vancomycin-unresponsive staphylococcus aureus bacteraemia in a daptomycin-naive patient-a review of the literature. Eur J Clin Microbiol Infect Dis 2011;30(5):603–10.
45. Liu C, Bayer A, Cosgrove SE, et al. Clinical practice guidelines by the infectious diseases society of america for the treatment of methicillin-resistant Staphylococcus aureus infections in adults and children. Clin Infect Dis 2011;52(3): e18–55.
46. Higuchi W, Takano T, Teng LJ, et al. Structure and specific detection of staphylococcal cassette chromosome mec type VII. Biochem Biophys Res Commun 2008;377(3):752–6.
47. Oliveira DC, Milheirico C, de Lencastre H. Redefining a structural variant of staphylococcal cassette chromosome mec, SCCmec type VI. Antimicrob Agents Chemother 2006;50(10):3457–9.
48. Zhang K, McClure JA, Elsayed S, et al. Novel staphylococcal cassette chromosome mec type carrying class A mec and type 4 ccr gene complexes in a Canadian epidemic strain of methicillin-resistant *Staphylococcus aureus*. Antimicrob Agents Chemother 2009;53(2):531–40.
49. Katayama Y, Ito T, Hiramatsu K. Genetic organization of the chromosome region surrounding mecA in clinical staphylococcal strains: role of IS431-mediated mecI deletion in expression of resistance in mecA-carrying, low-level methicillin-resistant *Staphylococcus haemolyticus*. Antimicrob Agents Chemother 2001;45(7):1955–63.
50. Nastaly P, Grinholc M, Bielawski KP. Molecular characteristics of community-associated methicillin-resistant staphylococcus aureus strains for clinical medicine. Arch Microbiol 2010;192(8):603–17.
51. Chua K, Laurent F, Coombs G, et al. Antimicrobial resistance: not community-associated methicillin-resistant staphylococcus aureus (ca-mrsa)! A clinician's guide to community MRSA - its evolving antimicrobial resistance and implications for therapy. Clin Infect Dis 2011;52(1):99–114.
52. Diep BA, Chambers HF, Graber CJ, et al. Emergence of multidrug-resistant, community-associated, methicillin-resistant staphylococcus aureus clone usa 300 in men who have sex with men. Ann Intern Med 2008;148(4):249–57.
53. CDC reminds clinical laboratories and healthcare infection preventionists of their role in the search and containment of vancomycin-resistant staphylococcus aureus (VRSA). Available at: http://www.cdc.gov/HAI/settings/lab/vrsa_lab_search_containment.html. Accessed April 12, 2011.
54. Weigel LM, Clewell DB, Gill SR, et al. Genetic analysis of a high-level vancomycin-resistant isolate of *Staphylococcus aureus*. Science 2003;302(5650):1569–71.
55. Zhu W, Murray PR, Huskins WC, et al. Dissemination of an enterococcus inc18-like vana plasmid associated with vancomycin-resistant *Staphylococcus aureus*. Antimicrob Agents Chemother 2010;54(10):4314–20.
56. de Niederhausern S, Bondi M, Messi P, et al. Vancomycin-resistance transferability from vana enterococci to *Staphylococcus aureus*. Curr Microbiol 2011; 62(5):1363–7.

57. Soriano A, Marco F, Martinez JA, et al. Influence of vancomycin minimum inhibitory concentration on the treatment of methicillin-resistant *Staphylococcus aureus* bacteremia. Clin Infect Dis 2008;46(2):193–200.

58. Sakoulas G, Moise-Broder PA, Schentag J, et al. Relationship of MIC and bactericidal activity to efficacy of vancomycin for treatment of methicillin-resistant *Staphylococcus aureus* bacteremia. J Clin Microbiol 2004;42(6):2398–402.

59. Steinkraus G, White R, Friedrich L. Vancomycin MIC creep in non-vancomycin-intermediate *Staphylococcus aureus* (VISA), vancomycin-susceptible clinical methicillin-resistant *S. aureus* (MRSA) blood isolates from 2001–05. J Antimicrob Chemother 2007;60(4):788–94.

60. Sader HS, Fey PD, Limaye AP, et al. Evaluation of vancomycin and daptomycin potency trends (MIC creep) against methicillin-resistant *Staphylococcus aureus* isolates collected in nine U.S. medical centers from 2002 to 2006. Antimicrob Agents Chemother 2009;53(10):4127–32.

61. Jones RN. Microbiological features of vancomycin in the 21st century: minimum inhibitory concentration creep, bactericidal/static activity, and applied breakpoints to predict clinical outcomes or detect resistant strains. Clin Infect Dis 2006;42(Suppl 1):S13–24.

62. Wang G, Hindler JF, Ward KW, et al. Increased vancomycin MICs for *Staphylococcus aureus* clinical isolates from a university hospital during a 5-year period. J Clin Microbiol 2006;44(11):3883–6.

63. Rybak M, Lomaestro B, Rotschafer JC, et al. Therapeutic monitoring of vancomycin in adult patients: a consensus review of the American Society of Health-System Pharmacists, the Infectious Diseases Society of America, and the Society of Infectious Diseases Pharmacists. Am J Health Syst Pharm 2009; 66(1):82–98.

64. Champney WS, Miller M. Linezolid is a specific inhibitor of 50S ribosomal subunit formation in *Staphylococcus aureus* cells. Curr Microbiol 2002;44(5): 350–6.

65. Tsiodras S, Gold HS, Sakoulas G, et al. Linezolid resistance in a clinical isolate of *Staphylococcus aureus*. Lancet 2001;358(9277):207–8.

66. Besier S, Ludwig A, Zander J, et al. Linezolid resistance in *Staphylococcus aureus*: gene dosage effect, stability, fitness costs, and cross-resistances. Antimicrob Agents Chemother 2008;52(4):1570–2.

67. Endimiani A, Blackford M, Dasenbrook EC, et al. Emergence of linezolid-resistant *Staphylococcus aureus* after prolonged treatment of cystic fibrosis patients in Cleveland, Ohio. Antimicrob Agents Chemother 2011;55(4):1684–92.

68. Hobbs JK, Miller K, O'Neill AJ, et al. Consequences of daptomycin-mediated membrane damage in *Staphylococcus aureus*. J Antimicrob 2008;62(5): 1003–8.

69. Silverman JA, Mortin LI, Vanpraagh AD, et al. Inhibition of daptomycin by pulmonary surfactant: in vitro modeling and clinical impact. J Infect Dis 2005;191(12):2149–52.

70. Skiest DJ. Treatment failure resulting from resistance of *Staphylococcus aureus* to daptomycin. J Clin Microbiol 2006;44(2):655–6.

71. Sakoulas G, Alder J, Thauvin-Eliopoulos C, et al. Induction of daptomycin heterogeneous susceptibility in *Staphylococcus aureus* by exposure to vancomycin. Antimicrob Agents Chemother 2006;50(4):1581–5.

72. Jones T, Yeaman MR, Sakoulas G, et al. Failures in clinical treatment of *Staphylococcus aureus* infection with daptomycin are associated with alterations in surface charge, membrane phospholipid asymmetry, and drug binding. Antimicrob Agents Chemother 2008;52(1):269–78.

73. Cui L, Tominaga E, Neoh HM, et al. Correlation between reduced daptomycin susceptibility and vancomycin resistance in vancomycin-intermediate *Staphylococcus aureus*. Antimicrob Agents Chemother 2006;50(3):1079–82.

74. Schmitz FJ, Witte W, Werner G, et al. Characterization of the translational attenuator of 20 methicillin-resistant, quinupristin/dalfopristin-resistant *Staphylococcus aureus* isolates with reduced susceptibility to glycopeptides. J Antimicrob Chemother 2001;48(6):939–41.

75. Drago L, Nicola L, De Vecchi E. A comparative in-vitro evaluation of resistance selection after exposure to teicoplanin, vancomycin, linezolid and quinupristin-dalfopristin in *Staphylococcus aureus* and *Enterococcus* spp. Clin Microbiol Infect 2008;14(6):608–11.

76. Allignet J, el Solh N. Diversity among the gram-positive acetyltransferases inactivating streptogramin A and structurally related compounds and characterization of a new staphylococcal determinant, vatB. Antimicrob Agents Chemother 1995;39(9):2027–36.

77. Markiewicz Z, Tomasz A. Variation in penicillin-binding protein patterns of penicillin-resistant clinical isolates of pneumococci. J Clin Microbiol 1989; 27(3):405–10.

78. Nagai K, Davies TA, Jacobs MR, et al. Effects of amino acid alterations in penicillin-binding proteins (PBPs) 1a, 2b, and 2x on PBP affinities of penicillin, ampicillin, amoxicillin, cefditoren, cefuroxime, cefprozil, and cefaclor in 18 clinical isolates of penicillin-susceptible, -intermediate, and -resistant pneumococci. Antimicrob Agents Chemother 2002;46(5):1273–80.

79. Zapun A, Contreras-Martel C, Vernet T. Penicillin-binding proteins and beta-lactam resistance. FEMS Microbiol Rev 2008;32(2):361–85.

80. Pernot L, Chesnel L, Le Gouellec A, et al. A PBP2x from a clinical isolate of *Streptococcus pneumoniae* exhibits an alternative mechanism for reduction of susceptibility to beta-lactam antibiotics. J Biol Chem 2004;279(16):16463–70.

81. Sahm DF, Brown NP, Draghi DC, et al. Tracking resistance among bacterial respiratory tract pathogens: summary of findings of the TRUST Surveillance Initiative, 2001–2005. Postgrad Med 2008;120(3 Suppl 1):8–15.

82. Chiu CH, Su LH, Huang YC, et al. Increasing ceftriaxone resistance and multiple alterations of penicillin-binding proteins among penicillin-resistant *Streptococcus pneumoniae* isolates in Taiwan. Antimicrob Agents Chemother 2007; 51(9):3404–6.

83. Gums JG, Boatwright DW, Camblin M, et al. Differences between ceftriaxone and cefotaxime: microbiological inconsistencies. Ann Pharmacother 2008; 42(1):71–9.

84. Cardoso MR, Nascimento-Carvalho CM, Ferrero F, et al. Penicillin-resistant pneumococcus and risk of treatment failure in pneumonia. Arch Dis Child 2008;93(3):221–5.

85. Sahm DF, Brown NP, Thornsberry C, et al. Antimicrobial susceptibility profiles among common respiratory tract pathogens: a GLOBAL perspective. Postgrad Med 2008;120(3 Suppl 1):16–24.

86. Rodriguez CA, Atkinson R, Bitar W, et al. Tolerance to vancomycin in pneumococci: detection with a molecular marker and assessment of clinical impact. J Infect Dis 2004;190(8):1481–7.

87. Low DE. Quinolone resistance among pneumococci: therapeutic and diagnostic implications. Clin Infect Dis 2004;38(Suppl 4):S357–62.

88. Bush K, Jacoby GA. Updated functional classification of beta-lactamases. Antimicrob Agents Chemother 2010;54(3):969–76.

89. Sirot DL, Goldstein FW, Soussy CJ, et al. Resistance to cefotaxime and seven other beta-lactams in members of the family Enterobacteriaceae: a 3-year survey in France. Antimicrob Agents Chemother 1992;36(8):1677–81.

90. Burwen DR, Banerjee SN, Gaynes RP. Ceftazidime resistance among selected nosocomial gram-negative bacilli in the United States. National Nosocomial Infections Surveillance System. J Infect Dis 1994;170(6):1622–5.

91. Edwards JR, Peterson KD, Andrus ML, et al. National Healthcare Safety Network (NHSN) Report, data summary for 2006 through 2007, issued November 2008. Am J Infect Control 2008;36(9):609–26.

92. Jacoby GA. Extended-spectrum beta-lactamases and other enzymes providing resistance to oxyimino-beta-lactams. Infect Dis Clin North Am 1997;11(4): 875–87.

93. Wiener J, Quinn JP, Bradford PA, et al. Multiple antibiotic-resistant Klebsiella and Escherichia coli in nursing homes [see comments]. JAMA 1999;281(6):517–23.

94. Montgomerie JZ. Epidemiology of Klebsiella and hospital-associated infections. Rev Infect Dis 1979;1(5):736–53.

95. Lin MF, Huang ML, Lai SH. Risk factors in the acquisition of extended-spectrum beta-lactamase Klebsiella pneumoniae: a case-control study in a district teaching hospital in Taiwan. J Hosp Infect 2003;53(1):39–45.

96. Lautenbach E, Patel JB, Bilker WB, et al. Extended-spectrum beta-lactamase-producing Escherichia coli and Klebsiella pneumoniae: risk factors for infection and impact of resistance on outcomes. Clin Infect Dis 2001;32(8):1162–71.

97. Du B, Long Y, Liu H, et al. Extended-spectrum beta-lactamase-producing Escherichia coli and Klebsiella pneumoniae bloodstream infection: risk factors and clinical outcome. Intensive Care Med 2002;28(12):1718–23.

98. D'Agata E, Venkataraman L, DeGirolami P, et al. The molecular and clinical epidemiology of enterobacteriaceae-producing extended-spectrum beta-lactamase in a tertiary care hospital. J Infect 1998;36(3):279–85.

99. Rahal JJ, Urban C, Horn D, et al. Class restriction of cephalosporin use to control total cephalosporin resistance in nosocomial Klebsiella [see comments]. JAMA 1998;280(14):1233–7.

100. Pena C, Pujol M, Ardanuy C, et al. Epidemiology and successful control of a large outbreak due to Klebsiella pneumoniae producing extended-spectrum beta-lactamases. Antimicrob Agents Chemother 1998;42(1):53–8.

101. Harris AD, McGregor JC, Johnson JA, et al. Risk factors for colonization with extended-spectrum beta-lactamase-producing bacteria and intensive care unit admission. Emerg Infect Dis 2007;13(8):1144–9.

102. Amino acid sequences for TEM, SHV and OXA extended-spectrum beta-lactamases. Available at: http://www.lahey.org/studies/inc_webt.asp. Accessed July, 2009.

103. Bonnet R. Growing group of extended-spectrum beta-lactamases: the CTX-M enzymes. Antimicrob Agents Chemother 2004;48(1):1–14.

104. Livermore DM. beta-Lactamases in laboratory and clinical resistance. Clin Microbiol Rev 1995;8(4):557–84.

105. Walsh TR. Emerging carbapenemases: a global perspective. Int J Antimicrob Agents 2010;36(Suppl 3):S8–14.

106. Patel G, Huprikar S, Factor SH, et al. Outcomes of carbapenem-resistant Klebsiella pneumoniae infection and the impact of antimicrobial and adjunctive therapies. Infect Control Hosp Epidemiol 2008;29(12):1099–106.

107. Martinez-Martinez L, Hernandez-Alles S, Alberti S, et al. In vivo selection of porin-deficient mutants of Klebsiella pneumoniae with increased resistance to

cefoxitin and expanded-spectrum-cephalosporins. Antimicrob Agents Chemother 1996;40(2):342–8.

108. Pangon B, Bizet C, Bure A, et al. In vivo selection of a cephamycin-resistant, porin-deficient mutant of *Klebsiella pneumoniae* producing a TEM-3 beta-lactamase. J Infect Dis 1989;159(5):1005–6.

109. Kaye KS, Gold HS, Schwaber MJ, et al. Variety of beta-lactamases produced by amoxicillin-clavulanate-resistant *Escherichia coli* isolated in the northeastern United States. Antimicrob Agents Chemother 2004;48(5):1520–5.

110. Coudron PE, Moland ES, Thomson KS. Occurrence and detection of AmpC beta-lactamases among *Escherichia coli*, *Klebsiella pneumoniae*, and *Proteus mirabilis* isolates at a veterans medical center. J Clin Microbiol 2000;38(5):1791–6.

111. Bell JM, Turnidge JD, Gales AC, et al. Prevalence of extended spectrum beta-lactamase (ESBL)-producing clinical isolates in the Asia-Pacific region and South Africa: regional results from SENTRY Antimicrobial Surveillance Program (1998–99). Diagn Microbiol Infect Dis 2002;42(3):193–8.

112. Urban C, Bradford PA, Tuckman M, et al. Carbapenem-resistant *Escherichia coli* harboring *Klebsiella pneumoniae* carbapenemase beta-lactamases associated with long-term care facilities. Clin Infect Dis 2008;46(11):e127–30.

113. Andriole VT. The quinolones. 2nd edition. New York: Academic Press; 1998.

114. Tian GB, Adams-Haduch JM, Bogdanovich T, et al. Identification of diverse OXA-40 group carbapenemases, including a novel variant, OXA-160, from *Acinetobacter baumannii* in Pennsylvania. Antimicrob Agents Chemother 2011; 55(1):429–32.

115. Walsh TR. Emerging carbapenemases: a global perspective. Int J Antimicrob Agents 2010;36(Suppl 3):S8–14.

116. Yang K, Guglielmo BJ. Diagnosis and treatment of extended-spectrum and AmpC beta-lactamase-producing organisms. Ann Pharmacother 2007;41(9): 1427–35.

117. Moellering RC Jr. Ndm-1–a cause for worldwide concern. N Engl J Med 2010; 363(25):2377–9.

118. Sanders WE Jr, Sanders CC. Inducible beta-lactamases: clinical and epidemiologic implications for use of newer cephalosporins. Rev Infect Dis 1988;10(4): 830–8.

119. Tenover FC, Emery SL, Spiegel CA, et al. Identification of plasmid-mediated AmpC {beta}-lactamases in *Escherichia coli*, *Klebsiella pneumoniae*, and *Proteus* species can potentially improve reporting of cephalosporin susceptibility testing results. J Clin Microbiol 2009;47(2):294–9.

120. Fakioglu E, Queenan AM, Bush K, et al. Amp C beta-lactamase-producing *Escherichia coli* in neonatal meningitis: diagnostic and therapeutic challenge. J Perinatol 2006;26(8):515–7.

121. Jacobs C, Frere JM, Normark S. Cytosolic intermediates for cell wall biosynthesis and degradation control inducible beta-lactam resistance in gram-negative bacteria. Cell 1997;88(6):823–32.

122. Korsak D, Liebscher S, Vollmer W. Susceptibility to antibiotics and beta-lactamase induction in murein hydrolase mutants of *Escherichia coli*. Antimicrob Agents Chemother 2005;49(4):1404–9.

123. Medeiros AA. Evolution and dissemination of beta-lactamases accelerated by generations of beta-lactam antibiotics. Clin Infect Dis 1997;24(Suppl 1):S19–45.

124. Kaye KS, Cosgrove S, Harris A, et al. Risk factors for emergence of resistance to broad-spectrum cephalosporins among *Enterobacter* spp. Antimicrob Agents Chemother 2001;45(9):2628–30.

125. Livermore DM, Warner M, Mushtaq S, et al. What remains against carbapenem-resistant Enterobacteriaceae? Evaluation of chloramphenicol, ciprofloxacin, colistin, fosfomycin, minocycline, nitrofurantoin, temocillin and tigecycline. Int J Antimicrob Agents 2011;37(5):415–9.

126. Metan G, Alp E, Yildiz O, et al. Clinical experience with tigecycline in the treatment of carbapenem-resistant Acinetobacter infections. J Chemother 2010; 22(2):110–4.

127. Ceccarelli M, Ruggerone P. Physical insights into permeation of and resistance to antibiotics in bacteria. Curr Drug Targets 2008;9(9):779–88.

128. Kessler RE. Cefepime microbiologic profile and update. Pediatr Infect Dis J 2001;20(3):331–6.

129. Ishii Y, Tateda K, Yamaguchi K. Evaluation of antimicrobial susceptibility for beta-lactams using the Etest method against clinical isolates from 100 medical centers in Japan (2006). Diagn Microbiol Infect Dis 2008;60(2):177–83.

130. Poirel L, Pitout JD, Nordmann P. Carbapenemases: molecular diversity and clinical consequences. Future Microbiol 2007;2(5):501–12.

131. Yigit H, Queenan AM, Anderson GJ, et al. Novel carbapenem-hydrolyzing beta-lactamase, KPC-1, from a carbapenem-resistant strain of *Klebsiella pneumoniae*. Antimicrob Agents Chemother 2001;45(4):1151–61.

132. Bratu S, Brooks S, Burney S, et al. Detection and spread of *Escherichia coli* possessing the plasmid-borne carbapenemase KPC-2 in Brooklyn, New York. Clin Infect Dis 2007;44(7):972–5.

133. Lomaestro BM, Tobin EH, Shang W, et al. The spread of *Klebsiella pneumoniae* carbapenemase-producing *K. pneumoniae* to upstate New York. Clin Infect Dis 2006;43(3):e26–8.

134. Bratu S, Mooty M, Nichani S, et al. Emergence of KPC-possessing *Klebsiella pneumoniae* in Brooklyn, New York: epidemiology and recommendations for detection. Antimicrob Agents Chemother 2005;49(7):3018–20.

135. Miriagou V, Tzouvelekis LS, Rossiter S, et al. Imipenem resistance in a *Salmonella* clinical strain due to plasmid-mediated class A carbapenemase KPC-2. Antimicrob Agents Chemother 2003;47(4):1297–300.

136. Villegas MV, Lolans K, Correa A, et al. First identification of *Pseudomonas aeruginosa* isolates producing a KPC-type carbapenem-hydrolyzing beta-lactamase. Antimicrob Agents Chemother 2007;51(4):1553–5.

137. Fung-Tomc J, Dougherty TJ, DeOrio FJ, et al. Activity of cefepime against ceftazidime- and cefotaxime-resistant gram-negative bacteria and its relationship to beta-lactamase levels. Antimicrob Agents Chemother 1989;33(4):498–502.

138. Choi SH, Lee JE, Park SJ, et al. Emergence of antibiotic resistance during therapy for infections caused by Enterobacteriaceae producing AmpC beta-lactamase: implications for antibiotic use. Antimicrob Agents Chemother 2008; 52(3):995–1000.

139. Danes C, Navia MM, Ruiz J, et al. Distribution of beta-lactamases in *Acinetobacter baumannii* clinical isolates and the effect of Syn 2190 (AmpC inhibitor) on the MICs of different beta-lactam antibiotics. J Antimicrob Chemother 2002;50(2):261–4.

140. Livermore DM. Acquired carbapenemases. J Antimicrob Chemother 1997; 39(6):673–6.

141. Afzal-Shah M, Woodford N, Livermore DM. Characterization of OXA-25, OXA-26, and OXA-27, molecular class D beta-lactamases associated with carbapenem resistance in clinical isolates of *Acinetobacter baumannii*. Antimicrob Agents Chemother 2001;45(2):583–8.

142. Bou G, Cervero G, Dominguez MA, et al. Characterization of a nosocomial outbreak caused by a multiresistant *Acinetobacter baumannii* strain with a carbapenem-hydrolyzing enzyme: high-level carbapenem resistance in *A. baumannii* is not due solely to the presence of beta-lactamases. J Clin Microbiol 2000;38(9):3299–305.

143. Quale J, Bratu S, Landman D, et al. Molecular epidemiology and mechanisms of carbapenem resistance in *Acinetobacter baumannii* endemic in New York City. Clin Infect Dis 2003;37(2):214–20.

144. Perez F, Hujer AM, Hujer KM, et al. Global challenge of multidrug-resistant *Acinetobacter baumannii*. Antimicrob Agents Chemother 2007;51(10):3471–84.

145. Miller GH, Sabatelli FJ, Hare RS, et al. The most frequent aminoglycoside resistance mechanisms–changes with time and geographic area: a reflection of aminoglycoside usage patterns? Aminoglycoside Resistance Study Groups. Clin Infect Dis 1997;24(Suppl 1):S46–62.

146. Vila J, Ruiz J, Goni P, et al. Quinolone-resistance mutations in the topoisomerase IV parC gene of *Acinetobacter baumannii*. J Antimicrob Chemother 1997;39(6):757–62.

147. Turner PJ, Greenhalgh JM. The activity of meropenem and comparators against *Acinetobacter* strains isolated from European hospitals, 1997–2000. Clin Microbiol Infect 2003;9(6):563–7.

148. Reddy T, Chopra T, Marchaim D, et al. Trends in antimicrobial resistance of acinetobacter baumannii isolates from a metropolitan detroit health system. Antimicrob Agents Chemother 2010;54(5):2235–8.

149. Landman D, Quale JM, Mayorga D, et al. Citywide clonal outbreak of multiresistant *Acinetobacter baumannii* and *Pseudomonas aeruginosa* in Brooklyn, NY: the preantibiotic era has returned. Arch Intern Med 2002;162(13):1515–20.

150. Landman D, Bratu S, Kochar S, et al. Evolution of antimicrobial resistance among Pseudomonas aeruginosa, Acinetobacter baumannii and Klebsiella pneumoniae in Brooklyn, NY. J Antimicrob Chemother 2007;60(1):78–82.

151. Seifert H, Strate A, Pulverer G. Nosocomial bacteremia due to *Acinetobacter baumannii*: clinical features, epidemiology, and predictors of mortality. Medicine (Baltimore) 1995;74(6):340–9.

152. Vila J, Ribera A, Marco F, et al. Activity of clinafloxacin, compared with six other quinolones, against *Acinetobacter baumannii* clinical isolates. J Antimicrob Chemother 2002;49(3):471–7.

153. Maragakis LL, Perl TM. *Acinetobacter baumannii*: epidemiology, antimicrobial resistance, and treatment options. Clin Infect Dis 2008;46(8):1254–63.

154. Nicodemo AC, Paez JI. Antimicrobial therapy for *Stenotrophomonas maltophilia* infections. Eur J Clin Microbiol Infect Dis 2007;26(4):229–37.

155. Denton M, Kerr KG. Microbiological and clinical aspects of infection associated with *Stenotrophomonas maltophilia*. Clin Microbiol Rev 1998;11(1):57–80.

156. Avison MB, von Heldreich CJ, Higgins CS, et al. A TEM-2 beta-lactamase encoded on an active Tn1-like transposon in the genome of a clinical isolate of *Stenotrophomonas maltophilia*. J Antimicrob Chemother 2000;46(6):879–84.

157. Cullmann W. Antibiotic susceptibility and outer membrane proteins of clinical *Xanthomonas maltophilia* isolates. Chemotherapy 1991;37(4):246–50.

158. Alonso A, Martinez JL. Expression of multidrug efflux pump SmeDEF by clinical isolates of *Stenotrophomonas maltophilia*. Antimicrob Agents Chemother 2001;45(6):1879–81.

159. Barbolla R, Catalano M, Orman BE, et al. Class 1 integrons increase trimethoprim-sulfamethoxazole MICs against epidemiologically unrelated

Stenotrophomonas maltophilia isolates. Antimicrob Agents Chemother 2004; 48(2):666–9.

160. Toleman MA, Bennett PM, Bennett DM, et al. Global emergence of trimethoprim/ sulfamethoxazole resistance in *Stenotrophomonas maltophilia* mediated by acquisition of sul genes. Emerg Infect Dis 2007;13(4):559–65.

161. Gales AC, Jones RN, Forward KR, et al. Emerging importance of multidrug-resistant *Acinetobacter* species and *Stenotrophomonas maltophilia* as pathogens in seriously ill patients: geographic patterns, epidemiological features, and trends in the SENTRY Antimicrobial Surveillance Program (1997–1999). Clin Infect Dis 2001;32(Suppl 2):S104–13.

162. Jones RN, Pfaller MA, Marshall SA, et al. Antimicrobial activity of 12 broad-spectrum agents tested against 270 nosocomial blood stream infection isolates caused by non-enteric gram-negative bacilli: occurrence of resistance, molecular epidemiology, and screening for metallo-enzymes. Diagn Microbiol Infect Dis 1997;29(3):187–92.

163. Canton R, Valdezate S, Vindel A, et al. Antimicrobial susceptibility profile of molecular typed cystic fibrosis *Stenotrophomonas maltophilia* isolates and differences with noncystic fibrosis isolates. Pediatr Pulmonol 2003;35(2): 99–107.

164. Insa R, Cercenado E, Goyanes MJ, et al. In vitro activity of tigecycline against clinical isolates of *Acinetobacter baumannii* and *Stenotrophomonas maltophilia*. J Antimicrob Chemother 2007;59(3):583–5.

165. Krueger TS, Clark EA, Nix DE. In vitro susceptibility of *Stenotrophomonas maltophilia* to various antimicrobial combinations. Diagn Microbiol Infect Dis 2001; 41(1/2):71–8.

166. Al-Jasser AM. *Stenotrophomonas maltophilia* resistant to trimethoprim-sulfamethoxazole: an increasing problem. Ann Clin Microbiol Antimicrob 2006;5:23.

167. Parry CM, Threlfall EJ. Antimicrobial resistance in typhoidal and nontyphoidal salmonellae. Curr Opin Infect Dis 2008;21(5):531–8.

168. Parry CM, Hien TT, Dougan G, et al. Typhoid fever. N Engl J Med 2002;347(22): 1770–82.

169. Taylor DE, Chumpitaz JC, Goldstein F. Variability of IncHI1 plasmids from *Salmonella typhi* with special reference to Peruvian plasmids encoding resistance to trimethoprim and other antibiotics. Antimicrob Agents Chemother 1985;28(3): 452–5.

170. Gilmour MW, Thomson NR, Sanders M, et al. The complete nucleotide sequence of the resistance plasmid R478: defining the backbone components of incompatibility group H conjugative plasmids through comparative genomics. Plasmid 2004;52(3):182–202.

171. Capoor MR, Nair D, Deb M, et al. Enteric fever perspective in India: emergence of high-level ciprofloxacin resistance and rising MIC to cephalosporins. J Med Microbiol 2007;56(Pt 8):1131–2.

172. Ko WC, Yan JJ, Yu WL, et al. A new therapeutic challenge for old pathogens: community-acquired invasive infections caused by ceftriaxone- and ciprofloxacin-resistant *Salmonella enterica* serotype choleraesuis. Clin Infect Dis 2005;40(2):315–8.

173. Shirakawa T, Acharya B, Kinoshita S, et al. Decreased susceptibility to fluoroquinolones and gyrA gene mutation in the *Salmonella enterica* serovar typhi and paratyphi A isolated in Katmandu, Nepal, in 2003. Diagn Microbiol Infect Dis 2006;54(4):299–303.

174. Crump JA, Kretsinger K, Gay K, et al. Clinical response and outcome of infection with *Salmonella enterica* serotype typhi with decreased susceptibility to fluoroquinolones: a United States foodnet multicenter retrospective cohort study. Antimicrob Agents Chemother 2008;52(4):1278–84.
175. Kownhar H, Shankar EM, Rajan R, et al. Emergence of nalidixic acid-resistant *Salmonella enterica* serovar typhi resistant to ciprofloxacin in India. J Med Microbiol 2007;56(Pt 1):136–7.
176. Crump JA, Barrett TJ, Nelson JT, et al. Reevaluating fluoroquinolone breakpoints for *Salmonella enterica* serotype typhi and for non-typhi salmonellae. Clin Infect Dis 2003;37(1):75–81.
177. Su LH, Wu TL, Chia JH, et al. Increasing ceftriaxone resistance in *Salmonella* isolates from a university hospital in Taiwan. J Antimicrob Chemother 2005; 55(6):846–52.
178. Thaver D, Zaidi AK, Critchley JA, et al. Fluoroquinolones for treating typhoid and paratyphoid fever (enteric fever). Cochrane Database Syst Rev 2008;4: CD004530.
179. Threlfall EJ, Ward LR. Decreased susceptibility to ciprofloxacin in *Salmonella enterica* serotype typhi, United Kingdom. Emerg Infect Dis 2001;7(3):448–50.
180. Connor BA, Schwartz E. Typhoid and paratyphoid fever in travellers. Lancet Infect Dis 2005;5(10):623–8.
181. Skov MN, Andersen JS, Baggesen DL. Occurrence and spread of multiresistant *Salmonella typhimurium* DT104 in Danish animal herds investigated by the use of DNA typing and spatio-temporal analysis. Epidemiol Infect 2008;136(8): 1124–30.
182. Meakins S, Fisher IS, Berghold C, et al. Antimicrobial drug resistance in human nontyphoidal *Salmonella* isolates in Europe 2000–2004: a report from the Enter-net International Surveillance Network. Microb Drug Resist 2008; 14(1):31–5.
183. Gay K, Robicsek A, Strahilevitz J, et al. Plasmid-mediated quinolone resistance in non-typhi serotypes of *Salmonella enterica*. Clin Infect Dis 2006;43(3): 297–304.
184. Li WC, Huang FY, Liu CP, et al. Ceftriaxone resistance of nontyphoidal *Salmonella enterica* isolates in Northern Taiwan attributable to production of CTX-M-14 and CMY-2 beta-lactamases. J Clin Microbiol 2005;43(7):3237–43.
185. Gupta A, Fontana J, Crowe C, et al. Emergence of multidrug-resistant *Salmonella enterica* serotype Newport infections resistant to expanded-spectrum cephalosporins in the United States. J Infect Dis 2003;188(11):1707–16.
186. Armand-Lefevre L, Leflon-Guibout V, Bredin J, et al. Imipenem resistance in *Salmonella enterica* serovar Wien related to porin loss and CMY-4 beta-lactamase production. Antimicrob Agents Chemother 2003;47(3):1165–8.
187. Shlim DR. Update in traveler's diarrhea. Infect Dis Clin North Am 2005;19(1): 137–49.
188. Little CL, Richardson JF, Owen RJ, et al. *Campylobacter* and *Salmonella* in raw red meats in the United Kingdom: prevalence, characterization and antimicrobial resistance pattern, 2003–2005. Food Microbiol 2008;25(3):538–43.
189. Ruiz J, Marco F, Oliveira I, et al. Trends in antimicrobial resistance in *Campylobacter* spp. causing traveler's diarrhea. APMIS 2007;115(3):218–24.
190. Serichantalergs O, Dalsgaard A, Bodhidatta L, et al. Emerging fluoroquinolone and macrolide resistance of *Campylobacter jejuni* and *Campylobacter coli* isolates and their serotypes in Thai children from 1991 to 2000. Epidemiol Infect 2007;135(8):1299–306.

191. Smith KE, Besser JM, Hedberg CW, et al. Quinolone-resistant *Campylobacter jejuni* infections in Minnesota, 1992–1998. Investigation team. N Engl J Med 1999;340(20):1525–32.

192. Gibreel A, Taylor DE. Macrolide resistance in *Campylobacter jejuni* and *Campylobacter coli*. J Antimicrob Chemother 2006;58(2):243–55.

193. Allos BM. *Campylobacter jejuni* infections: update on emerging issues and trends. Clin Infect Dis 2001;32(8):1201–6.

194. Engberg J, Aarestrup FM, Taylor DE, et al. Quinolone and macrolide resistance in *Campylobacter jejuni* and *C. coli*: resistance mechanisms and trends in human isolates. Emerg Infect Dis 2001;7(1):24–34.

195. Yan M, Sahin O, Lin J, et al. Role of the CmeABC efflux pump in the emergence of fluoroquinolone-resistant *Campylobacter* under selection pressure. J Antimicrob Chemother 2006;58(6):1154–9.

196. Centers for Disease Control and Prevention (CDC). Increases in fluoroquinolone-resistant *Neisseria gonorrhoeae*—Hawaii and California, 2001 [see comment]. MMWR Morb Mortal Wkly Rep 2002;51(46):1041–4.

197. Erbelding E, Quinn TC. The impact of antimicrobial resistance on the treatment of sexually transmitted diseases. Infect Dis Clin North Am 1997;11(4):889–903.

198. Ropp PA, Hu M, Olesky M, et al. Mutations in ponA, the gene encoding penicillin-binding protein 1, and a novel locus, penC, are required for high-level chromosomally mediated penicillin resistance in *Neisseria gonorrhoeae*. Antimicrob Agents Chemother 2002;46(3):769–77.

199. Ison CA, Dillon JA, Tapsall JW. The epidemiology of global antibiotic resistance among *Neisseria gonorrhoeae* and *Haemophilus ducreyi*. Lancet 1998; 351(Suppl 3):8–11 [erratum appears in Lancet 1998;352(9136):1316].

200. Gonococcal Isolate Surveillance Project (GISP) Annual Report. Centers for Disease Control and Prevention; 2006. Available at: http://www.cdc.gov/std/GISP2006/GISPSurvSupp2006Short.pdf. Accessed August 1, 2009.

201. Gill MJ, Simjee S, Al-Hattawi K, et al. Gonococcal resistance to beta-lactams and tetracycline involves mutation in loop 3 of the porin encoded at the penB locus. Antimicrob Agents Chemother 1998;42(11):2799–803.

202. Galimand M, Gerbaud G, Courvalin P. Spectinomycin resistance in *Neisseria* spp. due to mutations in 16S rRNA. Antimicrob Agents Chemother 2000;44(5):1365–6.

203. Cousin SL Jr, Whittington WL, Roberts MC. Acquired macrolide resistance genes and the 1 bp deletion in the mtrR promoter in *Neisseria gonorrhoeae*. J Antimicrob Chemother 2003;51(1):131–3.

204. Fenton KA, Ison C, Johnson AP, et al. Ciprofloxacin resistance in *Neisseria gonorrhoeae* in England and Wales in 2002 [see comment]. Lancet 2003;361(9372): 1867–9.

205. Anonymous. Surveillance of antibiotic resistance in *Neisseria gonorrhoeae* in the WHO Western Pacific Region, 2000. Commun Dis Intell 2001;25(4):274–6.

206. Kam KM, Kam SS, Cheung DT, et al. Molecular characterization of quinolone-resistant *Neisseria gonorrhoeae* in Hong Kong. Antimicrob Agents Chemother 2003;47(1):436–9.

207. Trees DL, Sandul AL, Neal SW, et al. Molecular epidemiology of *Neisseria gonorrhoeae* exhibiting decreased susceptibility and resistance to ciprofloxacin in Hawaii, 1991–1999. Sex Transm Dis 2001;28(6):309–14.

208. Coyne S, Courvalin P, Perichon B. Efflux-mediated antibiotic resistance in acinetobacter spp. Antimicrob Agents Chemother 2011;55(3):947–53.

209. Li XZ, Nikaido H. Efflux-mediated drug resistance in bacteria. Drugs 2004;64(2): 159–204.

Use of Antibacterial Agents in Renal Failure

Brett Gilbert, DO[a],*, Paul Robbins, DO[b],
Lawrence L. Livornese Jr, MD, FIDSA[c]

KEYWORDS

- Antibiotics • Renal failure • Volume of distribution • MDRD
- Dosing antibiotics with dialysis • Pharmacokinetics
- Dosing antibiotics with continuous renal replacement therapy
- Serum levels

The kidney is the major organ for maintaining fluid and electrolyte homeostasis. Changes in renal function, whether associated with normal aging or disease, can have profound effects on the pharmacology of antibacterial agents. It is imperative that clinicians have a basic understanding of these consequences to effectively prescribe antibacterial agents in the face of impaired or changing renal function.

This article reviews the pharmacokinetics of antibacterial agents in patients who have normal and decreased renal function. The concepts of volume of distribution, rate of elimination, loading and maintenance doses, and therapeutic drug monitoring are delineated. The recent controversy in the literature regarding proper vancomycin levels is reviewed. An updated formula to determine the glomerular filtration rate (GFR) is discussed. Comment is made about the use of intermittent dosing of cefazolin for patients who are receiving high-flux hemodialysis. The utility of once-daily aminoglycoside administration is reviewed. Newer and traditional methods of extracorporeal circulation and the resultant changes in the pharmacokinetics of antibacterial agents are discussed.

A version of this article appeared in the 23:4 issue of the *Infectious Disease Clinics of North America*.

B.G. is on the speakers' bureaus for Merck and Pfizer. No other potential conflicts of interest exist.

[a] Division of Infectious Diseases, Department of Medicine, Thomas Jefferson University Hospital, Lankenau Hospital, Lankenau Medical Building, Suite 164, Wynnewood, PA 19096, USA

[b] Division of Nephrology, Department of Medicine, Lankenau Hospital, Lankenau Medical Building, Suite 130, Wynnewood, PA 19096, USA

[c] Division of Infectious Diseases, Department of Medicine, Drexel University College of Medicine, Lankenau Hospital, Lankenau Medical Building, Suite 164, Wynnewood, PA 19096, USA

* Corresponding author.

E-mail address: santorow@mlhs.org

Med Clin N Am 95 (2011) 677–702
doi:10.1016/j.mcna.2011.03.010
0025-7125/11/$ – see front matter © 2011 Elsevier Inc. All rights reserved.

medical.theclinics.com

PHARMACOKINETICS
Bioavailability and Metabolism

Bioavailability refers to the degree that a drug is absorbed into the systemic circulation after extravascular administration. Relatively few studies have addressed this issue in patients who have renal failure. In chronic renal failure, numerous factors, such as nausea, vomiting, diabetic gastroparesis, and intestinal edema, may decrease gastrointestinal absorption. The conversion of urea to ammonia by gastric urease, antacids, or the use of alkalating agents such as bicarbonate and citrate increases gastric pH, thereby reducing the levels of drugs that require an acidic milieu for absorption.[1] Some drugs are bound by antacids and phosphate binders, which are commonly used in renal failure.[2] In chronic renal failure, bioavailability is further reduced as the result of decreased small bowel absorption.[3] First-pass hepatic metabolism may also be diminished in uremia, leading to increased serum levels of oral antibacterial agents. Impaired plasma protein binding increases the level of free drug; this permits more of a drug to bind to the site of action and, conversely, increases the amount of a drug available for elimination by dialysis or hepatic metabolism. Of note, the rates of glucuronidation, sulfated conjugation, and oxidation are generally unchanged in the presence of uremia.[4]

Distribution and Elimination

Plasma levels for a given drug are a function of the dose, bioavailability, volume of distribution, and rate of metabolism and excretion. The volume of distribution (V_d) is calculated by dividing the amount of drug in the body by the plasma concentration. In general, drugs that are highly protein bound are found mainly in the vascular space and have a small V_d. Those agents that are highly lipid soluble have a large V_d because they are able to penetrate body tissues more easily. Volumes of distribution can exceed the total volume of body water because the V_d is a mathematical construct that does not necessarily correspond to a distinct physiologic space. (This is why the term "apparent V_d" is often used.) The V_d is important in calculating the plasma half-life ($T_{1/2}$) of a drug and may also be used to determine the loading dose. The major routes of elimination of antibacterial agents and their metabolites are by way of the kidney and the liver. Small, generally inconsequential amounts are lost in sweat, saliva, expired air, and breast milk. The rate of elimination of most antibacterial agents follows first-order kinetics, that is, the rate of elimination is proportional to the amount of a drug in the body, and as the amount of a drug increases, so does the rate of elimination.

There is an elimination constant (K), such that:

Rate of elimination = K × amount of drug in body

Because the amount of a drug in the body can be calculated by multiplying the plasma concentration by the V_d, one can restate the equation:

Rate of elimination = K × V_d × plasma concentration

Plasma drug clearance is calculated by dividing the rate of elimination by the plasma concentration. Therefore:

Plasma drug clearance = K × V_d

It is traditional that the rate of plasma clearance is expressed as the time required for the concentration of a drug to decline by 50%, which is the $T_{1/2}$. The $T_{1/2}$ remains constant at all times for all drugs that follow first-order kinetics because as the concentration decreases, so does the rate of plasma clearance. Additionally, the $T_{1/2}$ is independent of the initial plasma concentration; it is purely a function of the elimination constant (K). Therefore:

$$T_{1/2} = \ln2/K = 0.693/K$$

By substituting for K from plasma drug clearance $= K \times V_d$:

$$T_{1/2} = (0.693)(V_d)/\text{plasma drug clearance}$$

Therefore, the $T_{1/2}$ is determined by using only the V_d and the plasma clearance. Any process that alters these will change the $T_{1/2}$. In renal insufficiency, the presence of edema or ascites will increase the V_d of highly protein-bound or water-soluble drugs, resulting in lower than expected plasma levels. However, muscle loss and dehydration can decrease V_d and lead to higher than expected concentrations of these same agents.

Renal Clearance

The rate of elimination of drugs by the kidneys depends on the GFR, a measure of kidney function that represents the filtration rates of all of the functioning nephrons and is a function of cardiac output. The renal clearance of antibiotics and other agents is determined by glomerular filtration along with renal tubular secretion and reabsorption. The glomerular filtration of a drug is influenced by its molecular size and protein-binding characteristics. When an increase in protein binding reduces glomerular filtration, elimination by way of renal tubular secretion may be enhanced. The proximal tubules have active transport systems that can secrete and reabsorb drugs. Beta-lactams are actively secreted by this system. In the setting of impaired renal function, whether as the result of normal aging or intrinsic renal disease, a reduction in both glomerular filtration and tubular secretion of drugs may occur, resulting in higher serum concentrations of these agents.

When considering the administration of an antibacterial agent that is excreted by the kidneys, determining the appropriate dosage requires that renal function be assessed. A 24-hour urine collection allows for accurate determination of the endogenous creatinine clearance, which is a close approximation of the GFR. (A small amount of creatinine is secreted in the proximal tubules.) In practice, it is often too time consuming or impractical to obtain a 24-hour urine collection to determine the GFR. The equation of Cockcroft and Gault[5] can be used to estimate creatinine clearance:

$$\text{Creatinine clearance in males} = \frac{(140 - \text{age}) \times \text{total body weight in KG}}{(72 \times \text{serum creatinine in mg/dl})}$$

In women, the clearance is 85% of this value.

Pesola and colleagues[6] suggest using ideal body weight (IBW) instead of total body weight. IBW can be calculated using height and gender, as stated by Devine.[7]

Male IBW = 50 kg + 2.3 kg for each inch of height more than 5 ft

Female IBW = 45.5 kg + 2.3 kg for each inch of height more than 5 ft

The above calculations are only valid when the renal function is stable and the serum creatinine is constant. When the patient is oliguric or the serum creatinine is rapidly rising, the creatinine clearance should be assumed to be less than 10 mL/min.

A newer equation has been developed as a method to estimate GFR based on data from the Modification of Diet in Renal Disease (MDRD) Study that uses six clinical and demographic variables, including serum creatinine.[8] The equation takes into account body-surface area and eliminates weight as a variable. In 2005, the MDRD equation was reformulated to use four variables rather than six for ease of clinical use, and it is used by many clinical laboratories to report estimated GFR.[9] This modification results in a 5% decrease in estimated GFR compared with the previous formula. The new formula is:

$$GFR = 175 \times \text{standardized(serum creatinine)} - 1 \cdot 154 \times (\text{age}) - 0 \cdot 203$$

$$\times 0.742(\text{if female}) \text{and} \times 1.212(\text{if black})$$

The MDRD formula[10,11] is probably most useful to assist the clinician for drug adjustment dosing decisions in patients who have relatively stable kidney function.[9] The formula, however, has not been validated for use in dosing all antibiotics, and many clinicians prefer the Cockcroft-Gault formula for its ease of use and because of their longer experience in using it for antibiotic dosing. In addition, one needs to keep in mind that when a patient is critically ill, elderly, malnourished, or obese and potentially nephrotoxic drugs are concurrently being used, so that the above equations used to estimate the GFR may be inaccurate, and an alternative method may need to be used to correctly adjust drug dosages.[12] A 24-hour urine collection should be obtained in this setting, using the midpoint between the creatinine and urea clearance.

Serum creatinine alone is not a reliable measure of creatinine clearance because it is a function of the GFR and muscle mass. In an elderly or debilitated patient, the serum creatinine may appear normal, even in the presence of significant renal insufficiency.

Trimethoprim and cimetidine compete with creatinine for secretory pathways in the proximal tubule and may cause an increase in serum creatinine without a change in the GFR.[13,14] A false elevation in serum creatinine, which is caused by interference with certain creatinine assays,[15,16] has been reported when using cefoxitin and cephalothin.

DOSING OF ANTIBACTERIAL AGENTS IN RENAL FAILURE
Initial Dose

The loading, or initial, dose is based on the extracellular fluid volume and is not altered in the presence of decreased renal function. The presence of ascites or edema may necessitate a larger dose, whereas dehydration may require a reduction in the dose. When a loading dose is not used, four maintenance doses are required to achieve a steady state. When antibacterial agents that have a short $T_{1/2}$ are used, each maintenance dose acts as a loading dose, and therefore no separate initial dose is used. A loading dose is generally used when it is necessary to achieve therapeutic plasma levels rapidly.

Maintenance Dose

After the loading dose, subsequent maintenance doses frequently require modification in patients who have decreased renal function.

Table 1 outlines specific dosing guidelines for the use of antibiotics in patients that are in renal failure. The classification is based on chemical class and then subdivided alphabetically.

The second through fifth columns indicate the percentage of drug excreted unchanged, the $T_{1/2}$ of each agent in normal patients and those who have end-stage renal disease, and the percentage of protein binding and V_d, respectively. The columns to the right provide recommendations for dosing schedules based on renal function. Modifications of doses are dictated by the severity of renal impairment as determined by the estimated GFR. The adjustments are labeled either "D" for dose reduction or "I" for interval extension. In the dose reduction method (D), a percentage of the usual dose of an antibacterial is given at the standard interval. In the interval extension method (I), the dose of an individual antibacterial agent remains constant, but the interval between doses is extended. Additional dosing requirements for various dialysis modalities, if available, are found in the last column to the right. If available, supplemental information for hemodialysis, continuous ambulatory peritoneal dialysis (CAPD), and continuous arteriovenous hemofiltration (CAVH) is indicated as well.

Once-Daily Aminoglycosides

In the era of antibiotic resistance, aminoglycoside antibiotics continue to play a critical role in the treatment of certain gram-negative bacterial infections. Because of the aminoglycosides' high side-effect profile and their prolonged postantibiotic effect, novel treatment approaches and dosing schedules have been implemented in an attempt to limit toxicity.[17,18] In the last 10 years, once-daily aminoglycoside therapy has been introduced to take advantage of aminoglycoside pharmacodynamics while attempting to reduce nephrotoxicity and ototoxicity.[19] Credence for this concept was supported by early animal studies that suggested that the incidence of acute renal failure could be reduced by using once-daily administration.[20] Nephrotoxicity in this class of antibiotics depends on the cumulative dose or concentrations that are greater than a critical level, so achieving the therapeutic goal quickly may allow for a shorter course of therapy.[21] Achieving increased periods of time in which the patient has a negligible serum concentration will reduce renal cortical and auditory exposure, potentially decreasing toxicity.[22] A meta-analysis performed by Hatala and colleagues[23] reviewed 13 studies, and the authors concluded that standard and once-daily regimens had similar bacteriologic cure rates and that once-daily dosing showed a trend toward reduced toxicity and mortality. Other benefits of once-daily dosing include reduced costs and prolonged postantibiotic effect. Lab draws will also be reduced because serum levels will have to be monitored less frequently.

Patient selection is important when considering a once-daily regimen. Only certain patient populations are appropriate for once-daily dosing; these include patients who have pelvic inflammatory disease, gram-negative bacteremia, urinary tract infections, febrile neutropenia, gynecologic infections, and respiratory infections.[24] Once-daily aminoglycoside dosing should not be used in cases for which little apparent benefit is expected, or for cases in which clinical evidence is lacking. There is little data for using once-daily aminoglycosides in the following situations: pregnancy, creatinine clearance less then 20 mL/min, bone and joint infections, central nervous system infections, infective endocarditis, obesity, burns, and solid organ transplantation.

Initial dosing for once-daily aminoglycosides should be based on creatinine clearance. **Table 2** provides dosage adjustments for patients who have renal insufficiency. Serum drug levels for patients who are receiving once-daily doses of gentamicin or tobramycin should achieve a peak concentration of 15 to 20 µg/mL. The trough concentration should be kept to less than 1 µg/ml.[25,26] Finally, the clinician should be comfortable using amikacin as a single daily dose. Fifteen mg/kg of amikacin should yield a peak of about 60 µg/mL. In the last five years, multidrug-resistant gram-negative organisms have become increasingly prevalent. These organisms often remain susceptible to amikacin as a result of the presence of different aminoglycoside modifying enzymes that render gentamicin and tobramycin resistant; therefore, amikacin is often the aminoglycoside of choice in many gram-negative infections.

Table 1
Recommended drug dosages and adjustments for patients in renal failure

Drug	Excreted, Unchanged %	T1/2 (Normal/ ESRD; Hours)	Plasma Protein Binding (%)	Vd (L/kg)	Dose for Normal Renal Function	Adjustment for Renal Function GFR, mL/min				Supplement for Dialysis
						Method	>50	10–50	<10	
Aminoglycoside antibiotics										
Amikacin	95	1.4–2.3/ 17–150	<5	0.22–0.29	5 mg/kg q8h	D and I	60%–90% q12h	30%–70% q12–18h	20%–30% q24–48h	IHD 2/3 normal dose after dialysis; CAPD 15–20 mg/L; CRRT Dose for GFR 10–50 and measure levels
Gentamicin	95	1.8/ 20–60	<5	0.23–0.26	1–1.7 mg/kg q8h	D and I	60%–90% q8–12h	30%–70% q12h	20%–30% q24–48h	IHD 2/3 normal dose after dialysis; CAPD 3–4 mg/L; CRRT Dose for GFR 10–50 and measure levels
Netilmicin	95	1–3/ 35–72	<5	0.19–0.23	2 mg/kg q8h	D and I	50%–90% q8–12h	20%–60% q12h	10%–20% q24–48h	IHD 2/3 normal dose after dialysis; CAPD 3–4 mg/L; CRRT Dose for GFR 10–50 and measure levels
Streptomycin	70	2.5/ 100	35	0.26	15 mg/kg q24h; 1 g max daily	I	q24h	q24–72h	q72–96h	IHD 1/2 normal dose after dialysis; CAPD 20–40 mg/L; CRRT Dose for GFR 10–50 and measure levels
Tobramycin	95	2.5/ 27–60	<5	0.22–0.33	1–1.7 mg/kg q8h	D and I	60%–90% q8–12h	30%–70% q12h	20%–30% q24–48	IHD 2/3 normal dose after dialysis; CAPD 3–4 mg/L; CRRT Dose for GFR 10–50 and measure levels

Carbapenems

Drug				Normal dose	Method	>50	10–50	<10	Supplement
Doripenem	70	1/18		8.1	500 mg q8h	D and I	100%	250 mg q8–12	No data	IHD No data CAPD No data CRRT No data
Ertapenem	38	4/6	85–95	8.2	1 g q24h	D	100%	100%	50%	IHD 150 mg after dialysis CAPD No data CRRT No data
Imipenem	20–70	1.0/4.0	13–21	0.17–0.30	0.25–1.0 g q6h	D	100%	50%	25%	IHD Dose after dialysis CAPD Dose for GFR <10 CRRT Dose for GFR 10–50
Meropenem	65	1.1/6–8	Low	0.35	0.5–1.0 g q6h	D and I	500 mg q6h	250–500 mg q12h	250–500 mg q24h	IHD Dose after dialysis CAPD Dose for GFR <10 CRRT Dose for GFR 10–50

Cephalosporin antibiotics

Drug				Normal dose	Method	>50	10–50	<10	Supplement
Cefaclor	70	1/3	25	0.24–0.35	250–500 mg q8h	D	100%	50%–100%	50%	IHD 250 mg after dialysis CAPD 250 mg q8–12h CRRT Not applicable
Cefadroxil	70–90	1.4/22	20	0.31	0.5–1.0 g q12h	I	q12h	q12–24h	q24–48h	IHD 0.5–1.0 g after dialysis CAPD 0.5 g/d CRRT Not applicable
Cefazolin	75–95	2/40–70	80	0.13–0.22	0.5–2.0 g q8h	I	q8h	q12h	q24–48h	IHD 0.5–1 g after dialysis[a] CAPD 0.5 g q12h CRRT Dose for GFR 10–50
Cefdinir	18	1.7/16	60–70	0.35	300 mg q12h	I	q12h	q12h	q24h	IHD 300 mg after dialysis CAPD Not applicable CRRT Not applicable
Cefditoren	99	1.6/4.7	88	9.3	200–400 mg q12h	D and I	100%	50%	50% q24h	IHD No data CAPD No data CRRT No data
Cefepime	85	2.2/18	16	0.3	0.25–2.0 g q8h	I	q12h	q16–24h	q24–48h	IHD 1 g after dialysis CAPD Dose for GFR <10 CRRT Not recommended

(continued on next page)

Table 1
(*continued*)

Drug	Excreted, Unchanged %	T1/2 (Normal/ESRD; Hours)	Plasma Protein Binding (%)	Vd (L/kg)	Dose for Normal Renal Function	Method	Adjustment for Renal Function GFR, mL/min			Supplement for Dialysis
							>50	10–50	<10	
Cefixime	18–50	3.1/12	50	0.6–1.1	250 mg q12h	D	100%	75%	50%	IHD 300 mg after dialysis CAPD 200 mg/day CRRT Not applicable
Cefotaxime	60	1/15	37	0.15–0.50	1 g q6h	I	q6h	q 8–12h	q24h	IHD 1 g after dialysis CAPD 1 g q24h CRRT 1 g q12h
Cefotetan	75	3.5/13–25	85	0.15	1–2 g q12h	D	100%	50%	25%	IHD 1 g after dialysis CAPD 1 g/d CRRT 750 mg q12h
Cefoxitin	80	1/13–23	41–75	0.2	1–2 g q6–8h	I	q8h	q8–12h	q24–48h	IHD 1 g after dialysis CAPD 1 g/d CRRT Dose for GFR 10–50
Cefpodoxime	30	2.5/26		0.6–1.2	200 mg q12h	I	q12h	q16h	q24–48h	IHD 200 mg after dialysis only CAPD Dose for GFR <10 CRRT Not applicable
Cefprozil	65	1.7/6		0.65	500 mg q12h	D and I	250 mg q12h	250 mg q12–16h	250 mg q24	IHD 250 mg after dialysis CAPD Dose for GFR <10 CRRT Dose for GFR <10
Ceftaroline	64	2.5/?	<20	20.3	600 mg iv q12h	D	100%	300–400 mg iv q12h	200 mg iv q12h	IHD Dose for GFR <10 CAPD No data CRRT No data
Ceftazidime	60–85	1.2/13–25	17	0.28–0.40	1–2 g q8h	I	q8–12h	q24–48h	q48h	IHD 1 g after dialysis CAPD 0.5 g q24h CRRT Dose for GFR 10–50

Drug	%	t½	PB	Vd	Dose	D/I	>50	10–50	<10	IHD	CAPD	CRRT
Ceftibuten	56	2/22	65	0.21	400 mg q24h	D	100%	50%	25%	400 mg after dialysis	Not applicable	Not applicable
Ceftizoxime	57–100	1.4/35	28–50	0.26–0.42	1–2 g q8–12h	I	q8–12h	q12–24h	q24h	1 g after dialysis	0.5–1.0 g q24h	Dose for GFR 10–50
Ceftriaxone	30–65	7–9/12–24	90	0.12–0.18	1–2 g q12–24h	—	100%	100%	100%	None	750 mg q12h	Dose for GFR 10–50
Ceftobiprole	?	3–4/no data	?	?	500 mg q8–12h	I	q8–12h	q12h	—	?	No data for GFR <30	?
Cefuroxime axetil	90	1.2/17	35–50	0.13–1.8	250–500 mg q12h	—	100%	100%	100%	Dose after dialysis	Dose for GFR <10	Not applicable
Cefuroxime sodium	90	1.2/17	33	0.13–1.8	0.75–1.5 g q8h	I	q8h	q8–12h	q24h	Dose after dialysis	Dose for GFR <10	1 g q12h
Cephalexin	98	0.7/16	20	0.35	250–500 mg q6h	I	q8h	q12h	q12h	Dose after dialysis	Dose for GFR <10	Not applicable
Macrolide antibiotics												
Azithromycin	6–12	10–60/?	10–50	18	250–500 mg q24h	—	100%	100%	100%	None	None	None
Clarithromycin	15	2.3–6/22	70	2.4	500 mg q12h	D	100%	75%	50%–75%	Dose after dialysis	None	None
Erythromycin	15	1.4/5.6	60–95	0.78	250–500 mg q6–12h	D	100%	100%	50%–75%	None	None	None

(continued on next page)

Table 1
(continued)

Drug	Excreted, Unchanged %	T1/2 (Normal/ESRD; Hours)	Plasma Protein Binding (%)	Vd (L/kg)	Dose for Normal Renal Function	Method	>50	10–50	<10	Supplement for Dialysis
								GFR, mL/min		
Miscellaneous antibacterials										
Aztreonam	75	1.7–2.9/6–8	55	0.1–2.0	1–2 g q8–12h	D	100%	50%–75%	25%	IHD 0.5g after dialysis CAPD Dose for GFR <10 CRRT Dose for GFR 10–50
Chloramphenicol	10	1.6–3.3/3–7	45–60	0.5–1.0	12.5 mg/kg q6h	—	100%	100%	100%	IHD None CAPD None CRRT None
Cilastin	60	1/12	44	0.22	With imipenem	D	100%	50%	Avoid	IHD Avoid CAPD Avoid CRRT Avoid
Clavulanic acid	40	1/3–4	30	0.3	100 mg q4–6h	D	100%	100%	50%–75%	IHD Dose after dialysis CAPD Dose for GFR <10 CRRT Dose for GFR 10–50
Clindamycin	10	2–4/3–5	60–95	0.6–1.2	150–900 mg q6–8h	—	100%	100%	100%	IHD None CAPD None CRRT None
Colistin	?	2–3/>48	Low	?	160mg q12h	D	100%	q24h	q36h	IHD 80 mg after dialysis
Daptomycin	78	9/28	92	0.1	4–6 mg/kg q24h	I	q24h	q24h	q48h	IHD Give after HD on HD days CAPD 4 mg/kg q48h CRRT 4 mg/kg q48h
Linezolid	30, 20	4.5/?	31	40–50	400–600 mg q12h	—	100%	100%	100%	IHD No data CAPD No data CRRT No data
Metronidazole	20	6–14/7–21	20	0.25–0.85	7.5 mg/kg q6–12h	D	100%	100%	75%	IHD Dose after dialysis CAPD Dose for GFR <10 CRRT Dose for GFR 10–50

Drug					Dose					Supplement
Nitrofurantoin	30–40	0.5/1	20–60	0.3–0.7	50–100 mg q6h	D	100%	Avoid	Avoid	IHD Not applicable CAPD Not applicable CRRT Not applicable
Sulbactam	50–80	1/10–21	30	0.25–0.50	0.75–1.5 g q6–8h	I	q6–8h	q12–24h	q12–48h	IHD Dose after dialysis CAPD 0.75–1.5 g/d CRRT 750 mg q12h
Sulfamethoxazole	70	10/20–50	50	0.28–0.38	1.0 g q8h	I	q12h	q18h	q24h	IHD 1 g after dialysis CAPD 1 g q24 CRRT Dose for GFR 10–50
Sulfisoxazole	70	3–7/6–12	85	0.14–0.28	1–2 g q6h	I	q6h	q8–12h	q12–24h	IHD 2g after dialysis CAPD 3 g/d CRRT Not applicable
Synercid Quinupristin	15	0.9/?	55–78	1	7.5 mg/kg q8–12h	—	100%	100%	100%	IHD None CAPD None CRRT None
Dalfopristin	19	0.75/?	11–26	1		—	—	—	—	
Tazobactam	65	1/17	22	0.21	1.5–2.25 g/d	D	100%	75%	50%	IHD 1/3 dose after dialysis CAPD Dose for GFR <10 CRRT Dose for GFR 10–50
Teicoplanin	40–60	33–190/62–230	60–90	0.5–1.2	6 mg/kg q24h	I	q24h	q48h	q72h	IHD Dose for GFR <10 CAPD Dose for GFR <10 CRRT Dose for GFR 10–50
Telavancin	76	8.0/19.7	90	0.14	10 mg/kg q24h	D and I	100%	7.5 mg/kg iv q24h	10 mg/kg iv q48h	IHD No data CAPD No data CRRT No data
Tigecycline	22	42	71–89	7–9	100 mg; then 50 mg q12h	—	100%	100%	100%	IHD None
Trimethoprim	40–70	9–13/20–49	30–70	1–2.2	100–200 mg q12h	I	q12h	q18h	q24h	IHD Dose after dialysis CAPD q24h

(continued on next page)

Table 1
(continued)

Drug	Excreted, Unchanged %	T1/2 (Normal/ESRD; Hours)	Plasma Protein Binding (%)	Vd (L/kg)	Dose for Normal Renal Function	Adjustment for Renal Function GFR, mL/min				Supplement for Dialysis
						Method	>50	10–50	<10	
Vancomycin	90–100	6–8/200–250	10–50	0.47–1.1	1 g q12h	D and I	500 mg q6–12h	500 mg q24–48h	500 mg q48–96h	IHD Dose for GFR <10 / CAPD Dose for GFR <10 / CRRT Dose for GFR 10–50
Penicillins										
Amoxicillin	50–70	0.9–23/5–20	15–25	0.26	250–500 mg q8h	I	q8h	q8–12h	q24h	IHD Dose after dialysis / CAPD 250 mg q12h / CRRT Not applicable
Ampicillin	30–90	0.8–1.5/7–20	20	0.17–0.31	250 mg–2 g q6h	I	q6h	q6–12h	q12–24h	IHD Dose after dialysis / CAPD 250 mg q12h / CRRT Dose for GFR 10–50
Dicloxacillin	35–70	0.7/1–2	95	0.16	250–500 mg q6h	—	100%	100%	100%	IHD None / CAPD None / CRRT Not applicable
Nafcillin	35	0.5/1.2	85	0.35	1–2 g q4–6h	—	100%	100%	100%	IHD None / CAPD None / CRRT None
Penicillin G	60–85	0.5/6–20	50	0.30–0.42	0.5–4 million U q4h	D	100%	75%	50%	IHD Dose after dialysis / CAPD Dose for GFR <10 / CRRT Dose for GFR 10–50
Penicillin VK	60–90	0.6/4.1	50–80	0.5	250 mg q6h	—	100%	100%	100%	IHD Dose after dialysis / CAPD Dose for GFR <10 / CRRT Not applicable
Piperacillin	75–90	0.8–1.5/3.3–5.1	30	0.18–0.30	3–4 g q4h	I	q4–6h	q6–8h	q8h	IHD Dose after dialysis / CAPD Dose for GFR <10 / CRRT Dose for GFR 10–50

Ticarcillin	85	1.2/11–16	45–60	0.14–0.21	3 g q4h	D and I	1–2 g q4h	1–2 g q8h	1–2 g q12h	IHD 3 g after dialysis CAPD Dose for GFR <10 CRRT Dose for GFR 10–50
Quinolone antibacterials										
Ciprofloxacin	50–70	3–6/6–9	20–40	2.5	400 mg IV or 500 mg orally	D	100%	50%–75%	50%	IHD 50% q12h CAPD 50% q8h CRRT 50% q12h
Levaquin	87	7	24–38	74–122	250–750 mg q24	D and I	100%	50% q24h	50% q48h	IHD Dose for GFR <10 CAPD Dose for GFR <10 CRRT 500 mg q48h
Moxifloxacin	96	12/14.5–16.2	40	2.0–3.5	400 mg q24h		100%	100%	100%	IHD No data CAPD No data CRRT No data
Norfloxacin	30	3.5–6.5/8	14	<0.5	400 mg q12h	I	q12h	q12–24h	Avoid	IHD Not applicable CAPD Not applicable CRRT Not applicable
Ofloxacin	68–80	5–8/28–37	25	1.5–2.5	400 mg q12h	D	100%	200 mg q12h	25%–50% q24h	IHD 100 mg q12h CAPD Dose for GFR <10 CRRT 300 mg q24h
Tetracycline antibacterials										
Doxycycline	33–45	15–24/18–25	80–93	0.75	100 mg q12h	—	100%	100%	100%	IHD None CAPD None CRRT None
Minocycline	6–10	12–16/12–18	70	1.0–1.5	100 mg q12h	—	100%	100%	100%	IHD None CAPD None CRRT None
Tetracycline	48–60	6–10/57–108	55–90	>0.7	250–500 mg qid	I	q8–12h	q12–24h	q24h	IHD None CAPD None CRRT None

Abbreviations: CRRT, continuous renal replacement therapy; D, dose reduction; ESRD, end-stage renal disease; HD, hemodialysis; I, interval increase; IHD, intermittent hemodialysis.

[a] See text for additional dosing comments.

Table 2
Suggested single daily dosage requirements of aminoglycosides adjustment for renal insufficiency

Estimated CRCL (mL/min)	Dosage Interval (h)	Dose (mg/kg)	Estimated Level (μg/mL) at Time Interval		
			1h	18h	24h
Gentamicin/tobramycin					
>80	24	5.0	20	<1	<1
70	24	4.0	16	<1	<1
60	24	4.0	16	1.5	<1
50	24	3.5	14	1.0	<1
40	24	2.5	10	1.5	<1
30	24	2.5	10	2.5	1.5
20	48	4.0	16	2.0	1.0
10	48	3.0	12	3.0	2.0
Hemodialysis[a]	48	2.0	8.0	6.0	5.0
Amikacin, kanamycin, streptomycin					
>80	24	15	60	<1	<1
70	24	12	48	2.5	<1
50	24	7.5	30	3.5	1.0
30	24	4.0	20	5.0	3.0
20	48	7.5	30	3.3	1.0
10	48	4.0	16	5.0	3.0
Hemodialysis[a]	48	3.0	20	15	12
Netilmicin					
>80	24	6.5	15	<1	<1
70	24	5.0	—	—	—
50	24	4.0	—	—	—
30	24	2.0	—	—	—
20	48	3.0	—	—	—
10	48	2.5	—	—	—
Hemodialysis[a]	48	2.0	—	—	—

Abbreviation: CRCL, creatinine clearance.
[a] Dose posthemodialysis.
Data from Gilbert DW, Bennett WM. Use of antimicrobial agents in renal failure. Infect Dis Clin North Am 1989;3:517–31; *Data from* Gilbert DN, Mollering RC, Sande MA. The Sanford guide to antimicrobial therapy 2008. Sperryville (VA): Antimicrobial Therapy Inc; 2008.

Intermittent-Dosing of Cefazolin with Hemodialysis

In hemodialysis patients who have suspected bloodstream or vascular infections, vancomycin and gentamicin are frequently given as empiric therapy. Often, when an isolate such as methicillin-susceptible *Staphylococcus aureus* (MSSA) is recovered, vancomycin is continued because doses of this drug may be given to patients who are undergoing hemodialysis, and there is no need for additional intravenous access. However, the emergence of vancomycin-resistant enterococcus and concerns about the increasing resistance of *S aureus* to glycopeptides has led to recommendations to limit the use of vancomycin when possible.[27] Stryjewski and colleagues[28] studied a group of long-term hemodialysis patients who had MSSA bacteremia and who were treated using either cefazolin or vancomycin over an 84-month period. Treatment failure, as defined by death or relapse of infection, was significantly higher in the vancomycin group, with an odds ratio of 3.53. The authors concluded that vancomycin was inferior to cefazolin for the treatment of MSSA bacteremia in hemodialysis patients and should not be continued after susceptibilities are known unless a patient has a beta-lactam allergy. This result is consistent with data from other clinical scenarios, demonstrating the superior efficacy of beta-lactam antibiotics compared with vancomycin when treating MSSA infections.

Sowinski and colleagues[29] studied the pharmacokinetics and clearance of cefazolin in 25 uninfected subjects undergoing thrice-weekly hemodialysis. Fifteen subjects underwent hemodialysis using high-efficiency hemodialyzers, and 10 using high-flux hemodialyzers. The subjects were given an intravenous dose of 15 mg/kg of cefazolin immediately after hemodialysis; both groups maintained cefazolin levels that were greater than the breakpoint for sensitive organisms (8 μg/mL), even with a 3-day interdialytic period.

In a previous study, Fogel and colleagues[30] concluded that for anuric hemodialysis patients, cefazolin can be effectively used at a dose of 1 g intravenously after each hemodialysis session. A number of nonanuric subjects were included in the study by Sowinski and colleagues. A total of 10 subjects produced enough urine to calculate cefazolin renal clearance, although only three could be considered nonoliguric (urine output >400 mL/day). All 25 subjects in this study maintained adequate cefazolin levels, despite the production of variable amounts of urine.

Kuypers and colleagues[31] used a fixed, postdialysis, 2-g dose of intravenous cefazolin in 15 uninfected hemodialysis patients, 14 of whom received dialysis using high-flux membranes. The weight-based range of doses for this group was from 19.2 to 37.7 mg/kg. Trough levels of cefazolin were obtained before subsequent dialysis sessions, and remained much greater than the MIC for susceptible organisms. However, a higher incidence of adverse effects was seen in this study than in the studies previously discussed, raising the concern that the higher serum levels of cefazolin achieved in this study led to undesirable side effects. The previously discussed studies demonstrated clearly that cefazolin can be administered on either a weight-based or fixed-dose schedule after each dialysis session and can provide a safe and effective alternative to vancomycin for susceptible organisms.

SERUM LEVELS

Because of potential toxicity, especially when vancomycin and aminoglycosides are combined, antimicrobial serum levels are most useful, and are generally obtained, when using either of these drugs. There is an increased incidence of nephrotoxicity when these agents are combined. Appropriate dosing requires the consideration of multiple factors, including patient weight, extracellular fluid shifts, renal function, hypoalbuminemia, location and severity of infection, and potential for toxicity. When administering aminoglycosides, it is even more important to establish safe serum levels in patients who have underlying renal failure because the potential for toxicity is greater.

Vancomycin drug levels have been reviewed extensively and are based on early reports of clinical observation and toxicity.[32] Vancomycin exhibits concentration-independent killing action in vitro, and its pharmacokinetics are affected by inoculum size. However, serum levels do not always correlate with a favorable microbiologic response.[33] In 2006, the Clinical and Laboratory Standards Institute modified vancomycin breakpoints for susceptible isolates to 2 μg/ml or less because of an increase of reports in the literature of vancomycin failures when the minimum inhibitory concentration approached 4 µg/ml. This modification was intended to increase detection of difficult-to-identify, heterogeneously resistant isolates that often result in clinical failure of vancomycin.[34] A significant number of vancomycin failures have been seen in the setting of methicillin-resistant *S aureus* pneumonia. This issue was addressed in a consensus statement by the American Society of Health-System Pharmacists, the Infectious Disease Society of America, and the Society of Infectious Disease Pharmacists.[35] They recommend that vancomycin serum-trough concentrations always be maintained at levels greater than 10 mg/L and that peak serum concentrations need not be checked. Additionally, they recommend that serum trough concentrations be maintained at between 15 and 20 mg/L for patients being treated for complicated infections such as bacteremia, endocarditis, osteomyelitis, meningitis, and hospital-acquired pneumonia. In contrast to aminoglycosides, vancomycin levels have not consistently been correlated with toxicity, and their utility continues to be debated in the literature.[36–39] Unlike vancomycin, aminoglycosides exhibit concentration-dependent killing action. This is important clinically because bactericidal activity is directly proportional to concentration levels.[18] Nevertheless, levels must be followed closely when using aminoglycosides because increased trough levels have been correlated with nephrotoxicity.[40]

Peak and trough concentrations are measured after achieving steady-state concentration. The latter correlates with the fourth dose in patients who have normal renal function, assuming that a loading dose has not been given. The peak concentration is measured approximately 30 to 60 min after completion of the infusion, rather than immediately following the dose, to allow for rapid-phase distribution to occur; otherwise, the measurement will reflect only the plasma volume and not the extracellular compartment. Trough levels are obtained immediately before the next scheduled dose. Random levels are obtained in patients who have underlying renal disease in cases in which the $T_{1/2}$ is sufficiently prolonged and intermittent dosing is being used.

DIALYSIS

When renal failure progresses to the point of uremia or inadequate urine output (oliguria), dialytic intervention is indicated. Typically, dialysis is begun when the GFR is less than 15 mL/min for patients who have diabetes or less than 10 mL/min for patients who do not have diabetes. There are a number of dialytic modalities used in both acute and chronic renal failure.

Hemodialysis

Standard, thrice-weekly, intermittent hemodialysis is the mainstay therapy for end-stage renal failure.[41] **Box 1** summarizes the factors affecting drug clearance by using hemodialysis. The clearance of low-molecular-weight antibiotics (<500 daltons [Da]) depends on blood flow rates, dialysate flow rates, and dialyzer surface area. As a rule, higher-molecular-weight drugs (>500–5,000 Da) are poorly dialyzed by conventional dialyzers. However, there is a trend toward using larger, more permeable (high-flux) membranes. These membranes have been shown to enhance the clearance of middle molecules, recently defined as being compounds that have a molecular weight of 500 to 12,000 Da, and to increase the removal of both low- and high-molecular-weight antibiotics.[29,42–44] To reduce the clearance of antibiotics during high-flux hemodialysis and avoid subtherapeutic drug levels, the administration of antibiotics at the end of a dialysis session or the use of higher intradialytic doses have been recommended.[43,45–47] For situations in which the transport properties of a drug or antibiotic are not known, Maher[48,49] proposed that the hemodialysis clearance of

---

Box 1
Factors affecting hemodialysis drug clearance

Drug properties

    Molecular weight

    Charge

    Lipid or water solubility

    V_d (tissue binding)

    Protein binding

    Other forms of steric hindrance

    Membrane binding

    Rapid excretion by another pathway

    Red blood cell partitioning

Hemodialyzer properties

    Blood flow

    Surface area

    Membrane permeability

    Pore size

    Fluid films (membrane geometry)

Dialysate properties

    Flow rate

    Solute concentration

    pH

    Temperature

Miscellaneous properties

    Convective transports during ultrafiltration

Data from Golper TA, Bennett WM. Drug usage in dialysis patients. In: Nissenson R, Fine RN, Gentile DE, editors. Clinical dialysis. 2nd edition. Norwalk (CT): Appleton and Lange; 1990. p. 608–30.

---

unbound drug can be estimated by multiplying the urea clearance by the ratio of the molecular weight of urea (60 Da) to the antibiotic's molecular weight (MW) (in which K = clearance and X is the antibiotic involved).

$$KX = Kurea \times 60/MWx$$

The nephrologist administering the dialysis therapy should be able to provide an estimate of the urea clearance for a given treatment. Fortunately, the clearance by dialysis of many antibiotics and postdialysis supplement requirements have been established for some time.[48–50] **Table 1** summarizes the data for those agents along with more recent additions.

Intermittent hemodialysis also remains the mainstay treatment of acute renal failure. In such a setting, however, it may be performed more or less often than thrice weekly. It therefore becomes very important to be aware of the dialysis schedule and to monitor antibiotic levels. Unfortunately, unless the laboratory's determination of the antibiotic level is performed and reported quickly, the next dose of antibiotic is likely to have been administered before the trough level is known. In fact, the trough level obtained prior to dialysis is obviously higher than the level at the end of dialysis, when the next dose is typically administered. Therefore, it is important to know when the trough level was obtained. If it was taken at the end of dialysis, there is no realistic opportunity for the level to be known by the time of dosing, unless administration is delayed.

Continuous Renal Replacement Therapy

Increasingly in acute renal failure, continuous methods of renal replacement therapy (CRRT) are being used. These include continuous arteriovenous hemofiltration (CAVH), continuous venovenous hemofiltration (CVVH), continuous arteriovenous hemodialysis (CAVHD), continuous venovenous hemodialysis (CVVHD) and in combination, continuous hemodiafiltration (CAVHDF, CVVHDF).

Hemofiltration (CAVH, CVVH) refers to the removal of an ultrafiltrate of plasma in which there is the solute loss only by convection or solvent drag, not diffusion. The plasma is filtered, but no dialysate is used, so the solute only moves along with plasma water. The efficiency of drug (or any solute) removal is related to the sieving coefficient (SC), which is the mathematical expression of the ability of a solute to cross a membrane convectively. The SC is determined by the ratio of the concentration of the substance in the ultrafiltrate to the plasma. When the patient is on CAVH, the concentration of the substance may be different in arterial and venous samples. For practical purposes of antibiotic or drug administration, the arterial and venous samples can be assumed to be equal, and therefore: SC = [UF]/[A], in which [UF] is the concentration of the antibiotic in the ultrafiltrate and A is arterial concentration. An SC of 1.0 means that a substance freely crosses the membrane and is removed in the same concentration as it exists in the plasma. An SC of zero means there is no removal (typically as the result of extensive size or protein-binding factors).

The rate of antibiotic clearance = SC × UFR (ultrafiltration rate)

Table 3 lists the SC for intravenous antibacterials commonly used to treat serious infections. Because CRRT is by definition continuous, antibiotic levels in this setting more accurately reflect true, real-time estimates of patient antibiotic levels than do levels for intermittent hemodialysis. The first of the two formulae used to determine the amount of antibiotic removed is: Amount antibiotic removed (in mg) = ultrafiltrate concentration (mg/L) × UFR (L/min) × time of procedure (min). This method depends on being able to obtain antibiotic levels in the ultrafiltrate. The second method is to extrapolate the ultrafiltrate concentration from the plasma sample, whereby: ultrafiltrate concentration = [plasma] × unbound fraction (because only the unbound fraction is filtered). The protein-bound fraction for commonly used antibiotics in the critical care setting is provided in **Table 1**. It should be noted that these protein-binding data are for healthy people and may be less reliable in critically ill patients. Nonetheless: amount of antibiotic removed (in mg) = [plasma] (mg/L) × unbound fraction × UFR (L/min) × time of procedure (min). Note that the plasma sample should reflect a steady-state level halfway between maintenance doses and after at least three $T_{1/2}$s.[41,51–53]

Continuous Hemodialysis

Removal of antibiotics during CAVHD or CVVHD occurs largely by diffusion across the dialyzer membrane into the drug-free dialysate on the other side of the membrane.

Table 3
Sieving coefficient

Antibacterials	SC
Amikacin	0.9
Amphotericin B	0.3
Amphotericin B, liposomal	0.10
Ampicillin	0.7
Cefoxitin	0.6
Ceftazidime	0.9
Ceftriaxone	0.2
Ciprofloxacin	0.8
Gentamicin	0.8
Imipenem	1.0
Levaquin	0.8
Linezolid	0.8
Metronidazole	0.8
Mezlocillin	0.7
Oxacillin	0.02
Penicillin	0.7
Piperacillin	0.7
Sulfamethoxazole	0.9
Vancomycin	0.8

There is usually a close correlation between the SC and unbound fraction because only the free or unbound drug is available for removal by hemofiltration.

Data from Golper TA. Drug removal during continuous renal replacement therapy. *In* Rose BD (ed): Nephrology Up-To-Date, vol 2, no 13. Wellesley, 1994.

Convective clearance, or solvent drag, is a less significant factor in drug removal in this modality. The two major limiting factors to antibiotic removal by diffusion are protein binding and molecular size. The type of membrane and its permeability characteristics are important determinants of antibiotic and drug removal. As a rule, the membranes used in CRRT are at least as permeable (and often more so) than those used in intermittent hemodialysis. Dosing for maintenance and additional or loading doses can be calculated when the desired plasma concentration of the antibiotic is known. The presently observed level is subtracted from the desired level. The difference in concentrations (in mg/L) $\times$ V_d (in L/kg) $\times$ body weight (kg) represents the amount of antibiotic necessary to achieve the desired antibiotic plasma level. This formula can be applied when the amount of antibiotic removal has not been directly measured or calculated.[41,52,54,55]

Sustained low-efficiency dialysis (SLED), a modified form of IHD, is being increasingly employed in the treatment of hemodynamically unstable patients with acute kidney injury. Using IHD equipment, extended treatment times of 6–12 hours or longer are utilized along with reduced blood and dialysate flow rates to achieve the hemodynamic stability of CRRT. Blood flow rates are usually set around 200 mL per minute and dialysate flow rates between 100–300 mL per minute.[56] Similar to IHD, solute and antimicrobial drug removal is completed primarily by diffusive clearance. Important factors influencing antimicrobial dosing during SLED include treatment length and dialysis membrane surface area with the extended duration possibly necessitating higher antimicrobial doses and more frequent monitoring of drug levels.[57]

Peritoneal Dialysis in End-Stage Renal Failure

Peritoneal dialysis as a chronic modality is performed with less than 15% of the end-stage renal disease population. The most common variety has been CAPD, in which the patient receives four exchanges per day (draining 2 L of dialysate, then instilling 2 L of fresh dialysate into the peritoneal cavity, where it dwells for 4–6 hours). The use of continuous-cycler peritoneal dialysis or automated peritoneal dialysis (APD) is becoming more prevalent. These modalities perform a number of exchanges using shorter dwell times during the night, allowing the patient to be free during the day. Often, the patient will receive an extra exchange during the day to enhance the adequacy of dialysis. For peritoneal dialysis, intraperitoneal (IP) antibiotic administration can be used to load, maintain, or reduce plasma levels. Dosing of IP antibiotics can be done once daily (intermittent dosing) or in each exchange (continuous dosing). For intermittent dosing, the dialysis solution that has the antibiotic added must dwell for at least 6 hours to insure adequate systemic absorption. Data support the contention that intermittent dosing is as effective as continuous dosing.[58] Heparin and insulin, which are common IP additives, do not affect the activity or stability of IP antibiotics.[59] The factors affecting peritoneal drug clearance are listed in **Box 2**. IP dosing guidelines for commonly used antibiotics used in CAPD are found in **Table 4**, and IV dosing and supplementation are described in **Table 1**.[41,59,60] In treating peritonitis, IP dosing is often preferred to IV dosing because IP absorption is increased when using many antibiotics for patients who have peritonitis, and higher IP antibiotic levels are achieved.[61] In contrast to CAPD, antibiotic dosing in APD has been less well studied. The use of shorter, more frequent exchanges in APD raises the concern of inadequate time for absorption to achieve therapeutic levels when using IP administration. Based on a randomized study that included children on APD, intermittent dosing of vancomycin in a long dwell is as effective as when it is administered in CAPD.[62] However a shorter dosing interval of 4 to 5 days is recommended to maintain serum trough levels that are greater than 15 μg/mL. Monitoring levels more frequently may be appropriate in the presence of residual renal function.

There is an inverse semilogarithmic relationship between peritoneal clearance and molecular weight. For most drugs, the peritoneal clearance of the unbound drug can be calculated by multiplying the urea clearance (20 mL/min) by the ratio of the square root of the weight of urea (60 Da) over the square root of the antibiotic's molecular weight. Charged antibiotics diffuse more slowly than neutral ones. As a rule, drugs that are not removed by hemodialysis are also not cleared by peritoneal dialysis.[63]

PERITONEAL DIALYSIS IN ACUTE RENAL FAILURE

Acute peritoneal dialysis may have variable dwell times, from no dwell time to 6 hours (similar to CAPD). In the setting of long dwell times (4–6 hours), the guidelines in **Table 4** cited should be appropriate for determining antibiotic dosing. In the setting of short dwell times, IP dosing may not be cost effective or as predictable in delivering or removing the antibiotic from the blood. In the critical care setting, multiple factors, such as hypotension or hypoperfusion of the mesenteric circulation, ileus, peristalsis, and dialysate temperature, may adversely affect clearance.[64,65] In patients receiving acute peritoneal dialysis with short dwells, it is recommended to administer antibiotics intravenously and exploit the peritoneal dialysis as a means of clearing the drug to allow trough levels to develop. As with any CRRT, continuous administration, whether IV or IP, can result in the absence of safe trough levels, with potential antibiotic-related toxicity. Because the number of exchanges per day (and hence, the degree of antibiotic clearance achieved) may change frequently in the critical care setting, it is

Box 2
Factors affecting peritoneal dialysis drug clearance

Drug properties

    Molecular weight

    Charge

    Lipid or water solubility

    V_d (tissue binding)

    Protein binding

    Other forms of steric hindrance

    Rapid excretion by another pathway

    Red cell partitioning

Intrinsic peritoneal membrane properties

    Surface blood flow

    Surface area

    Location

    Sclerosis

    Pore size

    Vascular disease

    Fluid films

Dialysate properties

    Flow rate

    Volume

    Chemical composition

    Distribution

    Temperature

Miscellaneous properties

    Ultrafiltration

    Clearance-raising additives

Data from Golper TA. Drugs and peritoneal dialysis. Dial Transplant 1979;8:41–3.

important to communicate closely with the nephrologist to appropriately adjust antibiotic loading, maintenance, and removal based on the amount of dialysis being prescribed.

ADVERSE EFFECTS OF ANTIBACTERIAL AGENTS IN RENAL FAILURE

Numerous adverse effects have been reported as resulting from the use of antibacterial agents in patients who have renal failure. Many of these effects are related to inappropriate dosing, whereas others stem from pathologic changes associated with uremia. A review of this topic has been published by Manian and colleagues.[66]

Neurologic toxicity, including psychosis, visual and auditory hallucinations, myoclonus, and seizures has been reported as the result of the use of penicillin, imipenem,

Table 4
Intraperitoneal antibiotic dosing guidelines for CAPD. Dosing of drugs with renal clearance in patients with residual renal function (defined as >100 mL/day urine output): dose should be empirically increased by 25%

Antibiotic	Intermittent (per Exchange, Once Daily)	Continuous (mg/L, All Exchanges)
Aminoglycosides		
Amikacin	2 mg/kg	LD 25, MD 12
Gentamicin	0.6 mg/kg	LD 8, MD 4
Netilmicin	0.6 mg/kg	LD 8, MD 4
Tobramycin	0.6 mg/kg	LD 8, MD 4
Cephalosporins		
Cefazolin	15 mg/kg	LD 500, MD 125
Cefepime	1 g	LD 500, MD 125
Cephalothin	15 mg/kg	LD 500, MD 125
Cephradine	15 mg/kg	LD 500, MD 125
Ceftazidime	1000–1500 mg	LD 500, MD 125
Ceftizoxime	1000 mg	LD 250, MD 125
Penicillins		
Azlocillin	ND	LD 500, MD 250
Ampicillin	ND	MD 125
Oxacillin	ND	MD 125
Nafcillin	ND	MD 125
Amoxacillin	ND	LD 250–500, MD 50
Penicillin G	ND	LD 50,000 units, MD 25,000 units
Quinolones		
Ciprofloxacin	ND	LD 50, MD 25
Others		
Vancomycin	15–30 mg/kg every 5–7 days	LD 1000, MD 25
Aztreonam	ND	LD 1000, MD 250
Antifungals		
Amphotericin	NA	1.5
Combinations		
Ampicillin/sulbactam	2 g every 12 h	LD 1000, MD 100
Imipenem/cilistatin	1 g b.i.d.	LD 500, MD 200
Quinupristin/dalfopristin	25 mg/L in alternate bags*	

Abbreviations: b.i.d., two times per day; LD, loading dose, in mg; MD, maintenance dose, in mg; NA, not applicable; ND, no data.
* Given in conjunction with 500 mg intravenous twice daily.
From Piraino B, Bailie GR, Bernardini J, et al. Peritoneal dialysis-related infections recommendations: 2005 update. Peritoneal Dialysis International 2005;25:107–31; with permission.

beta-lactams, acyclovir, amantadine, and quinolones.[67–70] Ototoxicity in the form of reversible auditory dysfunction can result from high dosages of erythromycin.[71] It remains unclear whether renal failure is an independent risk factor for aminoglycoside- or vancomycin-induced ototoxicity. Sulfonamide-induced hypoglycemia is believed to be the result of the structural similarity of sulfamethoxazole and hypoglycemic agents. Sulfamethoxazole may stimulate insulin secretion and can displace oral hypoglycemic agents from serum proteins, making more free drug available.[72,73] This interaction can be further exacerbated by the decreased clearance and protein binding of sulfamethoxazole in uremia. Platelet aggregation abnormalities induced by high doses of penicillins exacerbate the platelet dysfunction of uremia and vitamin K deficiency, and augment the effect of heparin when patients are on hemodialysis.[74–76] Renal failure does not appear to be an independent risk factor for the coagulopathy associated with cephalosporins containing the N-methyl-thiotetrazole side chain; vitamin K deficiency, which is often present in renal failure, seems to be the culprit.[77] The fluoroquinolones have been associated with increased risk for spontaneous Achilles tendon rupture in patients who have underlying renal failure, are over age 60, or with kidney, heart, or lung transplants.[78,79] The tetracycline antibiotics (with the exception of doxycyline) should be avoided in patients who have renal insufficiency because there has been an increased incidence of hepatotoxicity. Rarely, acute fatty necrosis of the liver can occur in patients who have underlying renal dysfunction.[80]

REFERENCES

1. Aronoff GR, Abel SR. Principles of administering drugs to patients with renal failure. In: Brenner BM, Stein JH, editors. Contemporary issues in nephrology. New York: Churchill-Livingstone; 1986. p. 77–82.
2. Hurwitz A. Antacid therapy in drug kinetics. Clin Pharm 1977;12:269–80.
3. Aronoff G, Bennett W, Berns J, et al. Drug prescribing in renal failure, dosing guidelines for adults. 5th edition. Philadelphia: American College of Physicians; 2007.
4. Reindenberg MM. The biotransformation of drugs in renal failure. Am J Med 1977; 62:482–5.
5. Cockcroft DW, Gault MH. Prediction of creatinine clearance from serum creatinine. Nephron 1976;16:31–41.
6. Pesola GR, Akhavan I, Madu A, et al. Prediction equation estimates of creatinine clearance in the intensive care unit. Intensive Care Med 1993;19:39–43.
7. Devine BJ. Gentamicin pharmacokinetics. Drug Intell Clin Pharm 1974;8:650–5.
8. Levey AS, Bosch JP, Lewis JB, et al. A more accurate method to estimate glomerular filtration rate from serum creatinine: a new prediction equation. Modification of Diet in Renal Disease Study Group. Ann Intern Med 1999;130:461–70.
9. Levey AS, Coresh J, Greene T, et al. Expressing the MDRD study equation for estimating GFR with IDMS traceable (gold standard) serum creatinine values [abstract]. J Am Soc Nephrol 2005;16:69A.
10. Stevens LA, Coresh J, Greene T, et al. Assessing kidney function—measured and estimated glomerular filtration rate. N Engl J Med 2006;354:2473–83.
11. Mathew TH, Johnson DW, Jones G. Chronic kidney disease and automatic reporting of estimated glomerular filtration rate: revised recommendations. Med J Aust 2007;187:459–63.
12. Froissart M, Rossert J, Jacquot C, et al. Predictive performance of the modification of diet in renal disease and Cockcroft-Gault equations for estimating renal function. J Am Soc Nephrol 2005;16:763–73.
13. Sher PP. Drug interferences with clinical laboratory tests. Drugs 1982;24: 24–63.
14. Sandburg T, Trollfors B. Effect of trimethoprim on serum creatinine in patients with acute cystitis. J Antimicrob Chemother 1986;17:123–4.
15. Harrington D, Drusano G, Smalls V, et al. False elevations of serum creatinine. JAMA 1984;252:2962–4.

16. Sherman RA, Eisenger RP, Weinstein MP, et al. Cefoxitin-induced pseudo acute renal failure. Clin Ther 1981;4:114–7.

17. Demczar DJ, Nafziger AN, Bertino JS. Pharmacokinetics of gentamicin at traditional versus high doses: implications for once-daily aminoglycoside dosing. Antimicrobial Agents Chemother 1997;41:1115–9.

18. Lacy MK, Nicolau DP, Nightingale CH, et al. The pharmacodynamics of aminoglycosides. Clin Infect Dis 1998;27:23–7.

19. Chuck SK, Raber SR, Rodvold KA, et al. National survey of extended-interval aminoglycoside dosing. Clin Infect Dis 2000;30:433–9.

20. Guiliano RA, Verpooten GA, DeBroe ME. The effect of dosing strategy on kidney cortical accumulation of aminoglycosides in rats. Am J Kidney Dis 1986;8:292–6.

21. Tam VH, Kabbara S, Vo G, et al. Comparative pharmacodynamics of gentamicin against *Staphylococcus aureus* and *Pseudomonas aeruginosa*. Antimicrobial Agents Chemother 2006;50:2626–31.

22. Edson RS, Terrell CL. The aminoglycosides. Mayo Clin Proc 1999;74:519–28.

23. Hatala R, Dinh T, CooK DJ. Once-daily aminoglycoside dosing in immunocompetent adults: a meta-analysis. Ann Intern Med 1996;124:717–25.

24. Freeman CD, Nicolau DP, Belliveau PP, et al. Once-daily dosing of aminoglycosides: review and recommendations for clinical practice. J Antimicrob Chemother 1997;39:677–86.

25. Rybak MJ, Abate BJ, Kang SL, et al. Prospective evaluation of the effect of an aminoglycoside dosing regimen on rates of observed nephrotoxicity and ototoxicity. Antimicrobial Agents Chemother 1999;43:1549–55.

26. Nicolau DP, Freeman CD, Belliveau PP, et al. Experience with a once-daily aminoglycoside program administered to 2,184 adult patients. Antimicrobial Agents Chemother 1995;39:650–5.

27. CDC, recommendations for preventing the spread of vancomycin resistance. MMWR 1994;44(RR-12):1–13.

28. Stryjewski ME, Szczech LA, Benjamin DK, et al. Use of vancomycin or first-generation cephalosporins for the treatment of hemodialysis-dependent patients with methicillin susceptible *Staphylococcus aureus* bacteremia. Clin Infect Dis 2007;44:190–6.

29. Sowinski KM, Mueller BA, Grabe DW, et al. Cefazolin dialytic clearance by high-efficiency and high-flux hemodialyzers. Am J Kidney Dis 2001;37:766–76.

30. Fogel MA, Nussbaum PB, Feintzeig ID, et al. Cefazolin in chronic hemodialysis patients: a safe, effective alternative to vancomycin. Am J Kidney Dis 1998;32:401–9.

31. Kuypers D, Vanwalleghem J, Maes B, et al. Cefazolin serum concentrations with fixed intravenous dosing in patients on chronic hemodialysis treatment. Nephrol Dial Transplant 1999;14:2050–1.

32. Geraci JE, Hermans PE. Vancomycin. Mayo Clin Proc 1983;58:88–91.

33. Ackerman BH, Vannier AM, Eudy EB. Analysis of vancomycin time-kill studies with *Staphylococcus* species by using a curve stripping program to describe the relationship between concentration and pharmacodynamic response. Antimicrobial Agents Chemother 1992;36:1766–9.

34. Tenover FC, Moellering RC. The rationale for revising the Clinical and Laboratory Standards Institute vancomycin minimal inhibitory concentration interpretive criteria for *Staphylococcus aureus*. Clin Infect Dis 2007;44:1208–15.

35. Rybak M, Lomaestro B, Rotschafer JC, et al. Therapeutic monitoring of vancomycin in adult patients: a consensus review of the American Society of Health-System

Pharmacists, the Infectious Disease Society of America, and the Society of Infectious Diseases Pharmacists. Am J Health Syst Pharm 2009;66:82–98.
36. Freeman CD, Quintiliani R, Nightingale CH. Vancomycin therapeutic drug monitoring: is it necessary? Ann Pharmocother 1993;27:594–8.
37. Saunders NJ. Vancomycin administration and monitoring reappraisal. J Antimicrob Chemother 1995;36:279–82.
38. Hammett-Stabler CA, Johns T. Laboratory guidelines for monitoring of antimicrobial drugs. Clin Chem 1998;44:1129–40.
39. Tobin CM, Darville JM, Thomson AH, et al. Vancomycin therapeutic drug monitoring: is there a consensus view? J Antimicrob Chemother 2002;50:713–8.
40. Raveh D, Kopyt M, Hite Y, et al. Risk factors for nephrotoxicity in elderly patients receiving once-daily aminoglycosides. QJM 2002;95:291–7.
41. Golper TA, Bennett WM. Drug usage in dialysis patients. In: Nissenson R, Fine RN, Gentile DE, editors. Clinical dialysis. 2nd edition. 2. Norwalk (CT): Appleton and Lange; 1990. p. 608–30.
42. Vanholder R, DeSmet R, Glorieux G, et al. Review on uremic toxins: classification, concentration, and interindividual variability. Kidney Int 2003;63:1934–43.
43. Marx MA, Frye RF, Matzke GR, et al. Cefazolin as empiric therapy in hemodialysis-related infections: efficacy and blood concentrations. Am J Kidney Dis 1998;32:410–4.
44. Barth RH, DeVincenzo N, Zara AC, et al. Vancomycin pharmacokinetics in high-flux hemodialysis [abstract]. J Am Soc Nephrol 1990;1:348.
45. Barth RH, DeVincenzo N. Use of vancomycin in high-flux hemodialysis: experience with 130 courses of therapy. Kidney Int 1996;50:929–36.
46. Foote EF, Dreitlein WB, Steward CA, et al. Pharmacokinetics of vancomycin when administered during high flux hemodialysis. Clin Nephrol 1998;50:51–5.
47. Mason NA, Neudeck BL, Welage LS, et al. Comparison of 3 vancomycin dosage regimens during hemodialysis with cellulose triacetate dialyzers: post-dialysis versus intradialytic administration. Clin Nephrol 2003;60:96–104.
48. Maher JF. Pharmacokinetics in patients with renal failure. Clin Nephrol 1984;21:39–46.
49. Maher JF. Principles of dialysis and dialysis of drugs. Am J Med 1977;62:475–81.
50. Kucers A, Crowe SM, Grayson ML, et al. The use of antibiotics: a clinical review of antibacterial, antifungal and antiviral drugs. London: Hodder Arnold; 1997.
51. Golper TA, Wedel SK, Kaplen AA, et al. Drug removal during continuous arteriovenous hemofiltration: theory and clinical observations. Int J Artif Organs 1985;8:307–12.
52. Golper TA. Drug removal during continuous renal replacement therapy. In: Rose BD, editor, Nephrology up-to-date, vol.6.3. Wellesley (MA); 1998.
53. Vincent HH, Vos MC, Akcahuseyin E, et al. Drug clearance by continuous hemodialfiltration (CAVHD). Analysis of sieving coefficients of diffusions. Blood Purif 1993;11:99–107.
54. Sigler MH, Teehan BP, Van Valkenbrugh D. Solute transport in continuous hemodialysis. A new treatment for acute renal failure. Kidney Int 1987;32:562–71.
55. Golper TA. Update on drug sieving coefficients and dosing adjustments during continuous renal replacement therapies. Contrib Nephrol 2001;132:349–53.
56. Marshall MR, Golper TA. Sustained low-efficiency dialysis for critically ill patients requiring renal replacement therapy. Kidney Int 2001;60:777–85.
57. Kielstein JT, Czock D, Schopke T, et al. Pharmacokinetics and total elimination of meropenem and vancomycin in intensive care unit patients undergoing extended daily dialysis. Crit Care Med 2006;34:51–6.

58. Wiggins KJ, Johnson DW, Craig JC, et al. Treatment of peritoneal dialysis-associated peritonitis: a systematic review of randomized controlled trials. Am J Kidney Dis 2007;50(6):967–88.
59. Sewell DL, Golper TA, Brown SD, et al. Stability of single and combination antimicrobial agents in various peritoneal dialysates in the presence of heparin and insulin. Am J Kidney Dis 1983;3:209–12.
60. Golper TA. Drugs and peritoneal dialysis. Dial Transplant 1979;8:41–3.
61. Piraino B, Bailie GR, Bernardini J, et al. Peritoneal dialysis-related infections recommendations: 2005 update. Perit Dial Int 2005;25(2):107–30.
62. Schaefer F, Klaus G, Muller-Wiefel DE, et al. Intermittent versus continuous intraperitoneal glycopeptide/ceftazidime treatment in children with peritoneal dialysis-associated peritonitis. J Am Soc Nephrol 1999;10(1):136–45.
63. Lasrich M, Maher JM, Hirszel P, et al. Correlation of peritoneal transport rates with molecular weight: a method for predicting clearances. ASAIO J 1979;2:107–13.
64. Gross M, McDonald HP. Effect of dialysate temperature and flow rate of peritoneal clearance. JAMA 1967;202:363–6.
65. Nolph KD, Popovich RP, Ghods AJ, et al. Determinants of low clearances of small solutes during peritoneal dialysis. Kidney Int 1978;13:117–23.
66. Manian F, Stone W, Alford R. Adverse antibiotic effects associated with renal insufficiency. Rev Infect Dis 1990;12:236–49.
67. Calandra G, Lydic E, Carrigan J, et al. Factors predisposing to seizures in seriously ill infected patients receiving antibiotics: experience with imipenem/cilastatin. Am J Med 1988;84:911–8.
68. Ing TS, Daugirdas JT, Soung LS, et al. Toxic effects of amantadine in patients with renal failure. Can Med Assoc J 1979;120:695–8.
69. Oldstone MB, Nelson E. Central nervous system manifestations of penicillin toxicity in man. Neurology 1966;16:693–700.
70. Wright AJ. The penicillins. Mayo Clin Proc 1999;74:290–307.
71. Kroboth PD, McNeil MA, Kreeger A, et al. Hearing loss and erythromycin pharmacokinetics in a patient receiving hemodialysis. Arch Intern Med 1983;143:1263–5.
72. Frankel MC, Leslie BR, Sax FL, et al. Trimethoprim-sulfamethoxazole–related hypoglycemia in a patient with renal failure. N Y State J Med 1984;84:30–1.
73. Lawson DH, Paice BJ. Adverse reactions to trimethoprim-sulfamethoxazole. Rev Infect Dis 1982;4:429–33.
74. Andrassy K, Scherz M, Ritz E, et al. Penicillin-induced coagulation disorder. Lancet 1976;2:1039–41.
75. McClure PD, Casserly JG, Monsier C, et al. Carbenicillin-induced bleeding disorder. Lancet 1970;2:1307–8.
76. Stuart JJ. Ticarcillin-induced hemorrhage in a patient with thrombocytosis. Southampt Med J 1980;73:1084–5.
77. Cohen H, Scott SD, Mackie IJ, et al. The development of hypoprothrombinaemia following antibiotic therapy in malnourished patients with low serum vitamin K1 levels. Br J Haemotol 1988;68:63–6.
78. Linden PD, Sturkenboom MC, Herings RM, et al. Increased risk of achilles tendon rupture with quinolone antibacterial use, especially in elderly patients taking oral corticosteroids. Arch Intern Med 2003;163:1801–7.
79. Levaquin Prescribing Information Revised September 2008.
80. Smilack JD. The tetracyclines. Mayo Clin Proc 1999;74:727–9.

Topical Antibacterial Agents

Peter A. Lio, MD[a],*, Elaine T. Kaye, MD[b]

KEYWORDS

- Antiseptics • Mupirocin • Neomycin • Gentamicin
- Bacitracin • Polymyxin

The skin presents a first line of defense against a wide range of bacterial invaders. When the integrity of the skin is compromised accidentally or intentionally, its natural defenses weaken and a role for antibacterials emerges. The topical route of application offers several advantages over systemic administration, including the avoidance of systemic toxicity and side effects, the decreased induction of bacterial resistance, and the high concentration of antibacterial agent at the site of infection. However, a treatment that must be physically applied to the skin is limited by patient compliance, local side effects such as allergic contact dermatitis, and the depth of penetration of the agent. Despite their shortcomings, topical antibacterial agents are highly versatile and can be used successfully for both prophylaxis and treatment of bacterial infections.

Outside of the hospital setting, *Staphylococcus aureus* and group A streptococci are classically considered the pathogens most often involved in infections of the skin. Recent data from hospitalized patients demonstrate that *S aureus*, *Enterococcus* spp, coagulase-negative staphylococci, *Escherichia coli* and *Pseudomonas aeruginosa* are the most prevalent pathogens involved in skin and soft tissue infections.[1]

These well-known offenders, as well as the panoply of more exotic pathogens that have been reported to cause skin infections, must be kept in mind while exploring the topical antibacterial agents at one's disposal.

PROFILES OF SELECTED ANTIBACTERIAL AGENTS
Antiseptics

Antiseptics, also known as disinfectants, are chemical agents primarily used to decrease the risk of infection in intact skin or in minor wounds. Alcohol and

---

A version of this article appeared in the 23:4 issue of the *Infectious Disease Clinics of North America*.
[a] Department of Dermatology, Northwestern University Feinberg School of Medicine, 676 North St Clair, Suite 1600, Chicago, IL 60611, USA
[b] Department of Dermatology, Harvard Medical School, Children's Hospital Medical Center, 65 Walnut Street, Wellesley Hills, Boston, MA 02481, USA
* Corresponding author.
E-mail address: p-lio@northwestern.edu

iodophors have rapid action against bacteria but little persistent activity, whereas chlorhexidine and triclosan are slower to act but persist on the stratum corneum for continued antimicrobial effects.[2,3] Most antiseptics are not suitable for open wounds as they may impede wound healing by direct cytotoxic effects to keratinocytes and fibroblasts.[4]

Hydrogen peroxide

Hydrogen peroxide is a common antiseptic agent used on intact skin and minor wounds. It is thought to kill bacteria in two distinct modes: rapidly by way of DNA damage from highly reactive hydroxyl radicals, and more slowly in a manner that may involve the inactivation of housekeeping enzymes.[5,6] It has limited bactericidal activity, however. In one study of mixed microorganism disinfection of a glass, it was found to be entirely ineffective.[7] A prospective study in human appendectomy wounds found that there was no statistical difference in the infection rate between a control group and a group receiving hydrogen peroxide.[8]

Hydrogen peroxide may be detrimental to wound healing, however, as it has been shown to be directly cytotoxic to keratinocytes, and even at very low concentrations inhibits keratinocyte migration and proliferation.[9]

Chlorhexidine

Chlorhexidine's role continues to expand as an effective and versatile antiseptic for both infection control and prevention.[10] Chlorhexidine gluconate is active against a wide range of gram-positive and gram-negative bacteria, yeast, and molds.[11] Chlorhexidine acts by disrupting cytoplasmic membranes and remains active for hours after application.[3,12,13] Its FDA indications are designated for general skin and wound cleansing, preoperative skin preparation, personnel hand wash and surgical hand scrub. Chlorhexidine is consistently superior to povidone-iodine and a number of other antiseptics in reducing colonizing flora immediately and several days after application.[2,14,15] While it is useful in decolonization of methicillin-resistant *Staphylococcus aureus* (MRSA) carriers, its ability to decrease skin and soft tissue infection is limited when used alone as a single agent, but it has been shown to reduce staphylococcal and streptococcal infections in marine recruits and MRSA infection in ICU patients when a combination of chlorhexidine bath is used along with intranasal mupirocin.[16–18] Daily chlorhexidine baths alone reduced contamination and acquisition of vancomycin-resistant enterococcus.[10,19] In addition, chlorhexidine is widely used for skin preparation before catheter insertion. More recent developments include chlorhexidine-impregnated dressings or sponges for maintenance of indwelling catheters and impregnated or coated catheters and catheter cuffs.[20,21] Finally, chlorhexidine is playing an emerging role in decontamination of the oropharynx as it impacts on nosocomial pneumonia. A meta-analysis found that chlorhexidine decontamination was responsible for a 30% decrease in the incidence of ventilator-associated pneumonia.[10,22]

Triclosan

Triclosan is a broad-spectrum cationic antimicrobial agent that is widely used in consumer products such as soaps, detergents, toothpastes, and cutting boards. Its mechanism of action is bacterial membrane disruption through blockade of lipid synthesis. This was elucidated recently when triclosan resistance was found in *E coli* strains. These strains were found to have a mutation in the *fabI* gene, which encodes an enzyme involved in fatty acid biosynthesis.[23] The emergence of resistance, although not yet clinically relevant, has sparked concern about the widespread use of this agent promoting resistance.

Iodophors

The iodophors are complexes of iodine and organic carrier compounds that have a broad spectrum of activity against bacteria and fungi. Its mechanism is thought to be by way of destroying microbial protein and DNA.[24] They were formulated to be less irritating and allergenic, but are also less active than pure iodine solutions.[25] Iodophors require at least 2 minutes of contact to release free iodine that exerts the antibacterial activity. In vitro data shows a large number of gram-positive isolates after exposure for 15 seconds but essentially none after 120 seconds of exposure.[26]

Iodophors are used most commonly for preoperative skin preparation. Povidone-iodine is a complex of the bactericidal iodine with the polymer polyvinylpyrrolidone (povidone). It is available in various commercial forms, including cleansers, surgical scrubs, and ointments. It is effective against MRSA and Enterococcus spp; clinically significant resistance to povidone-iodine has not been documented.[27]

The rate of adverse reactions with povidone-iodine is low although there are reports of contact dermatitis as well as metabolic acidosis with prolonged use.[28] In addition, iodine has been considered cytotoxic and deleterious to wound healing. One review concluded that in the majority of in vivo studies reviewed, povidone-iodine seemed to impair wound healing.[29]

Benzoyl peroxide and other antiacne agents

A powerful oxidizing agent, benzoyl peroxide has broad-spectrum bactericidal effects.[30] It is available in gels, creams, lotions, and washes and in various concentrations from 2.5% to 20%. Most commonly, benzoyl peroxide is used for the FDA-indicated treatment of acne vulgaris; however, in vitro tests confirm that it is effective against a wide range of organisms including Staphylococcus capitis, Staphylococcus epidermidis, Propionibacterium avidum, Propionibacterium granulosum, and Pityrosporum ovale, in addition to P acnes.[30]

Increasingly, benzoyl peroxide is being formulated in combination with antibiotics, such as clindamycin and erythromycin for the treatment of acne vulgaris. These topical combinations are more effective clinically and induce less resistance of P acnes.[31] Topical erythromycin alone is FDA-approved to treat acne vulgaris but has also been used in the treatment of erythrasma, pitted keratolysis, and trichomycosis axillaris caused by corynebacterium.[32]

Topical azelaic acid is a dicarboxylic acid that is used in both acne vulgaris and rosacea. It works by killing P acnes as well as decreasing keratin production.

Hypochlorite (Bleach)

Sodium hypochlorite (NaOCl) has historical significance as well as an emerging prominence because of its bleaching and disinfecting properties.[33] It was discovered in 1788 and used in 1820 to help embalm the decomposing body of Louis XVIII. Later, it was reformulated as Dakin's solution and used widely in World War II to treat both burns and wounds. Despite hypochlorite's broad spectrum activity against both gram-positive and gram-negative organisms, concerns have been raised about its potential for cytotoxicity.

More recently, NaOCl (bleach) has been used empirically in pediatric patients with impetiginized atopic dermatitis, most commonly in the proportion of one-half cup per full bath, for 15 minutes, twice weekly.[34,35] A series of in vitro experiments demonstrated that maximal killing of isolates of community-associated MRSA optimally requires a 5-minute exposure to hypochlorite at a concentration of 2.5 µl/mL.[36] This is equivalent to one-half cup of bleach in a quarter of a bathtubful of water. Perhaps the culmination of these findings lies in a newly released topical water-based gel containing 0.008% hypochlorous acid, and 0.002% sodium hypochlorite. This over-the-counter agent allegedly kills 99.99% of *S aureus* within 30 seconds of topical application. Although more studies are needed to confirm these findings, there is great promise in this very inexpensive, broad-spectrum and non-resistance inducing disinfectant in all its forms.[37]

Other antiseptic agents

A number of other antiseptics find service in more limited capacities. Benzalkonium chloride is a quaternary ammonium compound traditionally used for preparation of the urethral area for catheterization. It is thought to work by binding and disorganizing the bacterial membrane.[38]

Hexachlorophene is a chlorinated bisphenol compound with bacteriostatic activity against gram-positive bacteria. Its residue remains active for several days on skin. Neurotoxicity has resulted from excessive absorption and studies have also suggested a possible teratogenic effect.[39]

A number of botanic products such as thyme oil (thymol)[40] and clove oil (eugenol)[41] have been shown to have antibacterial properties. Undoubtedly, the list will continue to grow as new compounds are discovered and tested.

Antibiotic Agents

Mupirocin

Mupirocin, known formerly as pseudomonic acid A, is the major fermentation product of *Pseudomonas fluorescens*. It works by the reversible inhibition of bacterial isoleucyl-tRNA synthetase, thereby preventing protein and, subsequently, cell wall synthesis.[30] Mupirocin is highly effective against aerobic gram-positive cocci, especially *S aureus*, for which it is bactericidal at the concentrations present with the commonly used 2% ointment.[42] It is not effective against enterococci and generally has poor activity against gram-negative bacteria.[43]

Mupirocin is FDA-approved solely to treat impetigo in adults and children. However, it is a versatile agent that has also been used for treating secondarily infected lesions and for eradication of nasal staphylococcus carriage. It rarely causes local adverse effects, such as pruritus or contact dermatitis. Systemic absorption of mupirocin or its major metabolite, monic acid, has not been detected with short courses of administration.[42]

Despite mupirocin's unique mechanism of action, resistant strains have emerged.[44] In the context of widespread mupirocin use, rates have ranged from 11% to as high as 65%. In the absence of widespread use, one study still found 13% mupirocin resistance in MRSA isolates from SICU subjects, with 9% demonstrating high levels of resistance.[45] Such reports of mupirocin-resistant MRSA[46] argues for more judicious use of this important topical antibiotic.

Retapamulin

Retapamulin is one of a new class of antibiotics called pleuromutilins, which selectively inhibit the elongation phase of bacterial protein synthesis at a unique site on the ribosome.[47] Retapamulin is FDA-approved only for the topical treatment of impetigo caused by *S aureus* (MSSA) and *S pyogenes* in both adults and children. Retapamulin shows in vitro activity against *S aureus* and *S pyogenes*, including isolates resistant to β-lactams, macrolides, quinolones, and mupirocin. In 664 isolates of *S aureus*, including many with high levels of resistance to mupirocin and fusidic acid. and 448 (73%) MRSA isolates, retapamulin demonstrated excellent in vitro activity.[48] It is also promising that retapamulin shows a low propensity to developing resistance to *S aureus*.[49] More clinical studies of retapamulin in treatment of resistant *S aureus* are needed.

Dapsone

A sulfone synthesized initially in 1908, dapsone was initially put to use as an antileprosy medication.[50] Known for its powerful antiinflammatory effects in addition to its antimicrobial abilities, it was frequently used for severe inflammatory forms of acne before the advent of systemic retinoids but was limited by systemic toxicity. Recently, a 5% topical gel formulation has been FDA-approved for the treatment of mild-to-moderate acne.[51] Early studies suggest that the topical formulation is safe and that monitoring for hemolytic anemia is not necessary, even among these with known glucose 6-phosphate dehydrogenase deficiency. Although it is in the sulfa family, it appears that dapsone may not be very effective against the bacteria that are commonly treated with topical agents. In one study, the minimum inhibitory concentration (MIC) for dapsone was measured for *S pyogenes*, *S aureus*, and *E coli*, and found to have essentially no antibacterial effects against these pathogens.[52] Despite these negative findings, it is possible that other uses for topical dapsone will be uncovered as it becomes more widely available.

Neomycin and gentamicin

Neomycin is an aminoglycoside produced by *Streptomyces fradiae*. It is bactericidal by binding the 30s subunit of the bacterial ribosome to inhibit protein synthesis.[30] Neomycin is highly active against most gram-negative bacteria but is less active against *P aeruginosa* and anaerobic species such as *Bacteroides*. It is active against staphylococci but is not effective against other gram-positive bacteria such as streptococci.[43] Resistance has been reported in staphylococci and gram-negative bacilli including *E coli*, *Klebsiella*, and *Proteus*.

Neomycin is usually formulated as 20% neomycin sulfate in petrolatum, and is widely used by itself and in combination with other antibiotics, such as bacitracin and polymyxin B. One of the major drawbacks of neomycin is the perceived high prevalence of allergic contact dermatitis, estimated at 1%–6%, but perhaps higher still in patients who have a compromised skin barrier.[53,54] A recent review, however, highlights the fact that data from thousands of subjects show the actual incidence of allergic contact dermatitis to neomycin to be 1% or less in the general population.[54] Neomycin can be systemically absorbed if applied to large body surfaces in which skin is damaged, causing systemic toxicity such as ototoxicity and nephrotoxicity.[55]

Topical gentamicin is another aminoglycoside with the same mechanism of action as neomycin. It is highly active against gram-negative organisms such as *Pseudomonas* and some gram-positive bacteria, including some staphylococcal strains. It has been used to treat wounds, anogenital infections, and pseudomonas folliculitis. It should be applied with caution because of its history of causing ear and kidney toxicity when used on burn wounds, where it is rapidly absorbed.[32]

Polymyxin

Polymyxins are cationic decapeptides that are products of *Bacillus polymyxa*. Polymyxin acts as a surfactant that disrupts bacterial membranes. Polymyxins have bactericidal activity against some gram-negative organisms including *P aeruginosa*, *E coli*, *Enterobacter* sp and *Klebsiella* sp, but do not have activity against *Proteus*, most *Serratia*, or gram-positive bacteria.[43] Polymyxins only rarely cause allergic contact dermatitis, and are most often used in combination with bacitracin, zinc, and neomycin in a petrolatum base.

Bacitracin

Bacitracin is FDA-approved in adults for the treatment of superficial bacterial infections of the skin. Bacitracin is a polypeptide produced by *Bacillus subtilis*, named for Margaret Tracy, the 7-year-old girl from whose wound the strain was originally isolated.[33] Initially developed for systemic administration, nephrotoxicity limited its use.[30] Bacitracin A is the form most commonly used, often formulated as 20% bacitracin zinc in petrolatum. It exerts its antibacterial activity by complexing with C55-prenol pyrophosphate, a constituent of the bacterial cell wall, thus blocking cell wall formation.[30]

Bacitracin is primarily active against gram-positive organisms, including staphylococci, streptococci, clostridia, and corynebacteria. It is used for treatment of local infection and is a popular topical antibiotic for wound prophylaxis because of its low cost and low toxicity. Historically, bacitracin rarely caused sensitization[43] but, in recent years, it has become a frequent cause of allergic contact dermatitis.[56,57]

INTACT SKIN

Topical antibacterial agents can be used as prophylaxis against infection in a variety of inpatient and outpatient settings. In this capacity, antiseptics—chemicals used to disinfect, and antibiotics—biologically derived substances, serve this role.

Resident Skin Flora

The skin normally provides host to a number of bacteria, fungi, and even mites (ie, *Demodex* spp). Coagulase-negative staphylococci represent the dominant bacterial resident in the stratum corneum and on the skin surface, with a reservoir in the sebaceous glands. A number of agents successfully eradicate surface bacteria but are short-acting and are unable to clear bacteria that reside more deeply in the stratum corneum. A comparison of antiseptic agents and antimicrobial agents was performed on various sites in 14 healthy subjects.[58] The study results are summarized in **Table 1**.

Another study of 50 healthy subjects demonstrated that treatment with triple-antibiotic ointment (TAO) containing bacitracin, polysporin, and neomycin eradicated coagulase-negative staphylococci from 96% of skin surface sites versus mupirocin

Table 1 Eradication of coagulase-negative staphylococci by topical antibacterial agents			
Agent	**Sterilization of Skin Surface**	**Sterilization of Stratum Corneum**	**Prevention of Repopulation After 16 h**
10% povidone-iodine	Yes	No	—
2% aqueous iodine	Yes	Yes	—
2% tincture of iodine	Yes	Yes	No
70% ethanol	Yes	No	—
0.5% chlorhexidine-ethanol	Yes	No	—
Iodophor	Yes	Yes	No
Silver sulfadiazine	No	—	—
Mupirocin	Yes	Yes	No
TAO	Yes	Yes	Yes
Control	No	No	No

10% povidone-iodine, 2% aqueous iodine, 2% tincture of iodine, 70% ethanol, and 0.5% chlorhexidine-ethanol were applied for 15 seconds with a gauze sponge. Iodophor, silver sulfadiazine, mupirocin, and TAO were applied and covered for 6 hours with gauze. (*Based on data from* Hendley JO, Ashe KM. Effect of topical antimicrobial treatment on aerobic bacteria in the stratum corneum of human skin. Antimicrob Agents Chemother 1991;35(4):627–31.)

ointment, which eradicated the bacteria at 40% of the skin surface sites.[58] This study also showed that without neomycin, TAO was essentially equivalent to placebo.

Hand Hygiene

Alcohols are antiseptics that exhibit significant pan-antimicrobial and bactericidal activity,[59] predominantly by way of protein denaturation.[60] In concentrations ranging from 60% to 95%, alcohol-based hand washes (usually ethyl or isopropyl alcohol with emollients often added) safely, quickly, and effectively reduce microorganisms on the skin surface. For patients with recurrent skin and soft tissue infections, clinical guidelines include the use of alcohol-based cleansers as part of the personal hygiene measures recommended to prevent further episodes.[61] As a point of reference, a 62% gel preparation of ethyl alcohol exhibited a 99.99% reduction in bacteria from baseline levels after one application.[62] A number of studies in both clinical and nonclinical settings demonstrate significant decrease in bacterial counts on hands and in infection rates, significantly better than hand washing with antiseptic soap.[63–65]

A major limitation of alcohol is the transient effect of antibacterial action. Compounding alcohol with a preservative or another antibacterial agent can overcome this normally transient reduction of bacterial counts. In one study, 70% ethyl alcohol with 0.5% chlorhexidine gluconate was compared with 4% aqueous chlorhexidine, triclosan, 7.5% povidone-iodine or vehicle control for surgical scrubbing. Although all preparations reduced flora when compared with control on day 1, the combination of alcohol and chlorhexidine outperformed other preparations when evaluated on day 5.[2]

The powerful antimicrobial effect with relatively few drawbacks has led to rapid adoption of alcohol-based hand washes by numerous medical institutions and discussions of replacing traditional surgical scrubs with alcohol-based agents.[66]

Staphylococcal Colonization

Nasal colonization of *S aureus* predisposes the carrier to *S aureus* infections. Both logic and some clinical studies support the assertion that eradication of carriage results in significantly decreased rates of infection.[67,68] A number of techniques for eliminating the bacteria have been attempted, including systemic antibacterial agents, antiseptics, and topical antibacterials. Topical antibiotics such as bacitracin, tetracycline, and vancomycin applied to the nares have resulted in only temporary eradication of *S aureus*.[69]

Mupirocin demonstrates superior efficacy against a host of antibiotic-resistant strains and significant duration of clearing. A recent review of the evidence for mupirocin in treating *S aureus* colonization[67] highlighted some of the following results:

In one series, 5 days of intranasal mupirocin twice daily resulted in 13% positive culture results in the experimental group versus 93% in the placebo control group at 48 to 72 hours, 18% versus 88% at 4 weeks, and 53% versus 76% at 1 year.

A comparison between intranasal mupirocin and bacitracin in health care workers demonstrated 20% carriage for mupirocin recipients versus 77% carriage for the bacitracin group at 30 days follow-up.

Intranasal neomycin was compared with mupirocin (both thrice daily for 7 days) in a small study that showed 42% of the mupirocin group and 75% of the neomycin group had positive cultures at 3 months posttreatment.

While the data are convincing in terms of reducing carriage, subsequent differential infection rates are a more meaningful measure. Benefits of decolonization in reducing infection have been demonstrated in patients who are undergoing surgery as well as those receiving peritoneal dialysis and hemodialysis.[70] In one large study of 4030 subjects who received intranasal mupirocin twice daily for 5 days preoperatively, 4% of nasal carriers of S aureus in the treated group developed surgical site infection versus 7.7% of placebo-treated carriers.[71] A recent multicenter study demonstrated that a combination of intranasal mupirocin and chlorhexidine soap used in nasal carriers of S aureus reduced the risk of surgical-site infections.[72] A study of 267 nasal carriers of S aureus on peritoneal dialysis showed that the group treated with mupirocin twice daily for 5 days per month had 14 exit-site infections versus 44 in the placebo group.[73] Other types of infections such as peritonitis were not significantly reduced. Of note, the study revealed that treating large numbers of nonnasal carriers did not affect their infection rate.

Unlike the surgical and dialysis populations, however, nonsurgical subjects did not seem to clearly benefit from mupirocin prophylaxis. 1602 nonsurgical subjects were found to be nasal S aureus carriers at the time of admission and treated with mupirocin or placebo ointment twice daily for 5 days. Nosocomial S aureus infections did not differ between the two groups.[74] While mupirocin resistance and dosing regimen may be factors that affected the results, the study suggests that nonsurgical patients do not benefit from such screening and intervention.[75] Future studies may better define subsets of individuals with identifiable risk factors that may be appropriate candidates for decolonization.

MRSA

Although there was an overall decrease in Staphylococcal nasal colonization in the United States between 2001 and 2004, the prevalence of nasal colonization with MRSA has increased.[76] Individuals who have newly acquired MRSA as well as individuals who have harbored MRSA for greater than 1 year are at high risk for MRSA morbidity.[77]

Traditionally mupirocin has shown efficacy against MRSA. One study used mupirocin intranasally thrice weekly as a prophylatic regimen on a ward with endemic MRSA. This was effective at decreasing serious MRSA infection and resistance to mupirocin was not seen.[78] Mupirocin resistance has emerged, however, and there is speculation that this may be due to low concentrations of mupirocin in the pharynx during intranasal administration.[79,80] In one provocative study, mupirocin resistance was overcome by the use of intranasal TAO containing bacitracin, polymyxin B, and gramicidin.[81] With reports of high rates of mupirocin resistance (see above), including high-level resistance, infection control strategies for MRSA should not rely too heavily on mupirocin alone, especially as testing for mupirocin resistance is not routine at most institutions.[45]

MRSA decolonization as a strategy for infection control is controversial, primarily because there is no clear antibacterial regimen that succeeds in long-term eradication in hospitalized patients. Previous studies of mupirocin have focused on detection and treatment of MRSA carriage in the nose; however, there is ample evidence that MRSA colonizes multiple sites which, in addition to the nose, include the throat, axilla, groin, and rectal area.[82] Therefore, it follows that effective decolonization would need to address these broad anatomic sites.[83]

While systemic antimicrobials are not recommended routinely for decolonization, refractory cases of MRSA infection may respond to a combined strategy of oral and topical treatment. In one randomized study, hospitalized subjects who had MRSA received a 7-day course of chlorhexidine washes, intranasal mupirocin, rifampin and doxycycline.[84] 92% of these subjects were cleared of MRSA from all sites and 74% remained clear at 3 months. A previous study used a similar combined regimen of topical and oral antimicrobial agents and achieved 90% in the subjects followed up at 3 months.[85]

Although these studies imply that there may be effective regimens, likely including topical antibacterial agents, for long-term S aureus eradication there are still many important questions. The optimal dosing regimen remains unclear and its ability to alter infection rates needs to be better elucidated. It may even be argued that widespread MRSA decolonization may be detrimental as it might select for more virulent strains.

Although evidence is limited on methods to prevent CA-MRSA, the Infectious Diseases Society of America (IDSA) issued recommendations in 2011 for the practical management of recurrent skin and soft tissue infections. The society offers clinical guidelines on decolonization as a strategy to reduce recurrence of MRSA infections. These include a 5–10 day course of intranasal mupirocin which may be used alone or in combination with chlorhexidine or diluted bleach baths.[61] Newer agents such as lysostaphin, an endopeptidase, are being investigated in treating MRSA in animal models.[86] Less conventional antibacterial agents such as tea tree oil (*Melaleuca alternifolia*) have been studied as well. In one small study, tea tree oil was applied in a 4% nasal ointment with a 5% tea tree oil–based body wash and compared with mupirocin nasal ointment with triclosan body wash for MRSA eradication. The tea tree oil regimen was found to be more efficacious, although not significantly so.[87] Newer studies suggest that habituation may occur with tea tree oil and caution that this may decrease efficacy of other topical antibiotics.[88,89] The increasing importance of MRSA infections calls for more work in this area.

SUPERFICIAL WOUNDS

An Australian study of 177 superficial wounds in schoolchildren found infection rates of 8.5% and 12.5% by microbiologic and clinical criteria, respectively.[90] A landmark study on the natural history of superficial wound infection demonstrated a 47% streptococcal colonization rate of minor skin trauma (largely mosquito bites and abrasions) in a control group.[91] This same study showed that TAO containing bacitracin, polysporin, and neomycin decreased this rate to 15% when applied thrice daily.

Topical antibacterial agents also appear to have effects on wound healing in a manner seemingly unrelated to their antimicrobial properties. TAO has been shown to increase the reepithelialization rate of experimentally induced wounds by up to 25%[92] and minimize scarring and dyspigmentation compared with other agents and placebo.[93]

OPERATIVE WOUNDS
Preoperative Prophylaxis

Preoperative disinfection of the skin is widely accepted as the standard of care for decreasing postoperative wound infection.[94] Chlorhexidine and iodophors are generally accepted as among the most effective and widely used agents.[95] One prospective study found that preoperative showering with 4% chlorhexidine gluconate was more effective than povidone-iodine soap in reducing positive intraoperative wound cultures (4% vs 9%, respectively).[96] A more recent study suggested that a 2% chlorhexidine gluconate preparation with 70% isopropyl alcohol was more effective than either of the two constituents alone at reducing microbial counts at different time points.[12]

Postoperative Wound Care

Despite their excellent preoperative performance, disinfectants such as chlorhexidine, NaOCl, and povidone-iodine are generally not helpful in preventing infections in postoperative wounds; moreover, many experimental studies have demonstrated significant cytotoxicity from these agents.[4,97–99] Better suited for this task are the topical antibiotics such as bacitracin, mupirocin, and silver sulfadiazine (SSD), which appear to decrease infection rates and enhance wound healing.[92,100–102] In one large study of 6,000 surgical cases, neomycin-bacitracin-polymyxin spray was found to decrease infection rates.[103] Another trial of the neomycin-bacitracin-polymyxin spray versus no treatment of 851 surgical wounds demonstrated significant reduction in infection in the experimental group.[104]

In a mouse surgical wound model, mupirocin cream showed equal efficacy to the oral penicillin flucloxacillin and greater efficacy than oral erythromycin in reducing bacterial counts. It was also similar in efficacy to oral cephalexin against S pyogenes but superior against S aureus.[105]

Honey has been studied in a number of clinical settings, including as an agent for wound healing. The hyperosmolarity of honey impedes bacterial growth, whereas factors in honey called inhibines, which include hydrogen peroxide, flavonoids, and phenolic acids, appear to elicit antibacterial effects directly.[106] A systematic review of the data on honey concluded that, with some reservation due to study quality and small numbers, wound healing and infection rates were consistently better in those subjects treated with topical honey compared with several other active agents.[107]

BURNS

The moist, necrotic tissue in a burn patient is an ideal environment for bacterial growth. The large areas of ischemic tissue around the wounds may limit the availability and, thus, the usefulness of systemic antibiotics. Before 1965, the rate of burn wound sepsis was reported to be as high as 60%; this quickly fell to 28% after the widespread use of topical silver nitrate.[108] A 2008 review of wound management in the New England Journal of Medicine concluded that the optimal therapy for highly contaminated or infected burns with significant exudate is the application of topical antimicrobial agents and absorbent gauze dressings.[109]

Numerous topical agents and regimens have been proposed and tested, but SSD has long been recognized as the mainstay of topical burn therapy. With broad antimicrobial properties and a relatively small side-effect profile, it continues to be the standard by which other treatments are measured, especially for second- and third-degree burns.[109] Because SSD can cause cytotoxicity and thereby delay healing, newer synthetic dressings that release the silver slowly and reduce cytotoxicity are being developed.

A recent study demonstrates that the addition of 0.2% chlorhexidine digluconate to SSD results in superior antimicrobial effects against all bacteria studied in an in vitro model.[108] SSD has several documented side effects, however rare, including neutropenia, erythema multiforme, crystalluria, and methemoglobinemia.[110] These, in part, continue to drive the search for other agents.

Several studies have demonstrated the efficacy of mupirocin ointment for burn wounds, particularly those that are infected with MRSA. One such study of 45 children with burn wounds who developed MRSA infections despite treatment with SSD with chlorhexidine or povidone-iodine showed complete eradication of MRSA within 4 days of initiating mupirocin therapy.[111]

A large study compared 1053 burn subjects treated with povidone-iodine plus neomycin-framycetin-bacitracin ointment (PVP+N) with 1089 subjects treated with SSD and found that healing times and infection rates were statistically favorable for the PVP+N group.[112]

Honey has been studied as an alternative to SSD in burns. A 1998 study of 50 subjects, 25 of them treated with honey and 25 with SSD-impregnated gauze, showed that 100% of the honey-treated subjects showed evidence of wound healing by day 21 versus only 84% by day 21 in the SSD-treated group, although this was not statistically significant.[113] The study also found similar infection eradication rates in both groups. A systematic review of six studies with honey in burn wound treatment found that wound healing infection rates were consistently better in those subjects treated with topical honey compared with other active agents.[107] Recently, there has been some promising new data on honey. Using a standardized medical-grade honey, it was demonstrated that the bacteria on the arms of 42 healthy adults was reduced by 100-fold versus the placebo group, including multiple antibiotic-resistant strains.[114] The investigators suggest that with a more standardized honey preparation, future studies may show more consistent results and open the door for new possibilities for honey as a topical therapy.

The adverse effects associated with SSD are thought to be associated with the sulfa moiety; several attempts have been made to use silver alone. Silver is thought to exhibit its antibacterial properties by interacting with thiol groups in bacterial proteins, which leads to inactivation and by direct DNA condensation and loss of replication abilities.[115] Earlier studies demonstrated that coating nylon fibers with silver resulted in sustained broad bactericidal effects similar to those of SSD without the potential adverse effects of the sulfa moiety.[116] A modern version of this principle, in the form of a dressing of nanocrystalline silver (Acticoat, Smith & Nephew, London, England) was found nearly equivalent to SSD in terms of antimicrobial effects in an in vitro model.[108]

Despite great advances, burn management continues to be a highly challenging area. The authors follow the developments of some of these newer agents with great interest.

IMPETIGO

Impetigo is a superficial skin infection that can be divided into primary—arising in previously intact skin; and secondary—arising in skin that has had barrier damage, such as dermatitis. Whether primary or secondary, the skin manifestation is classically a superficial erosion and honey-colored crust. *S aureus* and *S pyogenes* are most often the causative agents. A Cochrane systematic review of impetigo[47] and a recent large systematic review[117] highlighted the following points:

- The peak incidence occurs between the ages of 2 and 6 years.
- Topical antibiotics are more effective than placebo.
- There is evidence that topical antibiotics are more effective than some systemic antibiotics for the treatment of impetigo.
- Topical antibiotics are the preferable first-line treatment.

One study compared oral erythromycin to topical mupirocin in 75 subjects who had impetigo. The mupirocin performed similarly on clinical grounds and superiorly on microbiological data.[118] Another more recent study in 159 subjects who had secondarily impetiginized eczema demonstrated that mupirocin cream applied thrice daily was bacteriologically superior to oral cephalexin.[119] Finally, experiments in a hamster impetigo model infected with *S aureus* demonstrated that mupirocin cream was significantly more effective than mupirocin ointment, not significantly different from neomycin-bacitracin cream, but significantly superior to oral erythromycin and cephalexin.[105]

More recently, retapamulin has been approved for use in impetigo caused by MSSA and S pyogenes, as described above.[47]

ULCERS

Preventing bacterial colonization and infection of deeper wounds likely depends on a number of factors, including debridement, active cleansing, and dressing choice. It is therefore difficult to evaluate the role of topical antibacterial agents when divorced from these other factors. A systematic review of topical antimicrobials in chronic wounds in 2001[120] and a more recent Cochrane review of antiseptics and antibiotics used for venous leg ulcers were inconclusive in terms of these agents' ability to promote ulcer healing, although the latter study offered evidence to support the use of cadexomer iodine.[121]

Daily application of gentian violet 0.1% solution and ointment (an antiseptic) was demonstrated to eradicate 18 cases of MRSA-infected ulcers that had failed previous treatment with povidone-iodine and systemic antibiotics.[122] The mechanism of gentian violet is not fully understood, but early studies demonstrated nonspecific protein and cell wall synthesis inhibition, as well as accumulation of cytidine diphosphoribitol and peptidoglycan precursors.[123]

Honey has also been used successfully for clearance of MRSA infection and improved healing in ulcers.[107,124]

Disinfectants are often empirically applied but may be too harsh for routine use in wounds. In vitro studies have demonstrated that antiseptics such as povidone-iodine and chlorhexidine show cytotoxic properties and may therefore delay healing of ulcers.[125]

INTRAVASCULAR CATHETERS

There is a 10%–20% mortality attributed to catheter-related bloodstream infection.[126] Appropriate antiseptic care of intravascular catheters should ideally decrease the incidence of infection and, thus, the risk of sepsis. Impregnation of central venous catheter cuffs with antibacterials is beyond the scope of this article.

A large meta-analysis involving a total of 4143 catheters concluded that chlorhexidine gluconate reduced the risk for catheter-related bloodstream infection by 49% compared with povidone-iodine.[126] The investigators hypothesized that chlorhexidine was more effective due to the fact that blood and serum can lessen the microbicidal effect of povidone-iodine but not chlorhexidine, and that chlorhexidine has both a more potent and a longer residual antimicrobial effect compared with povidone-iodine. A follow-up analysis by the same group calculated that the slightly higher cost of chlorhexidine compared with the decreased morbidity and mortality from its use in this clinical context resulted in a $113 savings per catheter used.[127]

Other topical antibiotics have been used for intravascular catheter care. A study of 709 consecutive subjects with venous catheters treated with neomycin-bacitracin-polymyxin spray or control demonstrated decreased colonization by more virulent potential pathogens such as E coli, Klebsiella, and Staphylococcus when the antibiotic spray was used.[128]

Despite decreasing colonization successfully, a prospective study of 827 catheters treated with neomycin-bacitracin-polymyxin ointment at the insertion of a catheter and every 48 hours thereafter failed to show a difference from placebo in the rate of local infection or catheter-associated sepsis.[129]

SUMMARY

Topical antibacterial agents have an important role in antimicrobial therapy. Antiseptics and antibiotic preparations offer important alternatives and supplements to systemic agents in a variety of clinical scenarios. These agents are highly versatile. Uses include prophylaxis of infection for traumatic and surgical wounds, S aureus decolonization, treatment of burns, and treatment of primary and secondary pyodermas. Although topical antibacterials are widely used in clinical practice, ongoing trials continue to elucidate their relative efficacies.

REFERENCES

1. Jones ME, Karlowsky JA, Draghi DC, et al. Epidemiology and antibiotic susceptibility of bacteria causing skin and soft tissue infections in the USA and Europe: a guide to appropriate antimicrobial therapy. Int J Antimicrob Agents 2003; 22(4):406–19.
2. Larson EL, Butz AM, Gullette DL, et al. Alcohol for surgical scrubbing? Infect Control Hosp Epidemiol 1990;11(3):139–43.
3. Fuursted K, Hjort A, Knudsen L. Evaluation of bactericidal activity and lag of regrowth (postantibiotic effect) of five antiseptics on nine bacterial pathogens. J Antimicrob Chemother 1997;40(2):221–6.
4. Tatnall FM, Leigh IM, Gibson JR. Comparative study of antiseptic toxicity on basal keratinocytes, transformed human keratinocytes and fibroblasts. Skin Pharmacol 1990;3(3):157–63.
5. Pericone CD, Park S, Imlay JA, et al. Factors contributing to hydrogen peroxide resistance in Streptococcus pneumoniae include pyruvate oxidase (spxb) and avoidance of the toxic effects of the Fenton reaction. J Bacteriol 2003; 185(23):6815–25.
6. Repine JE, Fox RB, Berger EM. Hydrogen peroxide kills Staphylococcus aureus by reacting with staphylococcal iron to form hydroxyl radical. J Biol Chem 1981; 256(14):7094–6.
7. Best M, Springthorpe VS, Sattar SA. Feasibility of a combined carrier test for disinfectants: studies with a mixture of five types of microorganisms. Am J Infect Control 1994;22(3):152–62.
8. Lau WY, Wong SH. Randomized, prospective trial of topical hydrogen peroxide in appendectomy wound infection. High risk factors. Am J Surg 1981;142(3): 393–7.
9. O'Toole EA, Goel M, Woodley DT. Hydrogen peroxide inhibits human keratinocyte migration. Dermatol Surg 1996;22(6):525–9.
10. Milstone AM, Passaretti CL, Perl TM. Chlorhexidine: expanding the armamentarium for infection control and prevention. Clin Infect Dis 2008;46(2):274–81.
11. Nicoletti G, Boghossian V, Gurevitch F, et al. The antimicrobial activity in vitro of chlorhexidine, a mixture of isothiazolinones ('kathon' cg) and cetyl trimethyl ammonium bromide (ctab). J Hosp Infect 1993;23(2):87–111.
12. Hibbard JS, Mulberry GK, Brady AR. A clinical study comparing the skin antisepsis and safety of chloraprep, 70% isopropyl alcohol, and 2% aqueous chlorhexidine. J Infus Nurs 2002;25(4):244–9.
13. Tattawasart U, Hann AC, Maillard JY, et al. Cytological changes in chlorhexidine-resistant isolates of Pseudomonas stutzeri. J Antimicrob Chemother 2000;45(2): 145–52.
14. Kaul AF, Jewett JF. Agents and techniques for disinfection of the skin. Surg Gynecol Obstet 1981;152(5):677–85.

15. Mermel L. Choice of disinfectants in obtaining blood cultures. Pediatr Infect Dis J 1994;13(5):425–6.
16. Whitman TJ, Herlihy RK, Schlett CD, et al. Chlorhexidine-impregnated cloths to prevent skin and soft-tissue infection in marine recruits: a cluster-randomized, double-blind, controlled effectiveness trial. Infect Control Hosp Epidemiol 2010;12:1207–15.
17. Sandri AM, Dalarosa MG, Ruschel de Alcantara L, et al. Reduction in incidence of nosocomial methicillin-resistant staphylococcus aureus (MRSA) infection in an intensive care unit: role of treatment with mupirocin ointment and chlorhexidine baths for nasal carriers of MRSA. Infect Control Hosp Epidemiol 2006; 27(2):185–7.
18. Wendt C, Schinke S, Wurttemberger M, et al. Value of whole-body washing with chlorhexidine for the eradication of methicillin-resistant *Staphylococcus aureus*: a randomized, placebo-controlled, double-blind clinical trial. Infect Control Hosp Epidemiol 2007;28(9):1036–43.
19. Vernon MO, Hayden MK, Trick WE, et al. Chlorhexidine gluconate to cleanse patients in a medical intensive care unit: the effectiveness of source control to reduce the bioburden of vancomycin-resistant enterococci. Arch Intern Med 2006;166(3):306–12.
20. Levy I, Katz J, Solter E, et al. Chlorhexidine-impregnated dressing for prevention of colonization of central venous catheters in infants and children: a randomized controlled study. Pediatr Infect Dis J 2005;24(8):676–9.
21. Rupp ME, Lisco SJ, Lipsett PA, et al. Effect of a second-generation venous catheter impregnated with chlorhexidine and silver sulfadiazine on central catheter-related infections: a randomized, controlled trial. Ann Intern Med 2005;143(8): 570–80.
22. Chlebicki MP, Safdar N. Topical chlorhexidine for prevention of ventilator-associated pneumonia: a meta-analysis. Crit Care Med 2007;35(2):595–602.
23. Heath RJ, Rubin JR, Holland DR, et al. Mechanism of triclosan inhibition of bacterial fatty acid synthesis. J Biol Chem 1999;274(16):11110–4.
24. Noronha C, Almeida A. Local burn treatments—topical antimicrobial agents. Ann Burn Fire Disasters 2000;8(4):216–9.
25. Ward RS, Saffle JR. Topical agents in burn and wound care. Phys Ther 1995; 75(6):526–38.
26. Gocke DJ, Ponticas S, Pollack W. In vitro studies of the killing of clinical isolates by povidone-iodine solutions. J Hosp Infect 1985;6(Suppl A):59–66.
27. Fleischer W, Reimer K. Povidone-iodine in antisepsis–state of the art. Dermatology 1997;195(Suppl 2):3–9.
28. Niedner R. Cytotoxicity and sensitization of povidone-iodine and other frequently used anti-infective agents. Dermatology 1997;195(Suppl 2):89–92.
29. Kramer SA. Effect of povidone-iodine on wound healing: a review. J Vasc Nurs 1999;17(1):17–23.
30. Hsu S, Quan L. Topical antibacterial agents. In: Wolverton SE, editor. Comprehenisve dermatologic drug therapy. Phildelphia: WB Saunders; 2001. p. 472–96.
31. Harkaway KS, McGinley KJ, Foglia AN, et al. Antibiotic resistance patterns in coagulase-negative staphylococci after treatment with topical erythromycin, benzoyl peroxide, and combination therapy. Br J Dermatol 1992;126(6): 586–90.
32. Gelmetti C. Local antibiotics in dermatology. Dermatol Ther 2008;21(3):187–95.
33. Barillo DJ. Topical antimicrobials in burn wound care: a recent history. Wounds 2008;20:192–8.

34. Huang JT, Abrams M, Tlougan B, et al. Treatment of *Staphylococcus aureus* colonization in atopic dermatitis decreases disease severity. Pediatrics 2009; 123(5):e808–14.
35. Kaplan SL. Commentary: prevention of recurrent staphylococcal infections. Pediatr Infect Dis J 2008;27(10):935–7.
36. Fisher RG, Chain RL, Hair PS, et al. Hypochlorite killing of community-associated methicillin-resistant *Staphylococcus aureus*. Pediatr Infect Dis J 2008;27(10):934–5.
37. Onset Dermatologics web site. Available at: http://www.onsetdermatologics. com/products/hylatopicplus-aurstat-kit. Accessed April 10, 2011.
38. Nagai K, Murata T, Ohta S, et al. Two different mechanisms are involved in the extremely high-level benzalkonium chloride resistance of a *Pseudomonas fluorescens* strain. Microbiol Immunol 2003;47(10):709–15.
39. Halling H. Suspected link between exposure to hexachlorophene and malformed infants. Ann N Y Acad Sci 1979;320:426–35.
40. Thuille N, Fille M, Nagl M. Bactericidal activity of herbal extracts. Int J Hyg Environ Health 2003;206(3):217–21.
41. Kalemba D, Kunicka A. Antibacterial and antifungal properties of essential oils. Curr Med Chem 2003;10(10):813–29.
42. Pappa KA. The clinical development of mupirocin. J Am Acad Dermatol 1990; 22(5 Pt 1):873–9.
43. Spann CT, Tutrone WD, Weinberg JM, et al. Topical antibacterial agents for wound care: a primer. Dermatol Surg 2003;29(6):620–6.
44. Antonio M, McFerran N, Pallen MJ. Mutations affecting the Rossman fold of isoleucyl-tRNA synthetase are correlated with low-level mupirocin resistance in *Staphylococcus aureus*. Antimicrob Agents Chemother 2002;46(2):438–42.
45. Jones JC, Rogers TJ, Brookmeyer P, et al. Mupirocin resistance in patients colonized with methicillin-resistant *Staphylococcus aureus* in a surgical intensive care unit. Clin Infect Dis 2007;45(5):541–7.
46. Walker ES, Vasquez JE, Dula R, et al. Mupirocin-resistant, methicillin-resistant *Staphylococcus aureus*: does mupirocin remain effective? Infect Control Hosp Epidemiol 2003;24(5):342–6.
47. Koning S, van der Wouden JC, Chosidow O, et al. Efficacy and safety of retapamulin ointment as treatment of impetigo: randomized double-blind multicentre placebo-controlled trial. Br J Dermatol 2008;158(5):1077–82.
48. Woodford N, Afzal-Shah M, Warner M, et al. In vitro activity of retapamulin against *Staphylococcus aureus* isolates resistant to fusidic acid and mupirocin. J Antimicrob Chemother 2008;62(4):766–8.
49. Weinberg JM, Tyring SK. Retapamulin: an antibacterial with a novel mode of action in an age of emerging resistance to *Staphylococcus aureus*. J Drugs Dermatol 2010;9(10):1198–204.
50. Wolf R, Matz H, Orion E, et al. Dapsone. Dermatol Online J 2002;8(1).
51. Draelos ZD, Carter E, Maloney JM, et al. Two randomized studies demonstrate the efficacy and safety of dapsone gel, 5% for the treatment of acne vulgaris. J Am Acad Dermatol 2007;56(3):439, e1–10.
52. Wolf R, Orni-Wasserlauf R. A century of the synthesis of dapsone: its anti-infective capacity now and then. Int J Dermatol 2000;39(10):779–83.
53. Gette MT, Marks JG Jr, Maloney ME. Frequency of postoperative allergic contact dermatitis to topical antibiotics. Arch Dermatol 1992;128(3):365–7.
54. Leyden JJ. The role of topical antibiotics in dermatologic practice. Medscape. Available at: http://www.medscape.com/viewprogram/2501. Accessed November 30, 2008.

55. Winkelman W, Gratton D. Topical antibacterials. Clin Dermatol 1989;7(3):156–62.
56. Kuznar W. Allergen of the year: reactions to common antibiotic bacitracin may be on the rise. Dermatology times 2003, June 1. Available at: http://www.modernmedicine. com/modernmedicine/article/articledetail.Jsp?Ts=1228065479155&id=60907. Accessed November 30, 2008.
57. Jacob SE, James WD. From road rash to top allergen in a flash: bacitracin. Dermatol Surg 2004;30(4 Pt 1):521–4.
58. Hendley JO, Ashe KM. Eradication of resident bacteria of normal human skin by antimicrobial ointment. Antimicrob Agents Chemother 2003;47(6):1988–90.
59. Hammond B, Ali Y, Fendler E, et al. Effect of hand sanitizer use on elementary school absenteeism. Am J Infect Control 2000;28(5):340–6.
60. Boyce JM. Using alcohol for hand antisepsis: dispelling old myths. Infect Control Hosp Epidemiol 2000;21(7):438–41.
61. Liu C, Bayer A, Cosgrove SE, et al. Clinical practice guidelines by the Infectious Diseases Society of America for the treatment of methicillin-resistant *Staphylococcus aureus* infections in adults and children. Clin Infect Dis 2011;52(3): e18–55.
62. Paulson DS, Fendler EJ, Dolan MJ, et al. A close look at alcohol gel as an antimicrobial sanitizing agent. Am J Infect Control 1999;27(4):332–8.
63. Girou E, Loyeau S, Legrand P, et al. Efficacy of handrubbing with alcohol-based solution versus standard handwashing with antiseptic soap: randomised clinical trial. BMJ 2002;325(7360):362.
64. Hilburn J, Hammond BS, Fendler EJ, et al. Use of alcohol hand sanitizer as an infection control strategy in an acute care facility. Am J Infect Control 2003; 31(2):109–16.
65. White C, Kolble R, Carlson R, et al. The effect of hand hygiene on illness rate among students in university residence halls. Am J Infect Control 2003;31(6):364–70.
66. Gruendemann BJ, Bjerke NB. Is it time for brushless scrubbing with an alcohol-based agent? AORN J 2001;74(6):859–73.
67. Laupland KB, Conly JM. Treatment of *Staphylococcus aureus* colonization and prophylaxis for infection with topical intranasal mupirocin: an evidence-based review. Clin Infect Dis 2003;37(7):933–8.
68. von Eiff C, Becker K, Machka K, et al. Nasal carriage as a source of *Staphylococcus aureus* bacteremia. Study group. N Engl J Med 2001;344(1):11–6.
69. Bradley SF. Effectiveness of mupirocin in the control of methicillin-resistant *Staphylococcus aureus*. Infect Med 1993;10:23–31.
70. van Rijen M, Bonten M, Wenzel R, et al. Mupirocin ointment for preventing Staphylococcus aureus infections in nasal carriers. Cochrane Database Syst Rev 2008;4:CD006216.
71. Perl TM, Cullen JJ, Wenzel RP, et al. Intranasal mupirocin to prevent postoperative *Staphylococcus aureus* infections. N Engl J Med 2002;346(24):1871–7.
72. Bode LG, Kluytmans JA, Wertheim HF, et al. Preventing surgical-site infections in nasal carriers of Staphylococcus aureus. N Engl J Med 2010;362:9–17.
73. Mupirocin Study Group. Nasal mupirocin prevents *Staphylococcus aureus* exit-site infection during peritoneal dialysis. Mupirocin Study Group. J Am Soc Nephrol 1996;7(11):2403–8.
74. Wertheim HF, Vos MC, Ott A, et al. Mupirocin prophylaxis against nosocomial *Staphylococcus aureus* infections in nonsurgical patients: a randomized study. Ann Intern Med 2004;140(6):419–25.
75. Chambers HF 3rd, Winston LG. Mupirocin prophylaxis misses by a nose. Ann Intern Med 2004;140(6):484–5.

76. Gorwitz RJ, Kruszon-Moran D, McAllister SK, et al. Changes in the prevalence of nasal colonization with *Staphylococcus aureus* in the United States, 2001–2004. J Infect Dis 2008;197(9):1226–34.

77. Datta R, Huang SS. Risk of infection and death due to methicillin-resistant *Staphylococcus aureus* in long-term carriers. Clin Infect Dis 2008;47(2):176–81.

78. Mayall B, Martin R, Keenan AM, et al. Blanket use of intranasal mupirocin for outbreak control and long-term prophylaxis of endemic methicillin-resistant *Staphylococcus aureus* in an open ward. J Hosp Infect 1996;32(4):257–66.

79. Watanabe H, Masaki H, Asoh N, et al. Low concentrations of mupirocin in the pharynx following intranasal application may contribute to mupirocin resistance in methicillin-resistant *Staphylococcus aureus*. J Clin Microbiol 2001;39(10):3775–7.

80. Patel JB, Gorwitz RJ, Jernigan JA. Mupirocin resistance. Clin Infect Dis 2009;49:935–41.

81. Fung S, O'Grady S, Kennedy C, et al. The utility of polysporin ointment in the eradication of methicillin-resistant *Staphylococcus aureus* colonization: a pilot study. Infect Control Hosp Epidemiol 2000;21(10):653–5.

82. Jeyaratnam D, Gottlieb A, Ajoku U, et al. Validation of the IDI-MRSA system for use on pooled nose, axilla, and groin swabs and single swabs from other screening sites. Diagn Microbiol Infect Dis 2008;61(1):1–5.

83. Yang ES, Tan J, Eells S, et al. Body site colonization in patients with community-associated methicillin-resistant *Staphylococcus aureus* and other types of *S aureus* skin infections. Clin Microbiol Infect 2010;16:425–31.

84. Simor AE, Phillips E, McGeer A, et al. Randomized controlled trial of chlorhexidine gluconate for washing, intranasal mupirocin, and rifampin and doxycycline versus no treatment for the eradication of methicillin-resistant *Staphylococcus aureus* colonization. Clin Infect Dis 2007;44(2):178–85.

85. Fung SK, Louie M, Simor AE. Combined topical and oral antimicrobial therapy for the eradication of methicillin-resistant *Staphylococcus aureus* (MRSA) colonization in hospitalized patients. Can J Infect Dis 2002;13(5):287–92.

86. Kokai-Kun JF, Walsh SM, Chanturiya T, et al. Lysostaphin cream eradicates *Staphylococcus aureus* nasal colonization in a cotton rat model. Antimicrob Agents Chemother 2003;47(5):1589–97.

87. Caelli M, Porteous J, Carson CF, et al. Tea tree oil as an alternative topical decolonization agent for methicillin-resistant *Staphylococcus aureus*. J Hosp Infect 2000;46(3):236–7.

88. McMahon MA, Blair IS, Moore JE, et al. Habituation to sub-lethal concentrations of tea tree oil (*Melaleuca alternifolia*) is associated with reduced susceptibility to antibiotics in human pathogens. J Antimicrob Chemother 2007;59(1):125–7.

89. McMahon MA, Tunney MM, Moore JE, et al. Changes in antibiotic susceptibility in staphylococci habituated to sub-lethal concentrations of tea tree oil (*Melaleuca alternifolia*). Lett Appl Microbiol 2008;47(4):263–8.

90. Langford JH, Artemi P, Benrimoj SI. Topical antimicrobial prophylaxis in minor wounds. Ann Pharmacother 1997;31(5):559–63.

91. Maddox JS, Ware JC, Dillon HC Jr. The natural history of streptococcal skin infection: prevention with topical antibiotics. J Am Acad Dermatol 1985;13(2 Pt 1):207–12.

92. Geronemus RG, Mertz PM, Eaglstein WH. Wound healing. The effects of topical antimicrobial agents. Arch Dermatol 1979;115(11):1311–4.

93. Berger RS, Pappert AS, Van Zile PS, et al. A newly formulated topical triple-antibiotic ointment minimizes scarring. Cutis 2000;65(6):401–4.

94. Proposed recommended practices for surgical skin preparation. Association of operating room nurses. AORN J 1996;63(1):221–7.

95. Gilmore OJ, Martin TD, Fletcher BN. Prevention of wound infection after appendicectomy. Lancet 1973;1(7797):220–2.

96. Garibaldi RA. Prevention of intraoperative wound contamination with chlorhexidine shower and scrub. J Hosp Infect 1988;11(Suppl B):5–9.

97. de Jong TE, Vierhout RJ, van Vroonhoven TJ. Povidone-iodine irrigation of the subcutaneous tissue to prevent surgical wound infections. Surg Gynecol Obstet 1982;155(2):221–4.

98. Rogers DM, Blouin GS, O'Leary JP. Povidone-iodine wound irrigation and wound sepsis. Surg Gynecol Obstet 1983;157(5):426–30.

99. Tatnall FM, Leigh IM, Gibson JR. Assay of antiseptic agents in cell culture: conditions affecting cytotoxicity. J Hosp Infect 1991;17(4):287–96.

100. Brown CD, Zitelli JA. A review of topical agents for wounds and methods of wounding. Guidelines for wound management. J Dermatol Surg Oncol 1993;19(8):732–7.

101. Leyden JJ, Kligman AM. Rationale for topical antibiotics. Cutis 1978;22(4):515–20, 22–8.

102. Watcher MA, Wheeland RG. The role of topical agents in the healing of full-thickness wounds. J Dermatol Surg Oncol 1989;15(11):1188–95.

103. Forbes GB. Staphylococcal infection of operation wounds with special reference to topical antibiotic prophylaxis. Lancet 1961;2:505.

104. Fielding G, Rao A, Davis NC, et al. Prophylactic topical use of antibiotics in surgical wounds: a controlled clinical trial using "Polybactrin". Med J Aust 1965;2(4):159–61.

105. Gisby J, Bryant J. Efficacy of a new cream formulation of mupirocin: comparison with oral and topical agents in experimental skin infections. Antimicrob Agents Chemother 2000;44(2):255–60.

106. Wahdan HA. Causes of the antimicrobial activity of honey. Infection 1998;26(1):26–31.

107. Moore OA, Smith LA, Campbell F, et al. Systematic review of the use of honey as a wound dressing. BMC Complement Altern Med 2001;1(2).

108. Fraser JF, Bodman J, Sturgess R, et al. An in vitro study of the anti-microbial efficacy of a 1% silver sulphadiazine and 0.2% chlorhexidine digluconate cream, 1% silver sulphadiazine cream and a silver coated dressing. Burns 2004;30(1):35–41.

109. Singer AJ, Dagum AB. Current management of acute cutaneous wounds. N Engl J Med 2008;359(10):1037–46.

110. Chung JY, Herbert ME. Myth: silver sulfadiazine is the best treatment for minor burns. West J Med 2001;175(3):205–6.

111. Rode H, Hanslo D, de Wet PM, et al. Efficacy of mupirocin in methicillin-resistant *Staphylococcus aureus* burn wound infection. Antimicrob Agents Chemother 1989;33(8):1358–61.

112. Sinha R, Agarwal RK, Agarwal M. Povidone iodine plus neosporin in superficial burns—a continuing study. Burns 1997;23(7/8):626–8.

113. Subrahmanyam M. A prospective randomised clinical and histological study of superficial burn wound healing with honey and silver sulfadiazine. Burns 1998;24(2):157–61.

114. Kwakman PH, Van den Akker JP, Guclu A, et al. Medical-grade honey kills antibiotic-resistant bacteria in vitro and eradicates skin colonization. Clin Infect Dis 2008;46(11):1677–82.

115. Feng QL, Wu J, Chen GQ, et al. A mechanistic study of the antibacterial effect of silver ions on *Escherichia coli* and *Staphylococcus aureus*. J Biomed Mater Res 2000;52(4):662–8.
116. MacKeen PC, Person S, Warner SC, et al. Silver-coated nylon fiber as an antibacterial agent. Antimicrob Agents Chemother 1987;31(1):93–9.
117. George A, Rubin G. A systematic review and meta-analysis of treatments for impetigo. Br J Gen Pract 2003;53(491):480–7.
118. Mertz PM, Marshall DA, Eaglstein WH, et al. Topical mupirocin treatment of impetigo is equal to oral erythromycin therapy. Arch Dermatol 1989;125(8): 1069–73.
119. Rist T, Parish LC, Capin LR, et al. A comparison of the efficacy and safety of mupirocin cream and cephalexin in the treatment of secondarily infected eczema. Clin Exp Dermatol 2002;27(1):14–20.
120. O'Meara SM, Cullum NA, Majid M, et al. Systematic review of antimicrobial agents used for chronic wounds. Br J Surg 2001;88(1):4–21.
121. O'Meara S, Al-Kurdi D, Ologun Y, et al. Antibiotics and antiseptics for venous leg ulcers. Cochrane Database Syst Rev 2010;(1):CD003557.
122. Saji M, Taguchi S, Uchiyama K, et al. Efficacy of gentian violet in the eradication of methicillin-resistant *Staphylococcus aureus* from skin lesions. J Hosp Infect 1995;31(3):225–8.
123. Walker JR, Shafiq NA, Allen RG. Bacterial cell division regulation: physiological effects of crystal violet on *Escherichia coli* lon + and lon − strains. J Bacteriol 1971;108(3):1296–303.
124. Natarajan S, Williamson D, Grey J, et al. Healing of an MRSA-colonized, hydroxyurea-induced leg ulcer with honey. J Dermatolog Treat 2001;12(1):33–6.
125. Kanj LF, Phillips TJ. Management of leg ulcers. Fitzpatrick's J Clin Dermatol 1994;52–60.
126. Chaiyakunapruk N, Veenstra DL, Lipsky BA, et al. Vascular catheter site care: the clinical and economic benefits of chlorhexidine gluconate compared with povidone iodine. Clin Infect Dis 2003;37(6):764–71.
127. Chaiyakunapruk N, Veenstra DL, Lipsky BA, et al. Chlorhexidine compared with povidone-iodine solution for vascular catheter-site care: a meta-analysis. Ann Intern Med 2002;136(11):792–801.
128. Zinner SH, Denny-Brown BC, Braun P, et al. Risk of infection with intravenous indwelling catheters: effect of application of antibiotic ointment. J Infect Dis 1969;120(5):616–9.
129. Maki DG, Band JD. A comparative study of polyantibiotic and iodophor ointments in prevention of vascular catheter-related infection. Am J Med 1981; 70(3):739–44.

Antibiotics for Gram-Positive Bacterial Infection: Vancomycin, Teicoplanin, Quinupristin/Dalfopristin, Oxazolidinones, Daptomycin, Telavancin, and Ceftaroline

Michael D. Nailor, PharmD[a,b,c], Jack D. Sobel, MD[c,*]

KEYWORDS
• Gram positive bacteria • Vancomycin • Daptomycin • Linezolid
• Quinupristin • Dalfopristin • MRSA • VRE

VANCOMYCIN

Vancomycin is a glycopeptide antibiotic that was isolated in 1956 from the actinomycete *Streptomyces orientalis*. It consists of a seven-membered peptide chain and two sugar moieties, vancosamine and glucose.[1] The clinical use of vancomycin became widespread in 1958 with the emergence of penicillinase-producing staphylococci, but the drug fell into disuse 2 years later with the advent of methicillin. Early preparations of vancomycin contained fermentation byproducts, resulting in marked toxicity. It is one of most widely used antibiotics in the United States for the treatment of

A version of this article appeared in the 23:4 issue of the *Infectious Disease Clinics of North America*.
[a] University of Connecticut School of Pharmacy, 69 North Eagleville Road Unit 3092, Storrs, CT 06269, USA
[b] Department of Pharmacy, Hartford Hospital, 80 Seymour Street, Hartford, CT 06102, USA
[c] Division of Infectious Diseases, Department of Internal Medicine, Wayne State University, 320 East Canfield, Detroit, MI 48201, USA
* Corresponding author. Harper University Hospital, 3990 John R Street, Detroit, MI 40201.
E-mail address: jsobel@intmed.wayne.edu

Med Clin N Am 95 (2011) 723–742
doi:10.1016/j.mcna.2011.03.011
0025-7125/11/$ – see front matter © 2011 Elsevier Inc. All rights reserved.

serious gram-positive infections, particularly those involving methicillin-resistant Staphylococcus aureus (MRSA).[2]

Mechanism of Action

Vancomycin exhibits concentration-independent bactericidal activity by the inhibition of bacterial cell wall synthesis. Specifically, it complexes with the D-alanyl-D-alanine portion of peptide precursor units, inhibiting peptidoglycan polymerase and transpeptidation reactions. This prevents the cross-linking of the cell wall peptidoglycan, which occurs during the second stage of cell wall synthesis. Because β-lactams inhibit cell wall biosynthesis in the third phase, there is no cross-resistance between the drugs and no competition for binding sites. Like penicillin, vancomycin requires actively growing bacteria to exert its effect. Also, vancomycin is capable of injuring protoplasts by altering the permeability of their cytoplasmic membrane and selectively inhibiting RNA synthesis.[3,4] Vancomycin exhibits minimal concentration-dependent killing action, but a moderately long in vitro postantibiotic effect.[5]

Antimicrobial Activity

Virtually all Staphylococcus aureus strains are susceptible to vancomycin. In addition, the vast majority of coagulase-negative staphylococci are susceptible. Vancomycin-resistant enterococci (VRE) bloodstream isolates have increased over the years, and in 2002, 17.7% of all enterococci isolates were resistant to vancomycin. Vancomycin resistance was more frequent among Enterococcus faecium isolates, at 60.9%, whereas in the more frequently isolated E. faecalis, resistance was detected in only 2.5% of cases.[6]

Vancomycin is bactericidal for most gram-positive organisms, with minimum inhibitory concentrations (MICs) in the range of 1 to 4 μg/mL.[2] However, against enterococci, vancomycin is only bacteriostatic.

Vancomycin-aminoglycoside combinations are synergistic for the majority of Staphylococcus aureus strains, whether they are methicillin susceptible or methicillin resistant.[7] In addition, substantial improvements in cure rates for Staphylococcus epidermidis prosthetic valve endocarditis are achieved by adding rifampin, gentamicin, or both to vancomycin.[8] Barring the presence of high-level gentamicin-resistant isolates (MIC >500 μg/mL), the combination of vancomycin-gentamicin is also synergistic for enterococci.

Vancomycin is bactericidal against a variety of other gram-positive aerobic and anaerobic organisms, including Corynebacterium spp, Bacillus spp, pneumococci, viridans streptococci, and clostridia, including Clostridium difficile. Most Listeria monocytogenes, lactobacilli, actinomycetes, and anaerobic streptococci are also susceptible.

Leuconostoc and Pediococcus species, which cause serious infections in immunocompromised patients, are resistant to vancomycin. Vancomycin has no activity against gram-negative organisms.

Pharmacokinetics, Dosing, and Administration

The 24-hour area under the curve (AUC)-MIC ratio is probably the most important pharmacokinetic (PK)-pharmacodynamic (PD) parameter correlating with the efficacy of vancomycin.[9] Vancomycin has a large volume of distribution, with therapeutic levels achievable in ascitic, pericardial, pleural, and synovial fluids. Vancomycin penetrates poorly into the aqueous humor and bile. Penetration into cerebrospinal fluid is poor, except for cases in which the meninges are inflamed, in cases in which cerebrospinal fluid concentrations range from 7% to 21% of concomitant serum levels.[10–12] The bone-to-serum ratio of vancomycin concentration is 10%, which increases to 20% to 30% in infected bone.[13] Relatively poor penetration of vancomycin into respiratory secretions (eg, epithelial lining fluid) is reported (25% of plasma concentrations in pneumonia), in part as a function of high protein binding (50%–60%).[14]

Vancomycin retains activity at a pH between 6.5 and 8, and concentrations achieved in abscess fluid approach those obtained in serum.[15] Vancomycin is eliminated by glomerular filtration, with 80% to 90% of an administered dose appearing in the urine within 24 hours. The serum half-life in adults who have normal renal function is 4 to 8 hours after intravenous injection.[11] Several nomograms exist for initiating vancomycin dosing and adjusting dosage in renal insufficiency.[16,17] However, because nomograms assume a fixed volume of distribution per kilogram of weight and wide variations can occur, serum levels should be monitored. Desired peak and trough levels have traditionally ranged from 30 to 40 µg/mL and 5 to 10 µg/mL, respectively; however, numerous recent guidelines advocate higher desired trough levels of from 15 to 20 µg/mL.[18–20] Unfortunately, there are limited human data that document superior efficacy for vancomycin and the possibility exists that increases in trough levels can result in increased toxicity. Vancomycin has an alpha-phase (mostly distribution) half-life of 30 minutes; therefore, if peaks are drawn, the samples should be collected approximately 1 hour postinfusion, using a 1-hour infusion.

Unlike previous recommendations of 1 g every 12 hours as a standard initiation dose, typical adult dosing is now highly variable as a result of variation in desired target trough concentrations. Vancomycin dosages should be calculated using actual body weight[20]; however, caution should be used for individuals weighing more than 120 kg. Elderly patients might only require 1 g every 24 hours, whereas younger patients might require 1.5 g every 8 hours or more to achieve serum trough concentrations of 15 to 20 µg/mL, depending on renal function and weight. Additionally, using loading doses (eg, 25 mg/kg) may also be helpful in quickly achieving desired trough levels that may prevent elevations in MRSA MICs, or tolerance, from occurring during therapy.[21] Although the AUC/MIC ratio is now considered the most predictive pharmacodynamic parameter for vancomycin, (specifically a target AUC/MIC ratio of ≥400), the ratio's clinical utility does not appear practical.[20] Continuous infusion regimens do not appear to offer any therapeutic advantage.[19] Regardless of the dosing interval selected, critically ill patients should have their trough concentrations measured within the first day of therapy, even if the levels are not believed to be at steady state, to ensure that adequate levels are achieved quickly. Determining trough serum vancomycin concentrations is the most practical and accurate method for monitoring vancomycin use.[20] The recommended intravenous dosing schedules for pediatric patients vary according to age and site of infection.[22] In newborns, vancomycin is given at a dosage of 15 mg/kg every 12 hours for the first week of life, or every 8 hours in newborns 8 to 30 days of age; 10–15 mg/kg every 6 hours is recommended for older infants and children. For central nervous system infections, 15 mg/kg every 6 hours is recommended. The volume of distribution is increased and the elimination phase is prolonged in adults compared with children.

Vancomycin cannot be administered intramuscularly because it causes severe pain at the injection site. Orally administered vancomycin is poorly absorbed from the gastrointestinal tract. However, patients who have renal impairment and inflamed bowel can have significant absorption.[23] The oral drug in a dosage of 125 to 500 mg every 6 hours is used to treat *C difficile* enterocolitis, with stool concentrations of vancomycin ranging from 100 to 800 µg/g for the 125-mg dose.[24] Vancomycin is rapidly absorbed into the general circulation after intraperitoneal administration and can be used to treat gram-positive bacterial infections related to continuous ambulatory peritoneal dialysis (CAPD). Therapeutic serum levels of vancomycin are attainable using this method.[25]

Hemodialytic removal of vancomycin depends on a variety of factors, including the filter being used, the flow rates, and the time on the dialysis circuit.[26] With the advent of high-flux filters, previous recommendations regarding vancomycin dosages of just 500 mg every week[5] may be outdated. Some patients now require 1 g of vancomycin after each dialysis session. Dosing recommendations at institutions should be individualized, and therapeutic drug monitoring should be used. Care should be taken so that levels are not obtained too soon after dialysis to avoid misinterpreting falsely low vancomycin levels. In such settings, falsely low vancomycin levels result from drug redistribution from tissues back into the serum after rapid removal of the drug in the serum during dialysis.[26]

Clinical Indications

Vancomycin remains a first line agent for methicillin-resistant strains of coagulase-negative and coagulase-positive staphylococcal infections, including bacteremia, endocarditis, pneumonia, cellulitis, and osteomyelitis.[27] For patients who are allergic to semisynthetic penicillins or cephalosporins, vancomycin is an alternative for methicillin-susceptible staphylococcal infections. However, in cases of serious infections caused by methicillin-susceptible organisms such as endocarditis, vancomycin is not as effective than semisynthetic antistaphylococcal penicillins or first generation cephalosporins and should not be used for convenience alone.[28,29] Some methicillin-susceptible strains that are deficient in autolysins may be tolerant to vancomycin, in which case the addition of gentamicin, rifampin, or both should be considered.

Vancomycin should be combined with gentamicin, rifampin, or both agents when treating prosthetic-device-related *Staphylococcus epidermidis* infections because cure rates are improved by using such combinations.[8] Foreign bodies may need to be removed if the patient has not responded to antibiotics or if infection relapses. *Staphylococcus epidermidis* infections of long-term intravenous catheters can usually be cured without removal of the device. Administration of the antibiotic should be rotated to alternating lumens in the case of multilumen catheters. Central nervous system shunt infections can often be treated using a combination of intravenous and intraventricular vancomycin, but in some cases, removal of the foreign body is necessary.[30] Vancomycin can be given intrathecally or intraventricularly at dosages of 3 to 5 mg per day in children if necessary.[31] In adults higher daily doses of 10 to 20 mg are needed.

Vancomycin is also the drug of choice for infections caused by penicillin-resistant streptococci, *Corynebacterium* group jeikeium, *Bacillus* spp, and penicillin-resistant enterococci. Accordingly, given the recent increased frequency of penicillin-resistant pneumococcal disease, vancomycin is now recommended as initial therapy for cases of proved, suspected, or possible pneumococcal meningitis, in combination with a third-generation cephalosporin, until susceptibility data are available. In cases of serious enterococcal infections, vancomycin should be combined with an aminoglycoside (gentamicin or streptomycin) unless high-level aminoglycoside resistance (MIC >500 or 2000 μg/mL, respectively) is present.

In the treatment of *C difficile* enterocolitis, the use of oral vancomycin should be reserved for patients who do not respond to therapy using metronidazole, for patients who have severe, life-threatening infections, for patients who cannot tolerate metronidazole, and for those who have relapsing disease and who require long courses or multiple repeated courses of therapy. Although vancomycin has the advantages of poor systemic absorption and fewer side effects, concern about the emergence of

VRE isolates should limit its use to treat this condition. If oral vancomycin is used, it should not be combined with cholestyramine because that agent binds vancomycin.

Resistance

VRE are becoming an alarming problem. In all National Nosocomial Infections Surveillance System–participating hospitals, resistance frequency has increased, regardless of the hospital's size or teaching affiliation.[32,33] The VanA phenotype (vancomycin MIC >256, teicoplanin resistant) is encoded by a gene located on a plasmid that is easily transferable to other enterococci using conjugation. The VanB phenotype is also transferable, and it codes for vancomycin resistance; however, these isolates retain susceptibility to teicoplanin. The transfer to and expression of enterococcal vancomycin-resistant genes in Staphylococcus aureus has been accomplished in the laboratory,[34] heightening concern that widespread vancomycin resistance in staphylococci will eventually emerge. The use of vancomycin and cephalosporin is a well-recognized risk factor for infection by VRE.[35] Thus, any program to control resistance must consider reducing unnecessary use of these antibiotics.

Reports to the US Centers for Disease Control and Prevention of glycopeptide-resistant enterococci (GRE) indicate an increase of more than 25 fold in the prevalence of GRE between 1989 and 1993.[27] The proportion of health care–associated GRE infections in intensive care units rose to 14%; although E faecalis is isolated at about four times the frequency of E faecium, the latter is responsible for most episodes of GRE.[27] Huycke and colleagues reported that although vancomycin resistance varied between 1.3% and 2.3% between the years 1995 and 1997 in cases of E faecalis infection, resistance increased from 28% to 52% in E faecium during the same period. Although carriage of these organisms by health care professionals has been described, most infections arise from the patient's own flora. As could be expected, vancomycin use is believed to contribute to the increase in GRE[36]; however, the use of other antibiotics, such as third-generation cephalosporins, also has contributed to GRE selection.[37] Additional factors associated with the emergence of GRE are shown in **Box 1**.

Selection pressure by overuse of vancomycin can be enormous. Ena and colleagues[39] described a 20-fold increase in the use of vancomycin between 1981 and 1991 in a 900-bed university teaching hospital. In only one-third of cases was

---

Box 1
Factors associated with emergence of glycopeptide-resistant enterococci[38]

1. Current or recent vancomycin use
2. Gastrointestinal tract colonization by GRE
3. Duration of hospital stay
4. Proximity to patients who are infected by GRE
5. Intrahospital transfer of patients between wards or floors
6. Prior use of certain broad spectrum antimicrobials (antianaerobes).
7. Location in an intensive care unit
8. Hemodialysis, ventilator, catheter, and other invasive device use.
9. Large hospital size
10. Intra-abdominal surgery.

vancomycin used for specific culture-directed therapy. The remainder of the cases were divided between prophylactic use and empiric therapy. In addition, the authors found a failure to make adjustments in therapy in the majority of cases in which vancomycin use for prophylactic or empiric reasons was initiated. Strong efforts should be made to control vancomycin use in all medical centers, as recommended by the US Centers for Disease Control and Prevention report from the Hospital Infection Control Practices Advisory Committee.[38]

Methicillin-resistant *Staphylococcus epidermidis* infections that are clinically unresponsive to vancomycin therapy have been described. One such infection occurred in a patient who was treated using vancomycin for more than two months for CAPD-associated peritonitis.[40] Heterogeneous resistance was found, with an MIC range to vancomycin of 2 to 16 μg/mL. Population analysis showed some colonies that had vancomycin MICs of 25 to 50 μg/mL.

An analysis of a large surveillance database of 35,458 *Staphylococcus aureus* strains by Jones[41] found that the MIC required to inhibit the growth of 90% of organisms (MIC_{90}) for vancomycin is 1 μg/mL. Some researchers are reporting that a greater percentage of their MRSA isolates have elevated MICs to vancomycin but are still within the susceptible range, a phenomenon known as MIC creep.[41,42] The most alarming aspect of these findings is that infections caused by MRSA that have vancomycin MICs of 2 μg/mL have worse surrogate outcomes.[43,44] Recently, a study showed that after adjusting for a number of variables, mortality was also worse in the elevated MIC group.[45] These reports have formed the basis for consensus recommendations that trough serum concentrations should always be maintained at greater than 10 μg/mL to avoid the development of resistance and possibly improve clinical outcome.[21] Accordingly, total trough serum vancomycin concentrations of 15 to 20 μg/mL are recommended.[20] Unfortunately, there is also a lack of data on antibiotic therapy that is superior to vancomycin for these infections. Although some experts recommend changing therapy on the basis of a vancomycin MIC of >1 μg/ml, recent guidelines continue to recommend vancomycin for organisms with an MIC to vancomycin of 2 μg/ml provided that the patient is making an appropriate response to therapy.[27] One center reported the emergence of daptomycin-nonsusceptible isolates when patients were switched to daptomycin as a result of elevated vancomycin MICs.[46] Patients in that report had a mean duration of vancomycin therapy of 4 days prior to switching to daptomycin, which may have contributed to the development of daptomycin-nonsusceptible isolates.

Glycopeptide-intermediate-resistant *Staphylococcus aureus* (GISA) was first described in Japan in May 1996, in a child who had an MRSA wound infection that was clinically unresponsive to vancomycin.[47–49] According to the National Committee for Clinical Laboratory Standards, vancomycin-susceptible strains of *Staphylococcus aureus* have MICs of 2 μg/mL or less, GISA strains of 4 to 8 μg/mL, and resistant strains of 16 μg/mL or greater.[50] Vancomycin should not be used when the MIC is 4 μg/ml or greater.[27]

Strains of apparently vancomycin-susceptible MRSA have also been detected that display subpopulations that have reduced sensitivity to vancomycin; they have been termed heterogeneous heteroresistant, vancomycin-intermediate *Staphylococcus aureus* (hVISA). Similar to cases of infection by MRSA that have MICs of 2 μg/mL to vancomycin, poor outcomes have been reported.[51] In some centers, rates of hVISA have been steadily rising since 1986, to as high as 8.3% between 2003 and 2007. However, there seems to be a lack of correlation between the trends for hVISA and vancomycin-intermediate *Staphylococcus aureus* (VISA) because the same researchers noted that the lowest rates of VISA, at 0.3%, were detected during the period from 2003 to 2007, which was down from 2.3% in the period preceding it.[52] Because this analysis was done retrospectively and vancomycin had been used as a mainstay of therapy in the hospitals reporting these results, it is unclear whether continued vancomycin use to treat infections caused by hVISA will promote the formation of VISA.

In 2002, the first naturally occurring vancomycin-resistant *Staphylococcus aureus* (VRSA) infection was described in a patient who had a nonhealing foot wound and who was receiving long-term hemodialysis in Michigan at an outpatient dialysis center.[53] Approximately 1 month later, an independent second case of VRSA was reported in an outpatient in Pennsylvania who also had nonhealing foot wounds.[54] Upon further analysis, it was determined that the VRSA from the Michigan patient carried the VanA gene coding for high-level vancomycin resistance and was most likely acquired from coexisting *E faecalis* present in the foot wound.[53] The first patient was cured of VRSA using a combination of antibiotic therapy (trimethoprim and sulfamethoxazole) and aggressive foot care.[53] The second patient was transiently colonized and did not require antimicrobial treatment. Common to both patients were repeated infections by *Staphylococcus aureus* and enterococci. An extensive contact tracing failed to show any spread beyond the index cases. However, if spread had occurred, the public health consequences of these difficult-to-treat, gram-positive infections would have been enormous.

Toxicity and Adverse Reactions

The "red man" syndrome is a nonimmunologically mediated histamine release associated with rapid infusion of vancomycin. Clinical signs and symptoms include pruritis, erythema and flushing of the upper torso, angioedema, and occasionally, hypotension. Slow administration (for at least 1 hour) and the administration of prophylactic antihistamines given two hours prior to infusion can protect against the development of this side effect.[55] A rapid bolus of vancomycin can also result in muscle spasms of the chest and back, which is known as the "pain and spasm" syndrome. Ototoxicity, which may continue to progress after discontinuation of therapy, may occur when serum levels of vancomycin are excessively high but rarely occurs when peak serum levels are 40 to 50 μg/mL or less. Deafness may be proceeded by tinnitus and high-tone hearing loss. Nephrotoxicity is similarly rare when vancomycin is used alone and at conventional dosages (eg, 1 g every 12 hours). Ototoxicity and nephrotoxicity may be potentiated when vancomycin and aminoglycosides are used in combination.[56] A recent retrospective report called into question the use of higher doses of vancomycin in light of the higher rates of nephrotoxicity seen in patients who received 4 g or more of vancomycin.[57] Care should be used when extrapolating these data because there may have been an unseen selection bias of giving patients higher doses of vancomycin when they were perceived by a clinician as having a more severe disease state, and the patients' underlying condition may have also contributed to the perceived toxicity.

Vancomycin-induced neutropenia is dose- and time-dependent, rare, and reversible after the drug is discontinued. It typically occurs when the duration of therapy exceeds 14 days.[58] Skin rash and drug fever occur in 4% to 5% of patients.[59]

TEICOPLANIN

Teicoplanin is a glycopeptide antibiotic with activity similar to that of vancomycin.[60] It is not commercially available in the United States.

QUINUPRISTIN/DALFOPRISTIN (SYNERCID)

Quinupristin-dalfopristin is a combination of two naturally occurring compounds isolated from *Streptomyces pristinaspiralis*.[61] This streptogramin class is water soluble[62] and contains quinupristin and dalfopristin in a 30:70 weight/weight ratio.[63]

Mechanism of Action

Quinupristin-dalfopristin exerts its activity through the inhibition of protein synthesis. Quinupristin and dalfopristin sequentially bind to different sites on the 50S ribosome, resulting in a stable, ternary drug-ribosome complex and interfering with different targets of 23S RNA. Newly synthesized peptide chains cannot be extruded from this complex.[61,64]

Pharmacokinetics, Dosing, and Administration

Quinupristin and dalfopristin are metabolized quickly after intravenous administration. Neither component is extensively protein bound. The recommended dosage is 7.5 mg/kg every 8 hours by the intravenous route for infections by VRE. The interval may be lengthened to every 12 hours for complicated skin and skin structure infections. There are no adjustments necessary for renal or hepatic impairment.[61] The combination has a postantibiotic effect for 6 to 8 hours. High intracellular concentrations are seen.[65] Excretion is primarily by way of the biliary tract. The drug combination is a potent inhibitor of the cytochrome P450 enzymes, with the potential for drug interactions.

Clinical Activity

The spectrum of activity of quinupristin-dalfopristin is similar to that of vancomycin. In a study of nearly 30,000 clinical isolates in the United States, susceptibility was seen for 97.7% of *Streptococcus pneumoniae* (including penicillin-resistant isolates), 97% of other streptococcal spp, 99% to 99.9% of *Staphylococcus aureus*, and 98% to 100% of coagulase-negative staphylococci. *E faecium* susceptibility varied by participating study region.[63] Overall, 0.2% of *E faecium* isolates were resistant to quinupristin/dalfopristin, with MICs greater than 4 μg/mL. The drug has no activity against *E faecalis*. It is bacteriostatic for *E faecium* and *Legionella* spp.[65] Gram-negative anaerobes such as *Fusobacterium* spp and *Bacteroides* spp are also susceptible.[61] VRSA isolates retained susceptibility to quinupristin-dalfopristin. In a study of 274 South African enterococcal isolates, 19.7% of *E faecium* strains were resistant. *Staphylococcus aureus* MICs were similar to those for vancomycin.[66] The main use for quinupristin-dalfopristin is in the treatment of vancomycin-resistant *E faecium*, and potentially for the treatment of GISA and VRSA. One case of successful therapy for VRE *faecium* prosthetic valve endocarditis has been described.[67] Superinfection by *E faecalis* during therapy has also been described.[68]

Resistance

Resistance may develop as the result of decreased ribosomal binding of either component, through enzymatic modification, or through efflux mechanisms and altered target.[61,69] A patient who developed quinupristin-dalfopristin–resistant *E faecium* bacteremia while receiving therapy using quinupristin-dalfopristin has been described.[70] In addition to clinical failures, resistant isolates have been recovered from human stool samples.[69] No cross-resistance to other currently available antimicrobials occurs. When used in combination with doxycycline, resistance to the streptogramin may be prevented.[71]

Toxicity and Adverse Events

Side effects of quinupristin-dalfopristin include venous irritation and elevation of conjugated bilirubin. The most troublesome side effect seen is the development of arthralgias and myalgias, which can be severe.

OXAZOLIDINONES

The oxazolidinones are a synthetic class of antimicrobial agents that were discovered in 1987. Although there are a number compounds in development, linezolid is the only commercially available product.

Mechanism of Action

Linezolid exerts its effect early in protein synthesis by inhibiting the initiation complex at the 30S ribosome.[72,73] The agent interacts with a translational component that is either directly or indirectly involved in binding mRNA during the start of translation.[73] Because of this unique action, no cross-resistance with other currently available antimicrobials occurs.

Antimicrobial Activity

The antimicrobial spectrum of the oxazolidinones is similar to that of vancomycin, with activity against most gram-positive organisms, including MRSA and penicillin-resistant pneumococci.[74,75] The compounds also have activity against gram-negative anaerobes and mycobacteria.[75] They are bacteriostatic for enterococci and staphylococci, but bactericidal for *Streptococcus pyogenes* and *Bacteroides fragilis*.[76]

Pharmacokinetics, Dosing, and Administration

Maximum peak plasma levels are achieved within 1 to 2 hours after administration. Linezolid has 100% oral bioavailability.[77,78] Linezolid differs from vancomycin by its enhanced penetration into respiratory secretions. Rapid penetration into bone, fat, and muscle is also reported, achieving levels of 4 μg/mL or greater in excess of the MIC of most susceptible organisms.[79] Urinary concentrations of linezolid are high, achieving bactericidal activity against urinary pathogens such as enterococci.[80] There is a short postantibiotic effect of about 1 hour; however, inhibition of virulence-factor expression by gram-positive cocci continues after exposure to subinhibitory concentrations of linezolid.[81] No synergy with aminoglycosides for gram-positive bacteria exists. Isolates of enterococci and streptococci are considered sensitive if their MICs are 2 μg/mL or less, and 4 μg/mL or less for staphylococci. The recommended dosage is 600 mg every 12 hours. The 24-hour AUC-MIC ratio is the pharmacodynamic parameter that bests predicts clinical efficacy.[9]

Clinical Indications

Although initially used to mainly treat patients who were infected by VRE, linezolid's role in treating MRSA infections has grown significantly. Linezolid is currently used for the treatment of pneumonia and skin and skin-structure infections caused by MRSA.[74,82] The high penetration of the drug into respiratory secretions is believed to contribute to linezolid being a very effective agent for the treatment of pneumonia caused by *Staphylococcus aureus* and *Streptococcus pneumoniae*.[83] A recent retrospective analysis of 339 patients who had documented *Staphylococcus aureus* pneumonia, including 160 patients who had MRSA pneumonia, suggested the superior efficacy of linezolid rather than vancomycin.[84] Additional prospective studies are required to confirm these findings. Similarly, several reports of superior activity in bacteremic pneumococcal pneumonia have been described.[85,86]

Given the excellent bioavailability of linezolid and its activity against MRSA and methicillin-resistant, coagulase-negative staphylococci, reports have appeared of efficacy and cost-savings accompanying the early switch and early discharge of patients who were treated using oral linezolid.[87-90] These studies, combined with the prevalence of community-acquired MRSA skin and skin-structure infections, have greatly increased the use of linezolid. It is apparent that parenteral linezolid is now being considered as a first-line therapy for multisite infections caused by MRSA organisms without vancomycin resistance. Although evidence of clinical equivalence has been published, many experts continue to reserve linezolid for vancomycin-resistant organisms, refractory infections, and vancomycin-intolerant patients.

Resistance

In gradient plate experiments, there was no increase in the MICs to linezolid upon serial passage of either MRSA or methicillin-resistant *Staphylococcus epidermidis* strains.[91-94] The previously described VRSA isolates retained susceptibility to linezolid. However, linezolid resistance has been described in enteroccci, even in patients who had no prior exposure to this novel antibiotic.[93,94] Additionally, reports of MRSA resistant to linezolid have emerged.[95-98] Resistance to linezolid has been described by two principle mechanisms. The most common mechanism is an alteration in domain V within the 23S rRNA gene. Up to six copies of this mutation can be present each leading to higher MICs. The second mechanism of resistance is the acquisition of a 23S rRNA methyltransferase endocded by the cfr (chloramphenicol-florfenicol resistance) gene.[99]

Toxicity and Adverse Events

Increases in the levels of hepatic enzymes and creatinine can occasionally occur. Skin rash has been reported. Linezolid has the potential for monoamine oxidase inhibition. In preclinical animal studies, reversible time- and dose-dependent myelosuppression occurred, particularly thrombocytopenia. Gerson and colleagues[100] concluded that hematological abnormalities associated with linezolid use were mild and reversible and not significantly different from those of comparator drugs. Thrombocytopenia occurred in 2.2% of patients, usually after 2 weeks of therapy. Long-term use is, however, associated with an incidence of up to 10%. In a study of 686 seriously ill patients who had nosocomial pneumonia, observed in multiple intensive care units, patients treated using linezolid rarely developed thrombocytopenia, which was no more frequent than with the use of vancomycin.[101]

DAPTOMYCIN

Daptomycin is a naturally occurring cyclic lipopeptide antibiotic that is a fermentation byproduct of *Streptomyces roseosporus*.[102] It consists of a 10-membered amino acid ring with a 10-carbon decanoic acid attached to a terminal L-tryptophan.[102]

Mechanism of Action

Daptomycin is rapidly bactericidal in a novel, concentration-dependent manner. It exhibits its action by binding to the cell membrane in a calcium-dependent manner, causing depolarization of the bacterial membrane potential, resulting in the termination of bacterial DNA, RNA, and protein synthesis and the termination of intracellular potassium release, thus causing cell death.[103]

Antimicrobial Activity

The spectrum of activity includes *Staphylococcus aureus*, streptococci, and enterococcal species, including those with multidrug resistance.[104,105] This includes vancomycin-, quinupristin-dalfopristin–, and linezolid-resistant gram-positive organisms. Daptomycin also demonstrates clinical activity against vancomycin-resistant *Leuconostoc* spp.[106] Neither *Listeria* nor *Clostridium* spp are susceptible. Daptomycin in combination with gentamicin is synergistic in killing staphylococci and enterococci.[103] Data regarding the addition of rifampin have been positive or indifferent.[107]

Pharmacokinetics, Dosing, and Administration

Daptomycin is available in intravenous form. It is administered once daily and exhibits linear pharmacokinetics at doses of up to 12 mg/kg.[103] Daptomycin is highly protein bound (92%) and is excreted in the kidney as intact drug.[103] Dosage adjustment for patients who have a creatinine clearance of less than 30 mL/min is recommended. It has a postantibiotic effect that lasts for about 2.5 to 5 hours.[108] Bactericidal activity is dose-dependent. Streptococci and staphylococci are considered sensitive if the MIC is 1 μg/mL or less, and enterococci are considered sensitive when the MIC is 4 μg/mL or less.

Clinical Indications

Daptomycin is approved by the US Food and Drug Administration for the treatment of complicated skin and soft-tissue infections caused by staphylococci (methicillin-susceptible *Staphylococcus aureus* and MRSA), *Streptococcus* spp, and E *faecalis*, at a dose of 4 mg/kg/day administered intravenously. A trial was completed that led to its approval for use in *Staphylococcus aureus* bloodstream infections, including right-sided endocarditis, using daptomycin at 6 mg/kg/day.[109] In the MRSA arm (99 patients) of this trial, success rates were numerically higher but not statistically significant in favor of daptomycin rather than the comparator vancomycin with 4 days of gentamicin. The toxicity of daptomycin was less than that of the vancomycin-gentamicin combination. Among patients who had treatment failure, six daptomycin-treated patients and one vancomycin-gentamicin–treated patient developed reduced susceptibility to their primary therapy. The length of bacteremia infection was similar between the two groups. Some experts have advocated for higher doses of daptomycin between 8 mg/kg and 10 mg/kg for serious infections, however further evidence is needed before this becomes a standard recommendation.[27] Patients should not be treated using daptomycin for pneumonia because the drug binds to surfactant, inhibiting its activity.

Resistance

VRSA and VRE isolates are susceptible to daptomycin. However, some hVISA and VISA isolates have shown reduced susceptibility to daptomycin without previous exposure to daptomycin but with exposure to vancomycin.[110–112] Resistance in MRSA has rarely been reported. However, only recently have the various automated systems used by many hospitals incorporated daptomycin into standard panels. One health system recently reported reduced susceptibility to daptomycin for MRSA isolates.[113] All of the isolates that showed reduced susceptibility had vancomycin MICs of 2 μg/mL. The correlation of MRSA with reduced susceptibility to vancomycin and reduced cross-susceptibility to daptomycin requires further study.

Toxicity and Adverse Events

Two major causes of toxicity for daptomycin are elevated levels of creatine phosphokinase and myopathy, both of which resolve after discontinuation of the drug. Weekly monitoring of creatine phosphokinase values during daptomycin therapy and discontinuation if creatine phosphokinase elevation is 5 times the upper limit of normal or greater is recommended. These effects are more common when divided doses are used compared with once-daily dosing.[114] Constipation and other gastrointestinal side effects have also been noted to occur.

TELAVANCIN

Telavancin is a lipoglycopeptide antibiotic newly approved for the treatment of gram-positive infections. It has activity against vancomycin susceptible enterococcus, many streptococcus species, and S aureus including MRSA. Telavancin retains potent activity against MRSA isolates with MICs of 2 μg/ml to vancomycin. It has recently gained FDA approval for complicated skin and skin structure infections caused by susceptible organisms. In the clinically evaluable population patients receiving telavancin with diminished renal function had a lower rate of clinical cure compared to patients with creatinine clearance estimates of >50 ml/min. The decrease was not significant in the all-treated populations and was not seen in the vancomycin comparator group. Additionally, the drug has been studied in hospital-acquired pneumonia and found to be non-inferior to vancomycin. Differences were not detected in the subgroups of patients with diminished renal function in the hospital acquired pneumonia trial. Dosing for telavancin is 10 mg/kg IV every 24 hours with adjustments made for patients with estimated creatinine clearance of <50 ml/min. Patients receiving telavancin have been more likely to experience increases in Scr than patients receiving vancomycin, 15% vs 7% respectfully. Additionally, 13% of patients have experienced foamy urine while receiving telavancin. The clinical significance of this reaction is not know. Lastly telavancin is known to falsely elevate coagulation test results such as the international normalized ratio (INR), activated partial thromboplastin test (aPTT), and factor Xa levels. The drug does not cause a coagulopathy. However, in patients in which coagulation testing is necessary it may be best to avoid the drug. Testing 18 or more hours after a dose of telavancin reduces the false positive reaction, but practically may not be feasible particularly for patients receiving intravenous heparin in which patients are often monitored every 6 hours.[115–117]

CEFTAROLINE

Ceftaroline is the most recent addition to the anti-MRSA armamentarium. It is also the first cephalosporin to be marketed in the United States with activity against MRSA. This unique aspect is a result of ceftaroline's ability to bind to penicillin binding protein 2a (PBP2a) encoded for by the mecA resistance gene that confers methicillin resistance. MICs of VISA and VRSA for ceftaroline are similar to MICs for MRSA. Additionally it is active against streptococci including most strains of penicillin resistant pneumococcus. In vitro activity suggest some affinity for E faecalis but not E faecium however there is limited clinical data to support its use against E faecalis. Unlike other advanced generation cephalosporins it does not have activity against Pseudomonas aeruginosa or gram negative organisms that harbor derepressed AMP C β-lactamases. It is supplied as ceftaroline fosamil a prodrug that is metabolized to the active form ceftaroline by serum phosphatase enzymes. Its other chemical properties are similar to other cephalosporins including a relatively short half-life (<3 hours) and time-dependent killing. Four phase 3 trials have been completed including 2 similarly designed trials in patients with community acquired pneumonia and 2 identically designed trials in patients with skin and skin structure infections. In each of the community acquired pneumonia trials and in the integrated (combining both studies together), ceftaroline met the non-inferiority end points. In one of the trials, success rates favored ceftaroline compared to ceftriaxone in the clinically evaluable, microbiologically evaluable, and microbiologically evaluable modified intent-to-treat populations. Ceftaroline is at least as efficacious as ceftriaxone, however costs concerns may limit its use. Unfortunately, there is a lack of data using ceftaroline for pneumonia caused by MRSA. Hence, ceftaroline's role as empiric therapy for community acquired pneumonia in patients with MRSA risk factors without vancomycin will be limited until further data are available. When compared to vancomycin for skin and soft tissue infections ceftaroline was shown to be non-inferior. The safety profile of ceftaroline seems similar to comparator drugs (vancomycin and ceftriaxone) with the exception of a greater proportion of patients receiving ceftaroline had a positive direct Coombs' test but there was not a higher incidence of hemolytic anemia. Ceftaroline dosing for all four of these trials was 600 mg IV every 12 hours. Renal adjustments are necessary for patients with creatinine clearances of less than 50 ml/min.[118–120]

SUMMARY

Gram-positive bacteria have shown a propensity to develop resistance to all of the available antibiotics in use. Additionally, the superiority data for any one agent rather than another is lacking, with the possible exception of linezolid, rather than vancomycin, for the treatment of MRSA pneumonia. Selecting the appropriate therapy is also complicated by differences in local susceptibility patterns, particularly as they relate to diminished susceptibility to vancomycin and daptomycin, site of infection, propensity to induce resistance, toxicity, dosage form availability, and only if the proceeding factors are similar, costs. Despite the increasing prevalence of gram-positive infections, judicious use of these agents and strict infection-control practices to preserve the activity of these agents is warranted.

REFERENCES

1. Pfeiffer RR. Structural features of vancomycin. Rev Infect Dis 1981; (Suppl 3):S205–9.
2. Moellering RC Jr. Vancomycin: a 50-year reassessment. Clin Infect Dis 2006; 42(Suppl 1):S3–4.
3. Jordan DC, Inniss WE. Selective inhibition of ribonucleic acid synthesis in Staphylococcus aureus by vancomycin. Nature 1959;184(Suppl 24):1894–5.
4. Jordan DC, Mallory HDC. Site of action of vancomycin on Staphylococcus aureus. Antimicrob Agents Chemother 1964;4:489–94.
5. Cunha BA, Quintiliani R, Deglin JM, et al. Pharmacokinetics of vancomycin in anuria. Rev Infect Dis 1981; (Suppl 3):S269–72.
6. Biedenbach DJ, Moet GJ, Jones RN. Occurrence and antimicrobial resistance pattern comparisons among bloodstream infection isolates from the SENTRY Antimicrobial Surveillance Program (1997–2002). Diagn Microbiol Infect Dis 2004;50:59–69.
7. Watanakunakorn C, Guerriero JC. Synergism between vancomycin and gentamicin or tobramycin for methicillin-susceptible and methicillin-resistant Staphylococcus aureus strains. Antimicrob Agents Chemother 1982;22:903–5.

8. Karchmer AW, Archer GC, Dismukes WE. *Staphylococcus epidermidis* causing prosthetic valve endocarditis: microbiologic and clinical observation as a guide to therapy. Ann Intern Med 1983;98:447–55.

9. Craig WA. Basic pharmacodynamics of antibacterials with clinical application to the use of ß-lactam, glycopeptides and linezolid. Infect Dis Clin North Am 2003; 17:479–501.

10. Hawley HB, Gump DW. Vancomycin therapy of bacterial meningitis. Am J Dis Child 1973;126:261–4.

11. Matzke GR, Zhanel GG, Guay DRP. Clinical pharmacokinetics of vancomycin. Clin Pharm 1986;11:257–82.

12. Redfield DC, Underman A, Norman D, et al. Cerebrospinal fluid penetration of vancomycin in bacterial meningitis. In: Nelson JD, Grassi C, editors, Current chemotherapy and infectious disease, vol. 1. Washington, DC: American Society for Microbiology; 1980. p. 638–41.

13. Graziani AL, Lawson LA, Gibson GA, et al. Vancomycin concentrations in infected and non-infected human bone. Antimicrob Agents Chemother 1988;32:1320–2.

14. Lamer C, de Beco V, Soler P, et al. Analysis of vancomycin entry into pulmonary lung fluid by bronchoalveolar lavage in critically ill patients. Antimicrob Agents Chemother 1993;37:281–6.

15. Torres JR, Sanders CV, Lewis AC. Vancomycin concentration in human tissues: preliminary report. J Antimicrob Chemother 1979;5:475–7.

16. Lake KD, Peterson CD. Evaluation of a method for initiating vancomycin therapy. Experience in 205 patients. Pharmacotherapy 1988;8:284–6.

17. Moellering RC Jr, Krogstad DJ, Greenblatt DJ. Vancomycin therapy in patients with impaired renal function: a nomogram for dosage. Ann Intern Med 1981; 94:343–6.

18. American Thoracic Society and Infectious Diseases Society of America. Guidelines for the management of adults with hospital-acquired, ventilator-associated, and healthcare-associated pneumonia. Am J Respir Crit Care Med 2005;171: 388–416.

19. Tunkel AR, Hartman BJ, Kaplan SL, et al. Practice guidelines for the management of bacterial meningitis. Clin Infect Dis 2004;39:1267–84.

20. Rybak M, Lomaestro B, Rotschafer JC, et al. Therapeutic monitoring of vancomycin in adult patients: a consensus review of the American Society of Health-System Pharmacists, the Infectious Diseases Society of America, and the Society of Infectious Diseases Pharmacists. Am J Health Syst Pharm 2009;66:82–98.

21. Rybak MJ. The pharmacokinetic and pharmacodynamic properties of vancomycin. Clin Infect Dis 2006;42:S35–9.

22. Schaad VB, McCracken GH, Nelson JD. Clinical pharmacology and efficacy of vancomycin in pediatric patients. J Pediatr 1980;96:119–26.

23. Spitzer PG, Eliopoulos GM. Systemic absorption on enteral vancomycin in a patient with pseudomembranous colitis. Ann Intern Med 1984;100(4):533–4.

24. Tedesco F, Markham R, Gurwith M, et al. Oral vancomycin for pseudomembranous colitis. Lancet 1978;2:226–8.

25. Morse GD, Nairn DK, Walshe JJ. Once weekly intraperitoneal therapy for gram-positive peritonitis. Am J Kidney Dis 1987;4:300–5.

26. Pallotta KE, Manley HJ. Vancomycin use in patients requiring hemodialysis: a literature review. Semin Dial 2008;21:63–70.

27. Liu C, Bayer A, Cosgrove S, et al. Clinical practice guidelines by the Infectious Diseases Society of America for the treatment of methicillin-resistant *Staphylococcus aureus* infections in adults and children. Clin Infect Dis 2011;52:1–38.

28. Small PM, Chambers HF. Vancomycin for *Staphylococcus aureus* endocarditis in intravenous drug abusers. Antimicrob Agents Chemother 1990;34:1227–31.
29. Stryjewski ME, Szczech LA, Benjamin DK Jr, et al. Use of vancomycin or first-generation cephalosporins for the treatment of hemodialysis-dependent patients with methicillin-susceptible *Staphylococcus aureus* bacteremia. Clin Infect Dis 2007;44:190–6.
30. Swayne R, Rampling A, Newsome SWB. Intraventricular vancomycin for treatment of shunt-associated ventriculitis. J Antimicrob Chemother 1987;19:249–53.
31. Gump DW. Vancomycin for treatment of bacterial meningitis. Rev Infect Dis 1981; (Suppl 3):S289–92.
32. National Nosocomial Infections Surveillance System (NNIS). Nosocomial enterococci resistant to vancomycin—United States, 1989–1993. Morb Mortal Wkly Rep 1993;42:597–9.
33. Moellering RC Jr. The enterococcus: a classic example of antimicrobial resistance on therapeutic options. J Antimicrob Chemother 1991;28:1–12.
34. Noble WC, Virani Z, Cree RGA. Co-transfer of vancomycin and other resistance genes from *Enterococcus faecalis* NCTC 12201 to *Staphylococcus aureus*. FEMS Microbiol Lett 1992;72:195–8.
35. Frieden TR, Munsiff SS, Low DE, et al. Emergence of vancomycin-resistant enterococci in New York City. Lancet 1993;342:76–9.
36. Boyce JM. Vancomycin-resistant enterococcus. Detection, epidemiology, and control measures. Infect Dis Clin North Am 1997;11:367–84.
37. Fridkin SK, Edwards JR, Courvall JM, et al. The effect of vancomycin and third-generation cephalosporins on prevalence of vancomycin-resistant enterococci in 126 U.S. adult intensive care units. Ann Intern Med 2001;135:175–83.
38. Centers for Disease Control and Prevention. Preventing the spread of vancomycin resistance—report from the Hospital Infection Control Practices Advisory Committee. Federal Register 1994.
39. Ena J, Dick RW, Jones RN. The epidemiology of intravenous vancomycin usage in a university hospital. JAMA 1993;269:598–602.
40. Sieradzki K, Roberts RB, Serur D, et al. Heterogeneously vancomycin-resistant *Staphylococcus epidermidis* strain causing recurrent peritonitis in a dialysis patient during vancomycin therapy. J Clin Microbiol 1999;37:39–44.
41. Jones RN. Microbiological features of vancomycin in the 21st century: minimum inhibitory concentration creep, bactericidal/static activity, and applied breakpoints to predict clinical outcomes or detect resistant strains. Clin Infect Dis 2006;42(Suppl 1):S13–24.
42. Steinkraus G, White R, Friedrich L. Vancomycin MIC creep in non-vancomycin–intermediate *Staphylococcus aureus* (VISA), vancomycin-susceptible clinical methicillin-resistant *S. aureus* (MRSA) blood isolates from 2001–05. J Antimicrob Chemother 2007;60:788–94.
43. Howden BP, Ward PB, Charles PG, et al. Treatment outcomes for serious infections caused by methicillin-resistant *Staphylococcus aureus* with reduced vancomycin susceptibility. Clin Infect Dis 2004;38:521–8.
44. Lodise TP, Graves J, Evans A, et al. Relationship between vancomycin MIC and failure among patients with methicillin-resistant *Staphylococcus aureus* bacteremia treated with vancomycin. Antimicrob Agents Chemother 2008;52:3315–20.
45. Soriano A, Marco F, Martinez JA, et al. Influence of vancomycin minimum inhibitory concentration on the treatment of methicillin-resistant *Staphylococcus aureus* bacteremia. Clin Infect Dis 2008;46(2):193–200.

46. Nailor MD, Zhao JJ, Salimnia H. Daptomycin for methicillin-resistant Staphylo-coccus aureus bacteremia with elevated vancomycin minimum inhibitory concentrations [abstract]. IDSA/ICAAC: K3488, 2008.

47. Centers for Disease Control and Prevention. Reduced susceptibility of *Staphylococcus aureus* to vancomycin—Japan, 1996. Morb Mortal Wkly Rep 1997;46: 624–6.

48. Hiramatsu K, Aritaka N, Hanaki H, et al. Dissemination in Japanese hospitals of strains of *Staphylococcus aureus* heterogeneously resistant to vancomycin. Lancet 1997;350:1670–3.

49. Smith TL, Pearson ML, Wilcox KR, et al. Emergence of vancomycin resistance in *Staphylococcus aureus*. N Engl J Med 1999;340:493–501.

50. Tenover FC, Moellering RC. The rationale for revising the clinical and laboratory standards institute vancomycin minimal inhibitory concentration interpretive criteria for *Staphylococcus aureus*. Clin Infect Dis 2007;44(9):1208–15.

51. Charles PG, Ward PB, Johnson PD, et al. Clinical features associated with bacteremia due to heterogeneous vancomycin-intermediate *Staphylococcus aureus*. Clin Infect Dis 2004;38:448–51.

52. Rybak MJ, Leonard SN, Rossi KL, et al. Characterization of vancomycin-heteroresistant *Staphylococcus aureus* from the metropolitan area of Detroit, Michigan, over a 22-year period (1986–2007). J Clin Microbiol 2008;46:2950–4.

53. Chang S, Sievert D, Hageman J, et al. Infection with vancomycin-resistant *Staphylococcus aureus* containing the vanA resistance gene. N Engl J Med 2003;348(14):1342–7.

54. Centers for Disease Control and Prevention Public Health Dispatch: vancomycin-resistant *Staphylococcus aureus*—Pennsylvania, 2002. 51(40), 2002.

55. Polk RE, Healy DP, Schwartz LP, et al. Vancomycin and the red man syndrome: pharmacodynamics of histamine release. J Infect Dis 1988;157:502–7.

56. Sorrell TC, Collignon PJ, et al. A prospective study of adverse reactions associated with vancomycin therapy. J Antimicrob Chemother 1985;16(2):235–41.

57. Lodise TP, Lomaestro B, Graves J, et al. Larger vancomycin doses are associated with an increased incidence of nephrotoxicitiy. Antimicrob Agents Chemother 2008;52:1330–6.

58. Adrouny A, Meguerditchian S, Koo CH, et al. Agranulocytosis related to vancomycin therapy. Am J Med 1986;81:1059–61.

59. Cook FV, Farrar WE. Vancomycin revisited. Ann Intern Med 1978;88:813–8.

60. Lundstrom TS, Sobel JD. Antibiotics for gram-positive bacterial infections: vancomycin, teicoplanin, quinupristin/dalfopristin and linezolid. In: Kaye D, editor. Philadelphia; WB Saunders Co. Infect Dis Clin North Am 2000;14(2):463–74

61. Chant C, Rybak MJ. Quinupristin/dalfopristin (RP 59500): a new streptogramin antibiotic. Ann Pharmacother 1995;29:1022–7.

62. Nichterlein T, Kretschmar M, Hof H. RP 59500, a streptogramin derivative, is effective in murine listeriosis. J Chemother 1996;8:107–12.

63. Jones RN, Ballow CH, Biedenbach DJ, et al. Antimicrobial activity of quinupristin-dalfopristin (RP 59500, Synercid) tested against over 28,000 recent clinical isolates from 200 medical centers in the United States and Canada. Diagn Microbiol Infect Dis 1998;30:437–51.

64. Hussain Qadri SM, Ueno Y, Abu Mostafa FM, et al. In vitro activity of quinupristin/dalfopristin, RP 59500, against gram-positive clinical isolates. Chemotherapy 1997;43:94–9.

65. Schulin T, Wennersten CB, Ferraro MJ, et al. Susceptibilities of *Legionella spp.* to newer antimicrobials in vitro. Antimicrob Agents Chemother 1998;42:1520–3.

66. Struwig MC, Botha PL, Chalkley LJ. In vitro activities of 15 antimicrobial agents against clinical isolates of South African enterococci. Antimicrob Agents Chemother 1998;42:2752–5.
67. Furlong WB, Rakowski TA. Therapy with RP 59500 (quinupristin/dalfopristin) for prosthetic valve endocarditis due to enterococci with VanA/VanB resistance patterns. Clin Infect Dis 1997;25:163–4.
68. Chow JW, Davidson A, Sanford E III, et al. Superinfection with *Enterococcus faecalis* during quinupristin/dalfopristin therapy. Clin Infect Dis 1997;24:91–2.
69. Hershberger E, Donabedian S, Konstantinou K, et al. Quinupristin-dalfopristin resistance in gram-positive bacteria: mechanism of resistance and epidemiology. Clin Infect Dis 2004;38:92–8.
70. Chow JW, Donabedian SM, Zervos MJ. Emergence of increased resistance to quinupristin/dalfopristin during therapy for *Enterococcus faecium* bacteremia. Clin Infect Dis 1997;24:90–1.
71. Aeschlimann JR, Zervos MJ, Rybak MJ. Treatment of vancomycin-resistant *Enterococcus faecium* with RP59500 (quinupristin-dalfopristin) administered by intermittent or continuous infusion, alone, or in combination with doxycycline, in an in vitro pharmacodynamic infection model with simulated endocardial vegetation. Antimicrob Agents Chemother 1998;42:2710–7.
72. Muller M, Sehimz KL. Oxazolidinones: a novel class of antibiotics. Cell Mol Life Sci 1999;56:280–5.
73. Tucker JA, Allwine DA, Grega KC, et al. Piperazinyl oxazolidinone antibacterial agents containing a pyridine, diazine, or triazene heteroaromatic ring. J Med Chem 1998;41:3727–35.
74. Clemett D, Markham A. Linezolid. Drugs 2000;59:815–27.
75. Dresser LD, Rybak MJ. The pharmacologic and bacteriologic properties of oxazolidinones, a new class of synthetic antimicrobials. Pharmacotherapy 1998;18:456–62.
76. Zurenko GE, Yagi BH, Schaadt RD, et al. In vitro activities of U-100592 and U-100766, novel oxazolidinone antibacterial agents. Antimicrob Agents Chemother 1996;40:839–45.
77. Patel R, Rouse MS, Piper KE, et al. In vitro activity of linezolid against vancomycin-resistant enterococci, methicillin-resistant *Staphylococcus aureus*, and penicillin-resistant *Streptococcus pneumoniae*. Diagn Microbiol Infect Dis 1999;34:119–22.
78. Pawsey SD, Dalry-Yates PT, Wajszczuk CP, et al. U-100766 safety, toleration and pharmacokinetics after oral and intravenous administration. In: Program and abstracts of the first European Congress of Infections [abstract]. Berlin. sy13.4, 1997.
79. Lovering AM, Zhang J, Bannister GC, et al. Penetration of linezolid into bone, fat, muscle and haematoma of patients undergoing routine hip replacement. J Antimicrob Chemother 2002;50:73–7.
80. Wagenlehner FME, Wydra S, Onda H, et al. Concentrations in plasma, urinary excretion, and bactericidal activity of linezolid (600 milligrams) versus those of ciprofloxacin (500 milligrams) in healthy volunteers receiving a single oral dose. Antimicrob Agents Chemother 2003;47:3789–94.
81. Gemmell CG, Ford CW. Virulence factor expression by gram-positive cocci exposed to subinhibitory concentrations of linezolid. J Antimicrob Chemother 2002;50:665–72.
82. Noskin G, Siddique F, Stosor V, et al. Successful treatment of persistent vancomycin-resistant *Enterococcus faecium* bacteremia with linezolid and gentamicin. Clin Infect Dis 1999;28:689–90.

83. Conte JE, Golden JA, Kipps J, et al. Intrapulmonary pharmacokinetics of linezolid. Antimicrob Agents Chemother 2002;46:1475–80.
84. Wunderink RG, Rello J, Cammarata SK, et al. Linezolid vs vancomycin: Analysis of two double-blind studies of patients with methicillin-resistant *Staphylococcus aureus* nosocomial pneumonia. Chest 2003;124:1789–97.
85. Birmingham MC, Rayner CR, Meagher AK, et al. Linezolid for the treatment of multidrug-resistant, gram-positive infections: experience from a compassionate use program. Clin Infect Dis 2003;36:159–68.
86. Moise PA, Forrest A, Birmingham MC, et al. The efficacy and safety of linezolid as treatment for *Staphylococcus aureus* infections in compassionate use patients who are intolerant of, or who have failed to respond to, vancomycin. J Antimicrob Chemother 2002;50:1017–26.
87. Lipsky BA, Itani K, Norden C, et al. Treating foot infections in diabetic patients: a randomized, multicenter; open-label trial of linezolid versus ampicillin-sulbactam/amoxicillin-clavulanate. Clin Infect Dis 2004;38(1):17–24.
88. Parodi S, Rhew DC, Goetz MB. Early switch and early discharge opportunities in intravenous vancomycin treatment of suspected methicillin-resistant staphylococcal species infections. J Manag Care Pharm 2003;9:317–26.
89. Shorr AF, Susla GM, Kollef MH. Linezolid for treatment of ventilator-associated pneumonia: a cost-effective alternative to vancomycin. Crit Care Med 2004; 32:137–43.
90. Li JZ, Willke RJ, Rittenhouse BE, et al. Effect of linezolid versus vancomycin on length of hospital stay in patients with complicated skin and soft tissue infections caused by known or suspected methicillin-resistant staphylococci: results from a randomized clinical trial. Surg Infect 2003;4(1):57–70.
91. Brickner SJ, Hutchinson DK, Burbachyn MR, et al. Synthesis and antibacterial activity of U-100592 and U-100766, two oxazolidinone antibacterial agents for the potential treatment of multidrug-resistant gram-positive bacterial infections. J Med Chem 1996;39:673–9.
92. Kaatz GW, Seo SM. In vitro activities of oxazolidinone compounds U-100592 and U-100766 against staphylococcus species. Antimicrob Agents Chemother 1996;40:799–801.
93. Rahim S, Pillai SK, Gold HS, et al. Linezolid-resistant, vancomycin-resistant *Enterococcus faecium* infection in patients without prior exposure to linezolid. Clin Infect Dis 2003;36:E146–8.
94. Schwartz MD, Shive DK, Sheikh ZHA. Delayed discovery of linezolid-resistant, vancomycin-resistant *Enterococcus faecium*: lessons learned. Clin Infect Dis 2004;38:155–6.
95. Wilson P, Andrews JA, Charlesworth R. Linezolid resistance in clinical isolates of *Staphylococcus aureus*. J Antimicrob Chemother 2003;51:186–8.
96. Garcia MS, De laa Torre MA, Morales G, et al. Clinical outbreak of linezolid-resistant *Staphylococcus aureus* in an intensive care unit. JAMA 2010;303:2260–4.
97. Ikeda-Dantsuji Y, Hanaki H, Sakai F, et al. Linezolid-resistant *Staphylococcus aureus* isolated from 2006 through 2008 at six hospitals in Japan. J Infect Chemother 2010;17:45–51.
98. Farrell DJ, Mendes RE, Ross JE, et al. Linezolid surveillance program results from 2008 (LEADER program for 2008). Diagn Microbiol Infect Dis 2009;65:392–403.
99. Nannini E, Murray BE, Arias CA. Resistance or decreased susceptibility to glycopeptides, daptomycin, and linezolid in methicillin-resistant *Staphylococcus aureus*. Curr Opin Pharmacol 2010;10:516–21.

100. Gerson SL, Kaplan SL, Bruss JB, et al. Hematologic effects of linezolid: summary of clinical experience. Antimicrob Agents Chemother 2002;46: 2723–6.
101. Nasraway SA, Shorr AF, Kuter DJ. Linezolid does not increase the risk of thrombocytopenia in patients with nosocomial pneumonia: comparative analysis of linezolid and vancomycin use. Clin Infect Dis 2003;37:1609–16.
102. Thorne GM, Adler J. Daptomycin: a novel lipopeptide antibiotic. Clin Microbiol Newslett 2002;24:33–40.
103. Tally FP, DeBruin MF. Development of daptomycin for gram-positive infections. J Antimicrob Chemother 2000;46:523–6.
104. Critchley IA, Draghi DC, Sahm DF, et al. Activity of daptomycin against susceptible and multidrug-resistant gram-positive pathogens collected in the SECURE study (Europe) during 2000–2001. J Antimicrob Chemother 2003;51:639–49.
105. Pankuch GA, Jacobs MR, Appelbaum PC. Bactericidal activity of daptomycin against *Streptococcus pneumoniae* compared with eight other antimicrobials. J Antimicrob Chemother 2003;51:443–6.
106. Golan Y, Poutsiaka D, Tozzi S, et al. Daptomycin for line-related *Leuconostoc* bacteremia. J Antimicrob Chemother 2001;47:364–5.
107. Credito K, Lin G, Appelbaum PC. Activity of daptomycin alone and in combination with rifampin and gentamicin against *Staphylococcus aureus* assessed with time-kill methodology. Antimicrob Agents Chemother 2007;51:1504–7.
108. Bush LM. In vitro post-antibiotic effect of daptomycin (LY-146032) against *Enterococcus faecalis* and methicillin-susceptible and methicillin-resistant *Staphylococcus aureus* strains. Antimicrob Agents Chemother 1989;33: 1198–2000.
109. Fowler VG, Boucher HW, Corey GR, et al. Daptomycin versus standard therapy for bacteremia and endocarditis caused by *Staphylococcus aureus*. N Engl J Med 2006;355:653–65.
110. Sakoulas G, Adler J, Thauvin-Eliopoulos C, et al. Induction of daptomycin heterogeneous susceptibility in *Staphylococcus aureus* by exposure to vancomycin. Antimicrob Agents Chemother 2006;50:1581–5.
111. Jevitt LA, Smith AJ, Williams PP, et al. In vitro activities of daptomycin, linezolid, and quinupristin-dalfopristin against a challenge panel of staphylococci and enterococci, including vancomycin-intermediate *Staphylococcus aureus* and vancomycin-resistant *Enterococcus faecium*. Microb Drug Resist 2003;9: 389–93.
112. Patel JB, Jevitt LA, Hagerman J, et al. An association between reduced susceptibility to daptomycin and reduced susceptibility to vancomycin in *Staphylococcus aureus*. Clin Infect Dis 2006;42(11):1652–3.
113. Fairfax MR, Nailor MD, Painter T. et al. Vancomycin and daptomycin susceptibility testing of Staphylococcus aureus in a clinical laboratory. IDSA/ICAAC C1–140, 2008.
114. Dvorchil BH, Brazier D, DeBruin MF, et al. Daptomycin pharmacokinetics and safety following administration of escalating doses once daily to healthy subjects. Antimicrob Agents Chemother 2003;47:1318–23.
115. Vibativ (telavancin) for injection. Package insert. Available at: http://www.astellas.us/docs/us/VIBATIV_PI_Final.pdf. Accessed April 2011.
116. Stryjewski ME, O'Riordan WD, Lau WK, et al. Telavancin versus standard therapy for treatment of complicated skin and soft-tissue infections due to gram-positive bacteria. Clin Infect Dis 2005;40:1601–7.

117. Rubinstein E, Lalani T, Corey GR, et al. Telavancin versus vancomycin for hospital-acquired pneumonia due to gram-positive pathogens. Clin Infect Dis 2011;52:31–40.
118. Saravolatz LD, Stein GE, Johnson LB. Ceftaroline: a novel cephalosporin with activity against methicillin-resistant *Staphylococcus aureus*. Clin Infect Dis 2011;52:1156–63.
119. File TM, Low DE, Eckburg PB, et al. Integrated analysis of FOCUS 1 and FOCUS 2: randomized, doubled-blinded, multicenter phase 3 trials of the efficacy and safety of ceftaroline fosamil versus ceftriaxone in patients with community-acquired pneumonia. Clin Infect Dis 2011;51:1395–405.
120. Corey GR, Wilcox M, Talbot G, et al. Integrated analysis of CANVAS 1 and 2: phase 3, multicenter, randomized, double-blind studies to evaluate the safety and efficacy of ceftaroline versus vancomycin plus aztreonam in complicated skin and skin-structure infection. Clin Infect Dis 2010;51:641–50.

Newer Beta-lactam Antibiotics: Doripenem, Ceftobiprole, Ceftaroline, and Cefepime

Jose A. Bazan, DO[a], Stanley I. Martin, MD[b],
Kenneth M. Kaye, MD[c],*

KEYWORDS

• Beta-lactam • Doripenem • Ceftobiprole
• Ceftaroline • Cefepime

Beta-lactam (β-lactam) antibiotics have been, and remain, the cornerstone of therapy for many life-threatening infections. Over the years, newer formulations have allowed clinicians to better provide broad empiric coverage and to use targeted therapy against commonly encountered gram-positive and gram-negative bacteria. For the most part, β-lactam antibiotics have evolved concomitantly with global antimicrobial resistance patterns. However, the emergence of pathogens like methicillin-resistant *Staphylococcus aureus* (MRSA), penicillin-intermediate and penicillin-resistant *Streptococcus pneumoniae*, multidrug-resistant (MDR) *Pseudomonas aeruginosa*, and extended-spectrum β-lactamase (ESBL)–producing gram-negative enteric organisms have provided new challenges, and the evolution of new β-lactams has slowed. This article focuses on the agents doripenem, ceftobiprole, and ceftaroline. In addition, this article summarizes recent developments regarding the potential increased mortality observed with the use of cefepime compared with that of other agents in the treatment of some infections.

A version of this article appeared in the 23:4 issue of the *Infectious Disease Clinics of North America*.
[a] Division of Infectious Diseases, The Ohio State University Medical Center, N1129 Doan Hall, 410 West 10th Avenue, Columbus, OH 43210, USA
[b] Division of Infectious Diseases, The Ohio State University Medical Center, N1148 Doan Hall, 410 West 10th Avenue, Columbus, OH 43210, USA
[c] Division of Infectious Diseases, Harvard Medical School, Channing Laboratory, Brigham and Women's Hospital, 181 Longwood Avenue, Boston, MA 02115, USA
* Corresponding author.
E-mail address: kkaye@rics.bwh.harvard.edu

Med Clin N Am 95 (2011) 743–760
doi:10.1016/j.mcna.2011.03.009
0025-7125/11/$ – see front matter © 2011 Elsevier Inc. All rights reserved.

medical.theclinics.com

DORIPENEM

Since the introduction of imipenem-cilastatin more than 20 years ago, the use of car-bapenems such as meropenem, ertapenem, and most recently doripenem has become more common in the face of infections caused by increasingly MDR bacteria. Doripenem (formerly S-4661), a parenteral 1-β-methyl carbapenem, is the newest agent in the family, and it received approval by the US Food and Drug Administration (FDA) in 2007 for the treatment of complicated intra-abdominal infections (IAIs) and complicated urinary tract infections (UTIs).[1] Doripenem binds to penicillin-binding proteins (PBPs) and leads to the inhibition of bacterial cell wall synthesis.[1,2] Similar to other β-lactams, its bactericidal activity is directly related to the time the concentra-tion of free drug exceeds the minimum inhibitory concentration (MIC) of the bacteria (% fT >MIC).[1,3] Unlike imipenem, its 1-β-methyl side chain confers stability in the face of renal dihydropeptidases.[4]

Similar to other carbapenems, doripenem exhibits a low degree of plasma protein binding. Imipenem-cilastatin, meropenem, and doripenem have ~20%, ~2%, and ~8% protein binding, respectively.[5–7] The metabolization of doripenem occurs through the actions of renal dihydropeptidase-I and undergoes renal excretion by a combination of glomerular filtration and active tubular secretion (78.7% unchanged drug and 18.5% inactive metabolites).[1,7,8] The normal plasma elimination half-life is approximately 1 hour, and the usual dose for patients who have normal renal func-tion is 500 mg infused intravenously (i.v.) for 1 hour every 8 hours.[1,3,7,8] This dosing regimen has been shown to achieve the fT >MIC target of 35% for susceptible organ-isms that have an MIC that is 1 μg/mL or less. For organisms that have an MIC that is 2 μg/mL or greater, the same target fT >MIC can be achieved by increasing the infu-sion time (>1 hour) without increasing the total daily dose, given the stability of the drug at room temperature.[3,7,9] Dosing requires adjustment in the setting of moderate renal dysfunction. For patients who have a creatinine clearance (CrCl) of 30 to 50 mL/min, 250 mg i.v. every 8 hours is recommended, and for a CrCl of 10 to 30 mL/min, 250 mg i.v. every 12 hours is recommended.[1,7] There are no established parameters at this time for dosing in patients who have a CrCl of less than 10 mL/min and those under-going hemodialysis.[1,7] Dosing of doripemen in the setting of renal replacement therapy (CRRT) is also not clearly defined. However, new data has recently emerged regarding the pharmacokinetic profile of doripemen in the setting of continuous venovenous hemofiltration and hemodiafiltration. According to Cirillo and colleagues, both types of CRRT significantly removed doripenem and its primary metabolite (M-1) when administered as a single 500 mg dose over 1 hour to patients with end-stage renal disease on hemodialysis. Nevertheless, these patients still demonstrated signif-icantly higher plasma drug concentrations, higher area under the plasma concentra-tion time curves (0–12 hour), and longer plasma elimination half lives compared to healthy individuals. These results demonstrate that commonly used CRRT modalities can have an additive effect on residual total body drug clearance.[10] Additional data is needed to help define optimal dosing strategies in patients with CrCl less than 10 mL/min, hemodialysis, and CRRT.

A number of studies have analyzed the in vitro activity of doripenem against bacte-rial isolates, using broth microdilution methods. The spectrum of antimicrobial activity of doripenem is similar to that of imipenem-cilastatin and meropenem for gram-positive and gram-negative bacteria.[11–14]

With regard to gram-positive bacteria, doripenem was the most active carbapenem against various isolates of methicillin-sensitive *Staphylococcus aureus* (MSSA) and methicillin-sensitive coagulase-negative staphylococci (MS-CoNS). It was twofold more active than meropenem or ertapenem against strains of *Enterococcus faecalis* and non-*faecium* enterococci, but twofold less active than imipenem-cilastatin.[10] On the other hand, vancomycin-resistant *Enterococcus faecium* isolates were uniformly resistant to doripenem.[11-15] Excellent in vitro activity has also been demonstrated against penicillin-susceptible, -intermediate, and -resistant *Streptococcus pneumoniae*, penicillin-susceptible and -resistant *Streptococcus viridans*, and the various β-hemolytic *Streptococcus* spp.[11-14]

Doripenem is active against Enterobacteriaceae. Its activity is similar to that of meropenem against wild-type (non-ESBL producing) and derepressed AmpC and ESBL-producing Enterobacteriaceae isolates.[11-15] Doripenem also displays excellent activity against common respiratory pathogens such as *Haemophilus influenzae* and *Moraxella catarrhalis* (including β-lactamase-producing strains).[11,13-15] With regard to the nonfermenting, aerobic, gram-negative bacteria, doripenem had the greatest activity against wild-type strains of *P aeruginosa* that had an MIC_{50} and MIC_{90} of 0.5 μg/mL and 8 μg/mL, respectively.[11] In addition, doripenem may still retain activity against strains of *P aeruginosa* that are resistant to other carbapenems. For instance, of 34 *P aeruginosa* strains resistant to carbapenems, 29.4% were susceptible to doripenem, whereas none were susceptible to imipenem-cilastatin, and 2.9% were susceptible to meropenem.[15] Notably, 44.1% of these same strains were sensitive to piperacillin-tazobactam, 29.4% were sensitive to cefepime, and 44.1% were sensitive to amikacin.[15] However, only 6.7% of Class B metallo-β-lactamase–producing strains of *P aeruginosa* strains were sensitive to doripenem.[15] Doripenem was active against 75.8% of wild-type *Acinetobacter baumanii* and 20.8% of carbapenem-resistant *Acinetobacter* spp (MIC_{90} of 16 μg/mL and >32 μg/mL, respectively).[14,15] *Aeromonas* spp isolates were sensitive to doripenem (MIC_{90} of 1 μg/mL), whereas doripenem's activity against strains of *Burkholderia cepacia* was variable and less than that of meropenem but similar to that of imipenem-cilastatin (MIC_{90} of 8 μg/mL). *Stenotrophomonas maltophilia* showed marked resistance to all carbapenems, including doripenem (MIC_{90} >16 μg/mL).[11] Finally, doripenem had good activity against anaerobic isolates of clinical importance such as *Bacteroides* spp, *Prevotella* spp, *Clostridium* spp, *Fusobacterium* spp, and anaerobic gram-positive cocci.[16]

Carbapenems as a class are generally resistant to hydrolysis by β-lactamases. Doripenem demonstrates enhanced stability and resistance to hydrolysis by derepressed AmpC β-lactamases and ESBLs.[17] Currently known mechanisms of decreased microbial susceptibility to doripenem include the production of metallo-β-lactamases such as IMP and VIM, decreased production or absence of the OprD outer membrane porin protein leading to decreased entry of the drug into the cell, and expression of multidrug efflux pumps that promote excretion of the drug out of the cell.[7,17-21] Compared with the other carbapenems, doripenem has a higher threshold for selection of nonsusceptible mutants in vitro, and it seems that high-level resistance may require the coexistence of more than one resistance mechanism.[7,17,18] At this time, some authors have suggested that it is unlikely that such complex alterations and multilevel mechanisms of resistance are selected in vivo during doripenem therapy.[7,17-19,22]

In a phase 3, prospective, multicenter, randomized, double-blind, noninferiority study, doripenem was found to have clinical cure rates comparable to those of meropenem for the treatment of complicated IAIs in the clinically evaluable (86.7% vs 86.6%) and microbiologically evaluable (85.9% vs 85.3%) cases at test-of-cure follow-up. In cases in which *P aeruginosa* was isolated (n = 19), microbial eradication was similar for doripenem and meropenem. Patients who had infected necrotizing pancreatitis and pancreatic abscesses were excluded from the study.[23] Another phase

3, randomized, double-blind, multicenter trial showed that doripenem was noninferior to levofloxacin for the treatment of complicated UTIs. Clinical cure rates in evaluable patients were 95.1% and 90.2% for the doripenem and levofloxacin groups, respectively.[24] Doripenem has also been studied for the treatment of hospital-acquired pneumonia (HAP) and ventilator-associated pneumonia (VAP) in two prospective, randomized, multicenter, and open-label studies.[25,26] Rea-Neto and colleagues[25] showed that doripenem was comparable and noninferior to piperacillin-tazobactam for the treatment of HAP and VAP. Cure rates for clinically evaluable patients were 81.3% and 79.8% for doripenem and piperacillin-tazobactam, respectively. Decreased susceptibility of P aeruginosa isolates was seen in 26.9% of patients treated using piperacillin-tazobactam and 7.7% of patients treated using doripenem. The authors acknowledged, however, a low rate of study-drug monotherapy when infection with P aeruginosa was suspected and severely ill and immunocompromised patients were excluded.[25] Chastre and colleagues[26] showed that doripenem was noninferior to imipenem-cilastatin in the treatment of VAP, with comparable cure rates of 68.3% versus 64.8% in clinically evaluable patients. All-cause mortality was similar for both treatment arms at 28 days (10.8% for doripenem vs 9.5% for imipenem-cilastatin). In cases in which P aeruginosa was isolated at baseline, both treatment arms had similar clinical cure and microbiological eradication rates. There was a trend toward better outcomes for patients who had higher baseline Acute Physiology and Chronic Health Evaluation II (APACHE II) scores, which were more than 20 points higher in the doripenem group than in the imipenem-cilistatin group (70.4% vs 57.7%).[26]

In previous studies, doripenem showed a good safety and tolerability profile compared with drugs studied in other arms. The incidence of study-drug-related adverse events (AEs) ranged from 16% to 32% for doripenem and from 18% to 27% for various comparators. The most commonly reported AEs were nausea, emesis, diarrhea, headaches, phlebitis, rash, and transaminitis. No seizure events that could be directly attributed to doripenem were reported.[23–26] Nevertheless, the epileptogenic potential of some carbapenems in patients who are at risk is a known potential side effect, particularly for imipenem-cilastatin.[27] Doripenem may not be exempt from this risk, according to some postmarketing reports from outside the United States.[1] However, a study evaluating the epileptogenic potential of doripenem administered i.v. or intracisternally in animal models failed to produce seizures.[28]

As the newest member of the carbapenem family, the role of doripenem may mirror that of meropenem more than any other carbapenem. They both have similar spectrums of antimicrobial activity and safety profiles. Based on the aforementioned non-inferiority comparative trials, doripenem has a place in the treatment of not only complicated IAIs and complicated UTIs but also other health-care-associated infections such as HAP and VAP that are caused by susceptible pathogens. In July 16, 2008, the FDA's Anti-Infective Drugs Advisory Committee voted in favor of doripenem's clinical efficacy and safety for the treament of HAP and VAP. At the time of writing, final FDA approval for these indications was pending.[29]

Finally, doripenem may play a important role in the treatment of serious infections due to MDR gram negative pathogens. The emergence of carbapenemase-producing strains of K pneumoniae (KPC) and carbapenem-resistant strains of P aeruginosa, presents a major challenge to clinicians given the limited antimicrobial options that are available to treat serious infections due to these organisms. New data are emerging about the potential utility of prolonged infusion doripenem to help treat such infections. Bulik and Nicolau analyzed the utility of prolonged infusion doripenem at doses known to simulate exposures in humans, for the treatment of thigh infection due to KPC-enzyme producing strains of K pneumoniae in immunocompetent and immunocompromised mice. Results demonstrated that in immunocompetent mice, 4-hour infusions of doripenem administered as 1 or 2 g every 8 hours, significantly decreased bacterial loads ($\sim$1 log CFU; $P<.05$), while in immunocompromised mice, bacteriostatic effects were noted in isolates with MICs up to 8 μg/mL and 16 μg/mL respectively.[30] Furthermore, a recent small retrospective study evaluated the use of doripenem 1 g i.v. every 8 hours infused over 4-hours combined with Fosfomycin 2 g i.v. every 8 hours for the treatment of HAP due to carbapenem-resistant *P aeruginosa* (doripenem MICs of 4–8 mg/L). Results demonstrated that 6 of 8 patients (75%) experienced clinical cure or improvement. In patients in which follow-up microbiological evaluation was performed, eradication was documented in 6 of 7 patients (87%). Overall, there were no significant AEs that could be attributed to therapy.[31] Additional clinical studies are needed to further define the role that extended-infusion doripenem will play in the treatment of infections due to MDR gram negatives, especially those that exhibit carbapenem resistance.

CEFTOBIPROLE

Since the emergence of the first MRSA isolate in the 1960s, the medical community has witnessed the widespread dissemination of MRSA and the burden that it can create in hospital wards and, most recently, surrounding communities.[32] It has been the rule that β-lactams as a class are ineffective against MRSA because of alterations in the target binding site PBP-2a that is coded by the *mec*A gene of the *mec* type IV staphylococcal cassette chromosome.[33,34] Ceftobiprole-medocaril (formerly BAL 5788, RO-5788) is a new, i.v.–administered, broad-spectrum pyrrolidinone cephalosporin that retains a high degree of affinity for PBP-2a.[35–37] In addition, ceftobiprole also has affinity for PBP-2x in penicillin-resistant *Streptococcus pneumoniae* and for PBP-3 in *Escherichia coli* and *P aeruginosa*.[35,37–39] Ceftobiprole was initially approved for use in Canada and Switzerland but has now been withdrawn for reasons discussed at the end of this section.[40–42]

Ceftobiprole-medocaril, the inactive prodrug, is cleaved to the active compound of ceftobiprole, diacetyl, and carbon dioxide by plasma esterases shortly after infusion. The degree of plasma protein binding has been reported to be $\sim$16% to 38%, whereas the volume of distribution is similar to that of the extracellular fluid compartment in adults at steady state. Ceftobiprole primarily undergoes renal excretion, and the majority of the drug is recovered in the urine ($\sim$83% unchanged drug, $\sim$0.3% prodrug, and $\sim$0.8% inactive metabolites). The activity of ceftobiprole depends on the length of time that the concentration of free drug is more than the MIC of the organism (% fT >MIC), and the mean serum half-life is approximately 3 to 4 hours.[35,43,44] Based on Monte Carlo simulation analysis, the likelihood of achieving the target fT >MIC of 30% and 50% for organisms with an MIC that is 2 μg/mL or less and 1 μg/mL or less, respectively, was greater than 90% with a dosage of 500 mg i.v. over 1 hour every 12-hours. Similarly, the likelihood of achieving the target fT >MIC of 40% and 60% for organisms with an MIC that is 4 μg/mL or less and 2 μg/mL or less, respectively, was greater than 90% with a dosage of 500 mg i.v. over 2 hours every 8 hours.[44,45] The current recommended dosage in the setting of normal renal function is 500 mg i.v. infused for 30 minutes to 2 hours every 8 to 12 hours, depending on the target percentage of fT >MIC desired and type of infection being treated. Thus, treatment of polymicrobial diabetic foot infections and gram-positive or gram-negative HAP or VAP may require 500 mg i.v. for 2 hours every 8 hours, versus treatment of a complicated skin and soft-tissue infection (SSTI) caused by a gram-positive bacteria, which may only require 500 mg i.v. for 1 hour every 12 hours.[35,44–48] Pharmacodynamic studies suggest that dose adjustments are required in the setting of mild to moderate renal dysfunction (CrCl ≤50 mL/min; 500 mg i.v. for 2 hours every 12 hours). Further data are needed regarding optimal dosing in the setting of severe renal dysfunction and hemodialysis.[44,45] Ceftobiprole does not undergo significant hepatic metabolism, and no dose adjustments appear to be required in the setting of hepatic dysfunction.[44]

The spectrum of antimicrobial activity of ceftobiprole is among the broadest of all currently available cephalosporins. As part of a longitudinal, global, resistance-surveillance program (SENTRY), Fritsche and colleagues[49] analyzed the in vitro activity of ceftobiprole using broth microdilution methods in 40,675 common bacterial isolates. With regard to gram-positive bacteria, ceftobiprole readily inhibited MSSA and MRSA at concentrations that are 4 μg/mL or less (MIC$_{90}$ 0.5 μg/mL and 2 μg/mL, respectively). The activity of ceftobiprole against MSSA isolates was equal to that of oxacillin and daptomycin, and eightfold greater than that of cefepime and ceftriaxone. Its activity was at least eightfold greater than that of any other β-lactam against MRSA and equal to that of linezolid, but twofold to fourfold less than that of vancomycin, TMP-SMX, or daptomycin. Ceftobiprole inhibited more than 99% of MS-CoNS and methicillin-resistant coagulase-negative staphylococci (MR-CoNS) isolates at concentrations of 0.5 μg/mL and 4 μg/mL, respectively. Its activity against MR-CoNS was comparable to that of vancomycin. Ceftobiprole showed good activity against ampicillin-sensitive, ampicillin-resistant, and vancomycin-resistant strains of Enterococcus faecalis, β-hemolytic Streptococcus spp, Streptococcus viridans Bacillus spp, Listeria spp, and Streptococcus pneumoniae. Ceftobiprole inhibited 100% of penicillin-susceptible and penicillin-resistant Streptococcus pneumoniae at concentrations of 0.25 μg/mL and 2 μg/mL respectively. Ceftobiprole, however, did not show significant activity against Corynebacterium spp. It also has no documented in vitro activity against Enterococcus faecium isolates regardless of their vancomycin or ampicillin susceptibility profiles.[49,50]

With regard to the Enterobacteriaceae, ceftobiprole showed good activity against non-ESBL–producing Escherichia coli, Proteus mirabilis, Citrobacter spp, Serratia spp, and Salmonella spp isolates. Ceftobiprole was less active than cefepime against non-ESBL–producing Klebsiella pneumoniae, Enterobacter spp, and indole-positive Proteus spp, with 76.9%, 85.4%, and 72.2% of respective isolates being inhibited by drug concentrations that were 8 μg/mL or less. Similar to other extended-spectrum cephalosporins, ceftobiprole showed limited activity against ESBL-producing strains of Escherichia coli and Klebsiella pneumoniae.[49]

The in vitro activity of ceftobiprole against nonfermenting, aerobic, gram-negative bacteria such as P aeruginosa was generally similar to other agents. Ceftobiprole inhibited 77.9% at concentrations that were 8 μg/mL or less, whereas the percentage susceptible to ceftazidime was 75.5%, imipenem 75.8%, cefepime 79.4%, meropenem 80.9%, piperacillin-tazobactam 84.8%, amikacin 87.4%, and polymixin B 99.8%. Ceftobiprole was active against Aeromonas spp, but not against Stenotrophomonas maltophilia, B cepacia, or Acinetobacter spp. It was readily active against wild-type and β-lactamase–producing strains of H influenzae and M catarrhalis.[49] Finally, it does have some activity against most anaerobic gram-positive cocci such as Propionibacterium acnes, non-difficile Clostridium spp, and Porphyromonas spp. However, Peptostreptococcus anaerobius, Clostridium difficile, Prevotella spp, and Bacteroides spp were generally tolerant or resistant.[51]

Ceftobiprole is generally resistant to hydrolysis by staphylococcal penicillinases, but not to ESBLs, carbapenemases, or OXA-10 β-lactamases produced by some MDR gram-negative bacteria. However, it is a poor substrate for Class A and

SHV-1, and class C AmpC β-lactamases, demonstrating low rates of hydrolysis on exposure.[52]

Ceftobiprole has been evaluated for the treatment of complicated SSTIs in phase 3 clinical trials. A randomized, double-blind, multicenter, noninferiority study compared ceftobiprole with vancomycin for the treatment of complicated SSTIs caused by gram-positive bacteria. The results showed comparable cure rates in clinically evaluable patients (93.3% for ceftobiprole vs 93.5% for vancomycin). In cases of documented MRSA infection, cure rates were similar for both treatment arms (91.8% for ceftobiprole vs 90.0% for vancomycin), including those caused by Panton-Valentin leukocidin (+) strains.[47] A second randomized, double-blind, multicenter, noninferiority trial compared ceftobiprole with vancomycin plus ceftazidime for the treatment of complicated SSTIs. In contrast with the first trial, patients who had diabetic foot infections were included in this study. Among the clinically evaluable patients, cure rates were 90.5% and 90.2% for the ceftobiprole and vancomycin/ceftazidime arms, respectively. Comparable clinical cure rates were found in patients who had documented infections caused by MRSA (89.7% for ceftobiprole vs 86.1% for vancomycin/ceftazidime) and P aeruginosa (86.7% for ceftobiprole vs 100% for vancomycin/ceftazidime). Similarly, cure rates for patients who had diabetic foot infections were 86.2% and 81.8% for ceftobiprole and vancomycin/ceftazidime, respectively.[48]

The incidence of at least one AE was 52% for ceftobiprole and 51% for vancomycin in the first study and 56% for ceftobiprole and 57% for vancomycin/ceftazidime group in the second. Nausea (14%), vomiting (7%), taste disturbance (8%), and infusion-site reactions (9%) were the most commonly reported AEs for the ceftobiprole arms.[47,48]

Laboratory studies using a rabbit model of MRSA aortic valve endocarditis and tibial osteomyelitis showed promising results with the use of ceftobiprole.[53,54] In addition, neutropenic-mouse-model studies have shown that ceftobiprole has excellent lung tissue penetration and achieves high concentrations in alveolar epithelial lining fluids that are much more than the MICs for various isolates of Staphylococcus aureus, including MRSA.[55]

Phase 3 clinical trials looking at the use of ceftobiprole for the treatment of community-acquired pneumonia, HAP, and neutropenic fever have been completed and we are awaiting their respective results.[56]

Ceftobiprole is the first available β-lactam to show bactericidal activity against MRSA in addition to a wide array of gram-negative pathogens. However, in November 28, 2008, the FDA notified the sponsor of ceftobiprole, Johnson & Johnson Pharmaceutical Research and Development, L.L.C. (J&JPRD), that it could not approve the drug for the treatment of complicated SSTI and diabetic foot infections. The FDA cited that irregularities had been found in 10 of 49 clinical trial sites when it reviewed data from two major studies (BAP00154 and BAP00414) that were presented by the company as part of its New Drug Application (NDA). The FDA concluded that J&JPRD had failed to adequately monitor the clinical investigators from the sites in question, thereby making the available data unreliable or unverifiable. The failure to adequately monitor could have affected safety and primary efficacy data from these sites. Furthermore, additional data was requested by the FDA regarding the conclusion that ceftobiprole was non-inferior to the comparator arm in subsets of patients that had skin and soft tissue abscesses that were drained or diabetic foot infections. The FDA did provide recommendations to the company regarding the design and conduct of two new clinical trials to re-evaluate the safety and efficacy of ceftobiprole for the treatment of complicated SSTI's.[57,58] In 2010, the European Committee for Medicinal Products for Human Use (CHMP) concluded that ceftobiprole should not be authorized for use.[59] Since then, both Canada and Switzerland have discontinued the sale and use of ceftobiprole.[60,61]

CEFTAROLINE

Ceftaroline is another β-lactam of the cephalosporin class that retains activity against MRSA. Ceftaroline fosamil (formerly PPI-0903M, formerly TAK-599) is a new, water-soluble, i.v.-administered, N-phosphono–type cephalosporin that undergoes hydrolysis of the phosphate group and is rapidly converted to its active compound in vivo after parenteral administration in animal models. In addition, it has a high degree of affinity for PBP-2a, with documented anti-MRSA activity.[62,63] The pharmacokinetic and pharmacodynamic profiles of ceftaroline have been analyzed in murine models of thigh, lung, and aortic valve infection, and in healthy human volunteers and patients who had complicated SSTIs. The results of these studies show that the mean serum half-life is ~2.6 hours, plasma protein binding is less than 20%, and drug clearance occurs mainly by way of renal excretion, with ~75% of the drug recovered in the urine.[64–68] The current dosing regimen used in patients who have normal renal function in phase 2 and 3 clinical trials is 600 mg i.v. infused for 1 hour every 12 hours.[69,70,72] Dosage adjustments are not required in the setting of mild renal dysfunction (CrCl >50–80 mL/min), but should be undertaken for patients who have more severe renal dysfunction (CrCl >30–50 mL/min; 400 mg i.v. for 1 hour every 12 hours, CrCl >=15 to <=30 mL/min 300 mg i.v. for 1 hour every 12 hours, end stage renal disease CrCl <15 mL/min including hemodialysis 200 mg i.v. over 1 hour every 12 hours [administer after hemodialysis on hemodialysis days]).[71]

Analysis of the in vitro activity of ceftaroline against various clinical and laboratory bacterial isolates from various parts of the world using broth microdilution methods showed that it has excellent activity against MSSA, MRSA, MS-CoNS, and MR-CoNS. Activity was fourfold greater than that of vancomycin and 16 fold greater than that of ceftriaxone or cefepime against MSSA isolates. When tested against 102 MRSA isolates, ceftaroline had an MIC_{90} of 2 μg/mL, which is similar to that of linezolid and slightly higher than that of vancomycin (MIC_{90} of 1 μg/mL). Activity was also documented against vancomycin-intermediate strains of *Staphylococcus aureus*. For 100 isolates of vancomycin-intermediate strains of *Staphylococcus aureus* tested, the ceftaroline MIC_{90} was 2 μg/mL, which is only slightly higher than that of linezolid, which had an MIC_{90} of 1 μg/mL.[73] Similar results were noted in clinical isolates from the United States, in which ceftaroline was the most active cephalosporin against all staphylococci tested.[74] Other gram-positive bacteria that showed susceptibility to ceftaroline included *Streptococcus pneumoniae* (ceftaroline MIC_{90}: penicillin-susceptible, ≤0.016 μg/mL; penicillin-intermediate, 0.06 μg/mL; penicillin-resistant, 0.25 μg/mL), β-hemolytic streptococci spp, and *Streptococcus viridans*. Ceftaroline was less active than vancomycin, imipenem-cilastatin, and levofloxacin against *Bacillus* spp. Ceftaroline showed only marginal activity against *Enterococcus faecalis* and was not effective against *Enterococcus faecium* (ceftaroline MIC_{90} for vancomycin-susceptible and vancomycin-resistant strains, >32 μg/mL).[73]

Ceftaroline displayed significant activity against the Enterobacteriaceae. Non-ESBL–producing strains were uniformly susceptible, whereas ESBL-producing strains of *Escherichia coli, K pneumoniae*, and *P mirabilis* were resistant. Among the nonfermenting, gram-negative bacteria, ceftaroline showed only minimal activity against certain isolates of *P aeruginosa* and *A baumanii* (ceftaroline MIC_{50} of 16 and MIC_{90} >32 μg/mL for both organisms) and was not active against *Alcaligenes* spp or *Stenotrophomonas maltophilia*. On the other hand, ceftaroline showed excellent activity against *Neisseria meningitidis*, *M catarrhalis*, and both β-lactamase–producing and non–β-lactamase–producing strains of *H influenzae*. In terms of anaerobic activity, it has significant effect against *Peptostreptococcus* spp, *Propionibacterium* spp, and non-*difficile Clostridium* spp. It has minimal to no activity against *Bacteroides fragilis* and *Prevotella* spp.[73]

Phase 2 and 3 clinical trials have been done to compare the safety and efficacy of ceftaroline with that of vancomycin with or without aztreonam for the treatment of complicated SSTIs in randomized and observer-blinded studies. In the phase 2 study, the clinical cure rate was 96.7% for ceftaroline and 88.9% for standard therapy.[57] In an integrated analysis of two phase 3 studies, the overall cure rates were 91.6% for ceftaroline and 92.7% for standard therapy in the clinically evaluable patient population. With respect to MRSA, similar clinical and microbiological cure rates were observed for both treatment arms (93.4% and 92.3% for ceftaroline vs 94.3% and 93.7% for vancomycin/aztreonam).[70]

In phase 2 and 3 comparative clinical trials for the treatment of complicated SSTIs, ceftaroline proved to be a well-tolerated drug and showed a good safety profile.[57,58] In the phase 2 study, the incidence of reported AEs was similar for both treatment groups (61.2% for ceftaroline vs 56.3% for standard therapy), with the great majority of AEs being mild in nature (87.9% for ceftaroline vs 70.8% for standard therapy). The most commonly reported ceftaroline-related AEs in this study were crystalluria (9% for ceftaroline vs 15.6% for standard therapy) and elevated serum creatinine phosphokinase levels (7.5% for ceftaroline and 6.3% for standard therapy).[57] In the phase 3 studies, both treatment arms had comparable rates of any reported AE after starting therapy (44.7% for ceftaroline vs 47.5% for standard therapy). Similar to the phase 2 study, the majority of AEs were mild in nature. The most commonly reported study-drug related AEs were nausea (5.9% vs 5.1%), diarrhea (4.9% vs 3.8%), and pruritus (3.5% vs 8.2%) in the ceftaroline and standard therapy arms respectively.[70]

An integrated analysis of two phase 3 clinical trials comparing ceftaroline to ceftriaxone for the treatment of community-acquired pneumonia (CAP) in hospitalized (non-ICU) patients, demonstrated that clinical cure rates were comparable between both treatment arms in the clinically evaluable patients (84.3% vs 77.7% respectively). The per-patient microbiological cure rates were 87% and 81% for ceftaroline and standad therapy respectively. Furthermore, clinical cure rates in microbiologically evaluable patients infected with non-MDR *Streptococcus pneumoniae*, MDR *Streptococcus pneumoniae*, or MSSA were 85.7%, 100%, and 72% for ceftaroline compared to 69.5%, 25%, and 55.6% for standard therapy respectively. No conclusions could be reached regarding efficacy of ceftaroline for the treatment of CAP due to MRSA as patients with suspected or documented infection with this pathogen were excluded from the study.[71]

Ceftaroline was well tolerated in both phase 3 CAP studies and had comparable incidence of any AE to ceftriaxone (47% vs 45.7%), most of which were mild in nature. The most commonly reported AEs in the ceftaroline arm compared to the standard therapy arm were diarrhea (4.2% vs 2.6%), headache (3.4% vs 1.5%), and insomnia (3.1% vs 2.3%). There were no differences between treatment arms with regards to other relatively infrequent AEs, including QT-interval, hepatobiliary, renal, and/or hematologic abnormalities.[71]

Based on the aforementioned studies, the FDA approved ceftaroline fosamil for the treatment of acute bacterial SSTI and CAP in adult patients ≥18 years-old. A prospective randomized study that will assess the efficacy of ceftaroline for the treatment of CAP in patients at high risk for MRSA should be scheduled to start by the end of

2011.[75] There is also preliminary in-vitro and in-vivo animal model data emerging on the potential use of NXL-104, a new experimental β-lactamase inhibitor, in combination with ceftaroline for the treatment of infections due to ESBL, AmpC β-lactamase, and KPC-enzyme producing Enterobacteriaceae.[76–81] Phase 1 trials using this combination are currently in development.[82]

CEFEPIME

This section on cefepime summarizes recent data from two comprehensive meta-analyses that put into question the safety and efficacy of cefepime and led to an FDA review regarding possible increased mortality risk from the use of cefepime.[83,84] This section also highlights reports of side effects such as neurotoxicity in the setting of renal failure.[85–87]

Since its introduction into clinical use more than a decade ago, cefepime, which is a broad-spectrum, antipseudomonal, fourth generation oxyimino-cephalosporin, has been one of the first-line agents for the empiric treatment of patients who have neutropenic fever. It is currently FDA approved for the treatment of moderate to severe pneumonia, uncomplicated and complicated UTIs, complicated IAIs, and uncomplicated SSTIs caused by susceptible bacteria.[87] Given its broad spectrum of antimicrobial activity, its stability in the face of inducible β-lactamases, and its higher threshold for selection of hyperproducing strains of chromosomally mediated β-lactamases, cefepime has been considered an appropriate agent for the treatment of severe gram-negative infections.[88–90] In addition, it also has superior activity against *Streptococcus pneumoniae* and staphylococci (methicillin-sensitive strains) compared with other extended-spectrum late-generation cephalosporins.[91–93] Cefepime has been for the most part a fairly well-tolerated drug, with most reported AEs being categorized as mild and statistically similar to those for the comparator arms in phase 3 clinical trials.[94] In addition, it has a low incidence of allergic cross-reactivity with penicillin and ceftazidime because of its unique side chain structure.[95] A comprehensive review of cefepime's dosing regimens, pharmacodynamic and pharmacokinetic properties, metabolism and elimination, and spectrum of antimicrobial coverage has been published in *Infectious Disease Clinics of North America*.[96]

In 2002, the FDA reviewed data submitted by the manufacturer of cefepime and approved an addition to cefepime's label warning about the increased risk for neurotoxicity, especially in the setting of renal failure.[86] The data were based on postmarketing reports that included episodes of encephalopathy, myoclonus, and seizures. Most of these cases were in patients who had renal dysfunction for whom administered doses exceeded recommendations. Some events, however, were also reported in patients who received renal-adjusted doses of cefepime. Discontinuation of the offending drug, or hemodialysis in some cases, led to resolution of symptoms in most patients.[85–87]

Recent data from two comprehensive systematic reviews and meta-analyses of randomized controlled trials, both from the same group, have put into question cefepime's efficacy and safety compared with that of other broad-spectrum β-lactams.[83,84] The first meta-analysis reviewed the results of 33 studies to determine if the outcomes of patients who had neutropenic fever were influenced by the choice of initial empiric β-lactam therapy.[83] The primary outcome was all-cause mortality assessed at 30 days posttreatment. The results showed that patients who received cefepime (17 trials, n = 3,123 patients) had a higher and more statistically significant 30 day all-cause mortality compared with patients who received other antipseudomonal β-lactams (*P* = .02). However, no significant differences were noted with regard to secondary outcomes analyzed, such as treatment failure, microbiological failure, infection-related mortality, antibiotic modification, addition of vancomycin, addition of antifungal agents, bacterial superinfections, any other superinfections, or AEs. The authors of that study compared piperacillin-tazobactam with cefepime (4 trials) and found no differences· in all-cause mortality. However, they stated that the latter results were hampered by a lack of substantial methodologic data that would allow definitive conclusions for this particular analysis.[83]

The second meta-analysis, by Yahav and colleagues,[84] reviewed the results of 57 studies in which cefepime was compared with other β-lactams to assess all-cause mortality at 30 days posttreatment as the primary outcome. Randomized trials were subdivided based on the comparator drug used and the type of infection for which the patient was being treated. Similar to the first meta-analysis, the authors found that in the 41 studies (38 of which were clinical trials) for which all-cause mortality was available, patients treated using cefepime had an overall higher and more statistically significant all-cause mortality compared with patients treated using other β-lactams, despite similar baseline risk factors for mortality ($P = .005$). This difference was most significant when cefepime was compared with piperacillin-tazobactam (relative risk [RR] 2.14; $P = .01$), but it was seen for all comparator drugs. The authors also concluded that except for cases of UTIs, all-cause mortality was higher for cefepime than for the comparator drugs with regard to the type of infection being treated.[84]

Yahav and colleagues offered some possible explanations for their findings. First, they stated that cefepime-induced neurotoxicity may have been underrecognized in the pool of patients that was analyzed, which in turn may have contributed to the overall higher all-cause mortality observed. Second, they argued that other factors such as inoculum, inadequate targeted-tissue concentrations, and pharmacodynamics (intermittent vs continuous cefepime dosing) may have played a role in the results.[83,84]

These reports have some limitations, however. In particular, complete all-cause mortality results were lacking in some of the trials analyzed, and potential patient selection bias might not have been fully accounted for in the meta-analysis. The FDA further reviewed the safety data on cefepime and requested support from Bristol-Meyers Squibb (BMS), the manufacturer of cefepime (Maxipime), with the goal of reaching a conclusion and releasing further recommendations to the public.[97,98] On June 17, 2009 the FDA released a communication stating its conclusions regarding the use of cefepime for its approved indications. The FDA performed its own meta-analysis that included both trial- and patient-level data from 88 clinical trials. This meta-analysis included the 38 clinical trials reported in the meta-analysis by Yahav et al, but also an additional 50 clinical trials which were not included in the latter. The total number of patients included in the FDA meta-analysis was 9,467 and 8,288 for the cefepime and comparator-treatment arms respectively. Results from the trial-level meta-analysis demonstrated that there was no statistically significant difference in the 30 day all cause mortality between cefepime and comparator-treated patients (6.21% vs 6.00%; adjusted risk difference 5.38 / 1000 population, 95% CI: −1.53 – 12.28). The FDA also found no statistically significant difference in 30 day all cause mortality when it analyzed patient-level data from 35 clinical trials (5.63% vs 5.68%; adjusted risk difference 4.83 / 1000 population, 95% CI: −4.72 – 14.38). Finally, a meta-analysis from trial-level data obtained from 24 febrile neutropenia trials failed to demonstrate a statistically significant increase in mortality associated with the use of cefepime (adjusted risk difference 9.67 / 1000 population, 95% CI: −2.87 – 22.21). Further investigations by the FDA revealed that according to patient-level data from 7 comparative febrile neutropenia trials, the majority of deaths in cefepime-treated patients could be attributed to underlying co-morbidities. Therefore, based on all these findings, the FDA concluded that cefepime should remain an appropriate treatment option for patients with approved indications for its use. Nevertheless, both the FDA and BMS will continue to perform independent safety reviews on the drug based on hospital utilization data.[99]

SUMMARY

The advent and approval of ceftaroline, a cephalosporin with anti-MRSA activity, is an exciting new development. MRSA is a major and growing problem in infectious diseases, and the addition of cephalosporins with activity against this organism will be greeted with high anticipation. The combination of ceftaroline with the new β-lactamase inhibitor NXL-104, also brings about much interest as it pertains to enhanced activity against ESBL and KPC-enzyme producing strains of Enterobacteriaceae. On the other hand, despite recent setbacks in its approval process at the FDA, ceftobiprole may one day still become available to clinicians and find its role in the treatment of serious infections due to MRSA and susceptible gram-negative organisms. Doripenem is also a welcome addition to the carbapenems, and its use will most likely mirror that of meropenem. Despite the fact the in vitro results seem to suggest that doripenem may retain activity against some carbapenem-resistant strains of P aeruginosa, it is not clear whether this has any in vivo clinical relevance. Nevertheless, more clinical data is needed regarding the use of prolonged-infusion doripenem for the treatment of serious infections due to MDR gram negative organisms, including carbapenem-resistant strains. Also, we are awaiting the final decision by the FDA regarding final approval of doripenem for the treatment of HAP and VAP. The authors of this article hope that future phase 3 clinical trials will help expand potential FDA-approved indications for these and any other upcoming β-lactams that might be in the early stages of development. Finally, the FDA updated its recommendations regarding cefepime. There were no statistically significant differences in 30 day all cause mortality between the cefepime and comparator treatment arms. Based on these findings, the FDA issued a statement that cefepime should retain its status as a treatment option for already approved indications, including the treatment of neutropenic fever.

REFERENCES

1. Ortho-McNeil Pharmaceutical. Doribax (doripenem) package insert. Raritan (NJ): Ortho-McNeil Pharmaceutical; 2007.
2. Davies T, Shang W, Bush K, et al. Affinity of doripenem and comparators to penicillin-binding proteins in Escherichia coli and Pseudomonas aeruginosa. Antimicrob Agents Chemother 2008;52:1510–2.
3. Bhavnani SM, Hammel JP, Cirincione BB, et al. Use of pharmacokinetic–pharmacodynamic target attainment analyses to support phase 2 and 3 dosing strategies for doripenem. Antimicrob Agents Chemother 2005;49:3944–7.
4. Iso Y, Irie T, Nishino Y, et al. A novel 1 ß-methylcarbapenem antibiotic, S-4661. Synthesis and structure-activity relationships of 2-(5-substituted pyrrolidin-3-ylthio)-1 ß-methylcarbapenems. J Antibiot 1996;49:199–209.
5. Rogers JD, Meisinger MA, Ferber F, et al. Pharmacokinetics of imipenem and cilastatin in volunteers. Rev Infect Dis 1985;7(Suppl 3):S435–46.
6. Moon YSK, Chung KC, Gill MA. Pharmacokinetics of meropenem in animals, healthy volunteers, and patients. Clin Infect Dis 1997;24(Suppl 2):S249–55.
7. Greer ND. Doripenem (Doribax): the newest addition to the carbapenems. Proc (Bayl Univ Med Cent) 2008;21:337–41.

8. Cirillo I, Mannens G, Janssen C, et al. The disposition, metabolism, and excretion of 14C-doripenem after a single 500-mg intravenous infusion in healthy men. Antimicrob Agents Chemother 2008;52:3478–83.

9. Lister PD. Carbapenems in the USA: focus on doripenem. Expert Rev Anti Infect Ther 2007;5:793–809.

10. Cirillo I, Vaccaro N, Balis D, et al. Influence of continuous venovenous hemofiltration and continuous venovenous hemodiafiltration on the disposition of doripenem. Antimicrob Agents Chemother 2011;55:1187–93.

11. Fritsche TR, Stilwell MG, Jones RN. Antimicrobial activity of doripenem (S-4661): a global surveillance report (2003). Clin Microbiol Infect 2005;11:974–84.

12. Ge Y, Wikler MA, Sahm DF, et al. In vitro antimicrobial activity of doripenem, a new carbapenem. Antimicrob Agents Chemother 2004;48:1384–96.

13. Tsuji M, Ishii Y, Ohno A, et al. In vitro and in vivo antibacterial activities of S-4661, a new carbapenem. Antimicrob Agents Chemother 1998;42:94–9.

14. Jones RN, Huynh HK, Biedenbach DJ, et al. Doripenem (S-4661), a novel carbapenem: comparative activity against contemporary pathogens including bactericidal action and preliminary in vitro methods evaluations. J Antimicrob Chemother 2004;54:144–54.

15. Jones RN, Huynh HK, Biedenbach DJ. Activities of doripenem (S-4661) against drug-resistant clinical pathogens. Antimicrob Agents Chemother 2004;48:3136–40.

16. Wexler HM, Engel AE, Glass D, et al. In vitro activities of doripenem and comparator agents against 364 anaerobic clinical isolates. Antimicrob Agents Chemother 2005;49:4413–7.

17. Mushtaq S, Ge Y, Livermore DM. Doripenem versus *Pseudomonas aeruginosa* in vitro: activity against characterized isolates, mutants, and transconjugants and resistance selection potential. Antimicrob Agents Chemother 2004;48:3086–92.

18. Sakyo S, Tomita H, Tanimoto K, et al. Potency of carbapenems for the prevention of carbapenem-resistant mutants of *Pseudomonas aeruginosa*. J Antibiot (Tokyo) 2006;59:220–8.

19. Kohler T, Michea-Hamzehpour M, Epp SF, et al. Carbapenem activities against *Pseudomonas aeruginosa*: respective contributions of OprD and efflux systems. Antimicrob Agents Chemother 1999;43:424–7.

20. Livermore DM. Of *Pseudomonas aeruginosa*, porins, pumps, and carbapenems. J Antimicrob Chemother 2001;47:247–50.

21. Masuda N, Sakagawa E, Ohya S, et al. Substrate specificities of MexAB-OprM, MexCD-OprJ, and MexXY-OprM efflux pumps in *Pseudomonas aeruginosa*. Antimicrob Agents Chemother 2000;44:3322–7.

22. Carmeli Y, Troillet N, Eliopoulos GM, et al. Emergence of antibiotic-resistant *Pseudomonas aeruginosa*: comparison of risks associated with different antipseudomonal agents. Antimicrob Agents Chemother 1999;43:1379–82.

23. Lucasti C, Jasovich A, Umeh O, et al. Efficacy and tolerability of IV doripenem versus meropenem in adults with complicated intra-abdominal infection: a phase III, prospective, multicenter, randomized, double-blind, noninferiority study. Clin Ther 2008;30:868–83.

24. Naber KG, Llorens L, Kaniga K, et al. Intravenous doripenem at 500 milligrams versus levofloxacin at 250 milligrams, with an option to switch to oral therapy, for treatment of complicated lower urinary tract infection and pyelonephritis. Antimicrob Agents Chemother 2009;53:3782–92.

25. Rea-Neto A, Niederman M, Lobo SM, et al. Efficacy and safety of intravenous doripenem vs piperacillin/tazobactam in nosocomial pneumonia: a randomized, open-label, multicenter study. Curr Med Res Opin 2008;24:2113–26.

26. Chastre J, Wunderink R, Prokocimer P, et al. Efficacy and safety of intravenous infusion of doripenem versus imipenem in ventilator-associated pneumonia: a multicenter, randomized study. Crit Care Med 2008;36:1089–96.
27. Norrby SR. Neurotoxicity of carbapenem antibacterials. Drug Saf 1996;15:87–90.
28. Horiuchi M, Kimura M, Tokumura M, et al. Absence of convulsive liability of doripenem, a new carbapenem antibiotic, in comparison with β-lactam antibiotics. Toxicology 2006;222:114–24.
29. U.S. Food and Drug Administration. Center for Drug Evaluation and Research. New Drug Application (NDA), Doripenem powder reconstitution and intravenous administration, Johnson & Johnson Pharmaceutical Research and Development, LLC., proposed for treatment of nosocomial pneumonia, including ventilator associated pneumonia. Available at: http://www.fda.gov/ohrms/dockets/ac/08/minutes/2008-4364m1-Final.pdf. Accessed April 11, 2011.
30. Bulik CC, Nicolau DP. In vivo efficacy of simulated human dosing regimens of prolonged-infusion doripenem against carbapenemase-producing Klebsiella pneumoniae. Antimicrob Agents Chemother 2010;54:4112–5.
31. Apisarnthanarak A, Mundy LM. Use of high-dose 4-hour infusion of doripenem, in combination with fosfomycin, for treatment of carbapenem-resistant Pseudomonas aeruginosa Pneumonia. Clin Infect Dis 2010;51:1352–4.
32. Chambers HF. The changing epidemiology of Staphylococcus aureus? Emerg Infect Dis 2001;7:178–82.
33. Livermore DM. Can beta-lactams be re-engineered to beat MRSA? Clin Microbiol Infect 2006;12(Suppl 2):11–6.
34. De Lecastre H, De Jonge BL, Matthews PR, et al. Molecular aspects of methicillin resistance in Staphylococcus aureus. J Antimicrob Chemother 1994;33:7–24.
35. Anderson SD, Gums JG. Ceftobiprole: an extended-spectrum anti-methicillin resistant Staphylococcus aureus cephalosporin. Ann Pharmacother 2008;42:806–16.
36. Adis R&D profile. Ceftobiprole medocaril. Drugs R D 2006;7:305–11.
37. Chambers HF. Solving staphylococcal resistance to beta-lactams. Trends Microbiol 2003;11:145–8.
38. Davies TA, Page MG, Shang W, et al. Binding of ceftobiprole and comparators to the penicillin-binding proteins of Escherichia coli, Pseudomonas aeruginosa, Staphylococcus aureus, and Streptococcus pneumoniae. Antimicrob Agents Chemother 2007;51:2621–4.
39. Georgopapadakou NH. Penicillin-binding proteins and bacterial resistance to β-lactams. Antimicrob Agents Chemother 1993;37:2045–53.
40. Basilea Pharmaceutica Ltd. Press Release: Ceftobiprole, a new anti-MRSA broad-spectrum antibiotic, receives its first marketing authorization by Health Canada. Available at: http://www.basilea.com/News-and-Media/Ceftobiprole-a-new-anti-MRSA-broad-spectrum-antibiotic-receives-its-first-marketing-authorization-by-Health-Canada/189. Accessed March 31, 2011.
41. Basilea Pharmaceutica Ltd. Press Release: Ceftobiprole, a new anti-MRSA broad-spectrum antibiotic, receives approval by Swissmedic. Available at: http://www.basilea.com/News-and-Media/Ceftobiprole-a-new-anti-MRSA-broad-spectrum-antibiotic-receives-approval-by-Swissmedic/219. Accessed March 31, 2011.
42. Basilea Pharmaceutica Ltd. Press Release: FDA issues Approvable Letter for ceftobiprole, a new anti-MRSA broad-spectrum antibiotic. Available at: http://www.basilea.com/News-and-Media/FDA-issues-Approvable-Letter-for-ceftobiprole-a-new-anti-MRSA-broad-spectrum-antibiotic/172. Accessed March 31, 2011.

43. Murthy B, Schmitt-Hoffman A. Pharmacokinetics and pharmacodynamics of ceftobiprole, an anti-MRSA cephalosporin with broad-spectrum activity. Clin Pharmacokinet 2008;47:21–33.
44. Lodise TP, Patel N, Renaud-Mutart A, et al. Pharmacokinetic and pharmacodynamic profile of ceftobiprole. Diagn Microbiol Infect Dis 2008;61:96–102.
45. Lodise TP, Pypstra R, Kahn JB, et al. Probability of target attainment for ceftobiprole as derived from a population pharmacokinetic analysis of 150 subjects. Antimicrob Agents Chemother 2007;51:2378–87.
46. Mouton JW, Schmitt-Hoffman A, Shapiro S, et al. Use of Monte Carlo simulations to select therapeutic doses and provisional breakpoints of BAL9141. Antimicrob Agents Chemother 2004;48:1713–8.
47. Noel GJ, Strauss RS, Amsler K, et al. Results of a double-blind, randomized trial of ceftobiprole treatment of complicated skin and skin structure infections caused by gram-positive bacteria. Antimicrob Agents Chemother 2008;52:37–44.
48. Noel GJ, Bush K, Bagchi P, et al. A randomized double-blind trial comparing ceftobiprole medocaril to vancomycin plus ceftazidime in the treatment of patients with complicated skin and skin structure infections. Clin Infect Dis 2008;46:647–55.
49. Fritsche TR, Sader HS, Jones RN. Antimicrobial activity of ceftobiprole, a novel anti-methicillin–resistant *Staphylococcus aureus* cephalosporin, tested against contemporary pathogens: results from the SENTRY antimicrobial surveillance program (2005–2006). Diagn Microbiol Infect Dis 2008;61:86–95.
50. Arias CA, Singh KV, Panesso D, et al. Time-kill and synergism studies of ceftobiprole against *Enterococcus faecalis*, including β-lactamase–producing and vancomycin-resistant isolates. Antimicrob Agents Chemother 2007;51:2043–7.
51. Goldstein EJ, Citron DM, Merriam CV, et al. In vitro activity of ceftobiprole against aerobic and anaerobic strains isolated from diabetic foot infections. Antimicrob Agents Chemother 2006;50:3959–62.
52. Queenan AM, Shang W, Kania M, et al. Interactions of ceftobiprole with β-lactamases from molecular classes A to D. Antimicrob Agents Chemother 2007;51:3089–95.
53. Chambers HF. Evaluation of ceftobiprole in a rabbit model of aortic valve endocarditis due to methicillin-resistant and vancomycin-intermediate *Staphylococcus aureus*. Antimicrob Agents Chemother 2005;49:884–8.
54. Yin LY, Calhoun JH, Thomas JK, et al. Efficacies of ceftobiprole medocaril and comparators in a rabbit model of osteomyelitis due to methicillin-resistant *Staphylococcus aureus*. Antimicrob Agents Chemother 2008;52:1618–22.
55. Laohavaleeson S, Tessier PR, Nicolau DP. Pharmacodynamic characterization of ceftobiprole in experimental pneumonia caused by phenotypically diverse *Staphylococcus aureus* strains. Antimicrob Agents Chemother 2008;52:2389–94.
56. National Institute of Health. ClinicalTrials.gov. Available at: http://clinicaltrials.gov/ct2/results?term=ceftobiprole&recr. Accessed April 12, 2011.
57. Johnson & Johnson Pharmaceutical Research & Development, L.L.C. Press Release: FDA Issues Complete Response Letter for Ceftobiprole for Treatment of Complicated Skin Infections. Available at: http://www.jnj.com/connect/news/all/20081126_011500. Accessed March 31,2011.
58. Basilea Pharmaceutica Ltd. Press Release: FDA issues ceftobiprole Complete Response Letter. Available at: http://www.basilea.com/News-and-Media/FDA-issues-ceftobiprole-complete-Response-letter/317. Accessed March 31, 2011.
59. Basilea Pharmaceutica Ltd. Press Release: European CHMP concludes re-examination of ceftobiprole. Available at: http://www.basilea.com/News-and-Media/

European-CHMP-concludes-re-examination-of-ceftobiprole/365. Accessed March 31, 2011.

60. Basilea Pharmaceutica Ltd. Press Release: Discontinuation of sale of ceftobiprole in Canada. Available at: http://www.basilea.com/News-and-Media/Discontinuation-of-the-sale-of-ceftobiprole-in-Canada/349. Accessed March 31, 2011.

61. Basilea Pharmaceutica Ltd. Press Release: Discontinuation of sale of ceftobiprole in Switzerland. Available at: http://www.basilea.com/News-and-Media/Discontinuation-of-sale-of-ceftobiprole-in-Switzerland/373. Accessed March 31, 2011.

62. Ishikawa T, Matsunaga N, Tawada H, et al. TAK-599, a novel n-phosphono type prodrug of anti-MRSA cephalosporin T-91825: synthesis, physicochemical and pharmacological properties. Bioorg Med Chem 2003;11:2427–37.

63. Iizawa Y, Nagai J, Ishikawa T, et al. In vitro antimicrobial activity of T-91825, a novel anti-MRSA cephalosporin, and in vivo anti-MRSA activity of its prodrug, TAK-599. J Infect Chemother 2004;10:146–56.

64. Andes D, Craig WA. Pharmacodynamics of a new cephalosporin, PPI-0903 (TAK-599), active against methicillin-resistant *Staphylococcus aureus* in murine thigh and lung infection models: identification of an in vivo pharmacokinetic–pharmacodynamic target. Antimicrob Agents Chemother 2006;50:1376–83.

65. Jacqueline C, Caillon J, Le Mabecque V, et al. In vivo efficacy of ceftaroline (PPI-0903), a new broad-spectrum cephalosporin, compared with linezolid and vancomycin against methicillin-resistant and vancomycin-intermediate *Staphylococcus aureus* in a rabbit endocarditis model. Antimicrob Agents Chemother 2007;51:3397–400.

66. Ge Y, Hubbel A. Poster A-1935, 46th Intersci Conf Antimicrob Agents Chemother 2006.

67. Ge Y, Liao S, Talbot GH. Poster A-34, 47th Intersci Conf Antimicrob Agents Chemother 2007.

68. Ge Y, Liao S, Thye DA, et al. Poster A-35, 47th Intersci Conf Antimicrob Agents Chemother 2007.

69. Talbot GH, Thye D, Das A, et al. Phase 2 study of ceftaroline versus standard therapy in treatment of complicated skin and skin structure infections. Antimicrob Agents Chemother 2007;51:3612–6.

70. Corey GR, Wilcox M, Talbot GH, et al. Integrated analysis of CANVAS 1 and 2: phase 3, multicenter, randomized, double-blind studies to evaluate the safety and efficacy of ceftaroline versus vancomycin plus Aztreonam in complicated skin and skin-structure infection. Clin Infect Dis 2010;51:641–50.

71. File TM Jr, Low DE, Eckburg PB, et al. Integrated Analysis of FOCUS 1 and FOCUS 2: randomized, double-blinded, multicenter Phase 3 Trials of the efficacy and safety of ceftaroline fosamil versus Ceftriaxone in patients with community-acquired pneumonia. Clin Infect Dis 2010;51:1395–405.

72. Physicians Desk Reference information for ceftaroline. Available at: http://www.pdr.net/drugpages/productlabeling.aspx?mpcode=30600138#section-3. Accessed April 14, 2011.

73. Sader HS, Fritsche TR, Kaniga K, et al. Antimicrobial activity and spectrum of PPI-0903M (T-91825), a novel cephalosporin, tested against a worldwide collection of clinical strains. Antimicrob Agents Chemother 2005;49:3501–12.

74. Ge Y, Biek D, Talbot GH, et al. In vitro profiling of ceftaroline against a collection of recent bacterial clinical isolates from across the United States. Antimicrob Agents Chemother 2008;52:3398–407.

75. U.S. Food and Drug Administration. Center for Drug Evaluation and Research. Application Number: 200327. NDA Approval Letter. Available at: http://www.accessdata.

fda.gov/drugsatfda_docs/appletter/2010/200327s000ltr.pdf. Accessed April 9, 2011.

76. Badal R, Bouchillon S, Hackel M, et al. Poster E-804, 50th Interscience Conference on Antimicrobial Agents and Chemotherapy 2010.

77. Sader HS, Castanheira M, Farrell DJ, et al. Poster E-821, 50th Interscience Conference on Antimicrobial Agents and Chemotherapy 2010.

78. Bowker K, Noel A, Elliott H, et al. Poster A1-1377, 50th Interscience Conference on Antimicrobial Agents and Chemotherapy 2010.

79. Craig WA, Andes DR. Poster A1-1378, 50th Intersci Conf Antimicrob Agents Chemother 2010.

80. Wiskirchen DE, Crandon JL, Furtado GH, et al. Poster A1-1379, 50th Interscience Conference on Antimicrobial Agents and Chemotherapy 2010.

81. Wiskirchen DE, Crandon JL, Williams G, et al. Poster A1-1380, 50th Interscience Conference on Antimicrobial Agents and Chemotherapy 2010.

82. National Institute of Health. ClinicalTrials.gov. Available at: http://www.clinicaltrials.gov/ct2/results?term=ceftaroline&recr. Accessed April 13, 2011.

83. Paul M, Yahav D, Fraser A, et al. Empirical antibiotic monotherapy for febrile neutropenia: systematic review and meta-analysis of randomized controlled trials. J Antimicrob Chemother 2006;57:176–89.

84. Yahav D, Paul M, Fraser A, et al. Efficacy and safety of cefepime: a systematic review and meta-analysis. Lancet Infect Dis 2007;7:338–48.

85. B. Braun Medical Inc. Y36-002-592: cefepime for injection; proposed package insert. issued:xxx. Available at: http://www.fda.gov/OHRMS/DOCKETS/dockets/06p0461/06p-0461-cp00001-04-attachment-03-vol1.pdf. Accessed December 7, 2008.

86. U.S. Food and Drug Administration. FDA drug warning. NDA 50–679/S-009, S-0014, and S-018. Available at: http://www.fda.gov/cder/foi/appletter/2002/50679slr009,014,018ltr.pdf. Accessed October 13, 2008.

87. Bristol-Myers Squibb. Maxipime (cefepime) package insert. Princeton (NJ): Bristol-Myers Squibb; 2007.

88. Sanders CC. Cefepime: the next generation? Clin Infect Dis 1993;17:369–79.

89. Sanders WE Jr, Tenney JH, Kessler RE. Efficacy of cefepime in the treatment of infections due to multiply resistant *Enterobacter* species. Clin Infect Dis 1996;23:454–61.

90. Acar J. Rapid emergence of resistance to cefepime during treatment. Clin Infect Dis 1998;26:1484–6.

91. Wynd MA, Paladino JA. Cefepime: a fourth generation parenteral cephalosporin. Ann Pharmacother 1996;30:1414–24.

92. Kessler RE, Bies M, Buck RE, et al. Comparison of a new cephalosporin, BMY-28142, with other broad spectrum beta-lactam antibiotics. Antimicrob Agents Chemother 1985;27:207–16.

93. Conrad DA, Scribner RK, Weber AH, et al. In vitro activity of BMY-28142 against pediatric pathogens, including isolates from cystic fibrosis sputum. Antimicrob Agents Chemother 1985;28:58–63.

94. Neu HC. Safety of cefepime: a new extended-spectrum parenteral cephalosporin. Am J Med 1996;100(6A):68S–75S.

95. Pichichero ME. Use of selected cephalosporins in penicillin-allergic patients: a paradigm shift. Diagn Microbiol Infect Dis 2007;57(Suppl 3):S13–8.

96. Martin SI, Kaye KM. Beta-lactam antibiotics: newer formulations and newer agents. Infect Dis Clin North Am 2004;18:603–19.

97. U.S. Food and Drug Administration. Early communication about ongoing safety review: cefepime (marketed as Maxipime). Available at: http://www.fda.gov/cder/drug/early_comm/cefepime.htm. Accessed October 19, 2008.

98. U.S. Food and Drug Administration. Update of safety review: follow-up to the November 14, 2007, communication about the ongoing safety review of cefepime (marketed as Maxipime). Available at: http://www.fda.gov/cder/drug/early_comm/cefepime_update_200805.htm. Accessed October 19, 2008.

99. U.S. Food and Drug Administration. FDA Alert June 17, 2009; Information for Healthcare Professionals: Cefepime (marketed as Maxipime). Available at: http://www.fda.gov/Drugs/DrugSafety/PostmarketDrugSafetyInformationforPatientsandProviders/DrugSafetyInformationforHeathcareProfessionals/ucm167254.htm. Accessed April 15, 2011.

Review of Macrolides (Azithromycin, Clarithromycin), Ketolids (Telithromycin) and Glycylcyclines (Tigecycline)

Jerry M. Zuckerman, MD[a,b,*], Fozia Qamar, MD[c,d],
Bartholomew R. Bono, MD[a,e]

KEYWORDS

- Macrolides • Ketolides • Glycylcyclines
- Antimicrobials • Review

Erythromycin, the first macrolide antibiotic discovered, has been used since the early 1950s for the treatment of upper respiratory tract and skin and soft tissue infections caused by susceptible organisms, especially in patients who are allergic to penicillin. Several drawbacks, however, have limited the use of erythromycin, including frequent gastrointestinal intolerance and a short serum half-life. Advanced macrolide antimicrobials synthesized by altering the erythromycin base have resulted in compounds with broader activity, more favorable pharmacokinetics and pharmacodynamics, and better tolerability. Two of these agents, clarithromycin (Biaxin) and azithromycin (Zithromax) have been used extensively for the treatment of respiratory tract

A version of this article appeared in the 23:4 issue of the *Infectious Disease Clinics of North America*.
[a] Jefferson Medical College, 1025 Walnut Street, Philadelphia, PA 19107, USA
[b] Division of Infectious Diseases, Department of Medicine, Albert Einstein Medical Center, Klein Building, Suite 331, 5501 Old York Road, Philadelphia, PA 19141, USA
[c] University of Massachusetts Medical School, 55 Lake Avenue North, Worcester, MA 01655, USA
[d] Department of Medicine, UMass Medical Memorial Center, Benedict Building, 55 Lake Avenue North, Worcester, MA 01655, USA
[e] Bryn Mawr Medical Specialists Association, 933 Haverford Road, Bryn Mawr, PA 19010, USA
* Corresponding author. Division of Infectious Diseases, Department of Medicine, Albert Einstein Medical Center, Klein Building, Suite 331, 5501 Old York Road, Philadelphia, PA 19141.
E-mail address: zuckermj@einstein.edu

Med Clin N Am 95 (2011) 761–791
doi:10.1016/j.mcna.2011.03.012
0025-7125/11/$ – see front matter © 2011 Elsevier Inc. All rights reserved.

medical.theclinics.com

infections, sexually transmitted diseases, and infections caused by *Helicobacter pylori* and *Mycobacterium avium* complex (MAC).

Ketolides share many of the characteristics of the advanced macrolides. Their in vitro spectrum of activity also includes gram-positive organisms (*Streptococcus pneumoniae, Streptococcus pyogenes*) that are macrolide resistant. Telithromycin (Ketek), specifically developed for the treatment of respiratory tract infections, received FDA approval in 2004. In 2007, because of increasing reports of hepatotoxicity, the FDA withdrew two of telithromycin's treatment indications, limiting its approval to the treatment of mild to moderate community-acquired pneumonia.

Glycylcyclines are a class of antimicrobial agents developed to overcome tetracycline-specific resistance mechanisms (efflux pumps and ribosomal protection). Tigecycline (Tygacil), a derivative of minocycline, is the first antimicrobial in this class to receive FDA approval. Tigecycline is active in vitro against a broad spectrum of bacteria, including multidrug-resistant (MDR) organisms, and is indicated for the treatment of complicated skin and skin structure infections, complicated intra-abdominal infections and community-acquired pneumonia. This article reviews the pharmacokinetics, antimicrobial activity, clinical use, and adverse effects of these antimicrobial agents.

CHEMISTRY

Erythromycin's structure consists of a macrocyclic 14-membered lactone ring attached to two sugar moieties (a neutral sugar, cladinose, and an amino sugar, desosamine). In the acidic environment of the stomach, it is rapidly degraded to the 8,9-anhydro-6,9-hemiketal and then to the 6,9,9,12-spiroketal form. The hemiketal intermediate may be responsible for the gastrointestinal adverse effects associated with erythromycin.[1]

Clarithromycin (6-O-methylerythromycin) is synthesized by substituting a methoxy group for the C-6 hydroxyl group of erythromycin. This substitution creates a more acid-stable antimicrobial and prevents the degradation of the erythromycin base to the hemiketal intermediate, which results in improved oral bioavailability and reduced gastrointestinal intolerance.[2] Clarithromycin is available as immediate-release tablets (250 or 500 mg), extended-release tablets (500 mg), and granules for oral suspension (125 or 250 mg/5 mL).

Azithromycin (9-deoxo-9a-aza-9a-methyl-9a-homoerythromycin) is formed by inserting a methyl-substituted nitrogen in place of the carbonyl group at the 9a position of the aglycone ring. The resulting dibasic 15-membered ring macrolide derivative is more appropriately referred to as an azalide. This change produces a compound that is more acid stable and has a longer serum half-life ($t_{1/2}$), increased tissue penetration, and greater activity against gram-negative organisms compared with erythromycin.[2] Azithromycin is available as 250-, 500- or 600-mg immediate-release tablets, 2-g microsphere extended-release powder, oral suspension (100–200 mg/5 mL), and intravenous preparation (lypholized 500 mg/10 mL vial).

Ketolides are synthesized by two changes in the 14-membered erythronolide A ring: substituting a keto function for the alpha-L-cladinose moiety at position 3 and replacing the hydroxyl group at position 6 with a methoxy group.[3] These changes promote greater acid stability and prevent induction of macrolide-lincosamide-streptogramin B (MLS$_B$) resistance.[4] Telithromycin is synthesized by cycling of the C11-12 positions to form a carbamate ring with an imidazo-pyridyl group attachment that enhances binding to the bacterial ribosome and in vitro activity.[5] Telithromycin is available in 300- or 400-mg tablets.

Tigecycline is synthesized by the addition of a *tert*-butyl-glycylamido group to the C-9 position of minocycline. This addition overcomes the efflux pump and ribosomal protection mechanisms that confer resistance to tetracycline and extends its antimicrobial activity against a variety of bacteria.[6] Tigecycline is only available as an intravenous preparation (lyophilized 50 mg/vial).

MECHANISM OF ACTION AND RESISTANCE

The macrolides and ketolides are bacteriostatic antimicrobials. They reversibly bind to domain V of 23S ribosomal RNA (rRNA) of the 50s subunit of the bacterial ribosome inhibiting RNA-dependent protein synthesis.[7,8] The ketolides bind with a 10- to 100-fold higher affinity to the ribosome than erythromycin. The ketolides also have a greater affinity for binding to domain II of the 23S rRNA.[4]

Macrolide resistance in streptococci arises from either an alteration of the drug-binding site on the ribosome by methylation (MLS$_B$ resistance) or by active drug efflux. The efflux mechanism is mediated by the macrolide efflux (*mef*) genes and is specific for 14- and 15-membered macrolides.[3] Macrolide resistance is usually low level (minimum inhibitory concentrations [MICs] 1–32 mg/L), and in vitro susceptibility to ketolides, lincosamides, and streptogramins is maintained.[9] Methylation of an adenine residue in domain V of the 23S rRNA, mediated by the erythromycin ribosome methylase (*erm*) genes, prevents binding of the macrolides and ketolides to domain V and results in high level macrolide resistance (MIC $\geq$64 mg/L). Ketolides presumably maintain their antimicrobial activity by virtue of their ability to bind to an alternative site — domain II of the 23S rRNA.[10] Methylase may be either induced or constitutively expressed, and resistance to erythromycin implies cross-resistance to clarithromycin and azithromycin. Clarithromycin and azithromycin can induce methylase production but telithromycin does not.[11] Decreased susceptibility to telithromycin in streptococci has been associated with a variety of mutations in the *erm*(B) gene and its promoter region, ribosomal proteins L4 and L22, and in the 23S rRNA.[12–14]

Tigecycline is also a bacteriostatic antibiotic. It reversibly binds to the 30S ribosomal subunit inhibiting protein synthesis. Glycylcyclines bind with a fivefold higher affinity to the ribosome compared with tetracyclines.[15] This enhanced ribosomal binding enables tigecycline to overcome resistance caused by ribosomal protection. Tigecycline also maintains activity against bacteria-containing tetracycline-specific efflux pumps by failing to be recognized as a substrate.[16] Susceptibility to tigecycline is reduced, however, by the overexpression of multidrug efflux pumps (eg, MexXY, AcrAB) that may be found in gram-negative organisms. These multidrug efflux pumps are naturally expressed in *Pseudomonas aeruginosa*.[16,17] Reduced susceptibility of *Acinetobacter* spp to tigecycline has been reported in isolates with a resistance-nodulation-division-type multicomponent efflux transporter.[18]

PHARMACOKINETICS

The structural alterations to the erythromycin base used to synthesize the advanced macrolides and ketolides result in improved pharmacokinetic properties. Compared with erythromycin, clarithromycin and azithromycin are more acid stable and have greater oral bioavailability (55% and 37%, respectively).[2] The peak plasma concentration of clarithromycin immediate-release tablets is increased by 24% when administered with food, but the overall bioavailability is unchanged.[19] The bioavailability of the extended-release formulation, however, is decreased by 30% when administered in the fasting state and should be administered with food.[20] The bioavailabilities of the tablet, sachet, or suspension formulations of azithromycin are not affected by meals.[21] The absorption of azithromycin 2-g extended-release microsphere formulation is increased with food and should be administered on an empty stomach to ensure appropriate (slower) absorption from the gastrointestinal tract.[22] Oral absorption of an 800-mg dose of telithromycin is excellent (90%); however, 33% of the dose undergoes first-pass hepatic metabolism, which results in an absolute oral bioavailability of 57%.[23] The bioavailability, rate, and extent of absorption of telithromycin are unaffected by food.[24]

The single-dose pharmacokinetics of erythromycin, clarithromycin, azithromycin, and telithromycin are summarized in **Table 1**. Several differences between the pharmacokinetics of these antimicrobials are apparent. First, the peak serum concentration (C_{max}) of azithromycin after a 500-mg dose is fivefold lower than that achieved with a comparable dose of clarithromycin or telithromycin. Although azithromycin concentrations are low in the serum, tissue concentrations are significantly higher, as discussed later. Second, the terminal half-life of azithromycin and telithromycin are long enough to allow once-daily dosing. Twice-daily dosing of the immediate-release formulation of clarithromycin is necessary based on the terminal half-life of 4 to 5 hours.[2] Protein binding is higher for clarithromycin and telithromycin (60%–70%) compared with azithromycin (7%–50%).

Clarithromycin is metabolized to an active metabolite, 14-hydroxyclarithromycin. Larger doses of clarithromycin result in nonlinear increases in the $t_{1/2}$ and in the area under the plasma concentration-time curve (AUC) of clarithromycin because of saturation of the metabolic pathway.[25] Steady-state peak plasma concentrations of 3 to 4 mg/L are achieved within 3 days with clarithromycin, 500 mg, every 8 to 12 hours and the elimination half-life increases to 5 to 7 hours.[19] Although steady-state peak plasma concentrations are lower and achieved later with the extended-release formulation of clarithromycin than a comparable daily dose of the immediate-release formulations, the 24-hour AUC is equivalent between the two formulations, supporting the once-daily dosing of the extended-release formulation.[20]

The azithromycin 2-g extended-release microsphere formulation has a slower rate of absorption compared with an equivalent dose of the immediate-release tablet, which results in a mean peak serum concentration that is 57% lower and a t_{max} that is 2.5 hours later.[22] The mean relative bioavailability of the extended-release form was 82.8%. When compared with a 3-day regimen of 500-mg azithromycin immediate-release tablets in healthy subjects, a 2-g single dose of extended-release azithromycin on day 1 had a C_{max} and 24-hour AUC that were two- and threefold higher, respectively. Overall AUC for the 5-day study period was equivalent for the two dosing regimens.[26] Daily doses of telithromycin, 800 mg, result in a steady-state peak plasma concentration of 2.27 mg/L and a terminal half-life of 9.81 hours.[27]

Table 1
Comparative pharmacokinetics of macrolide antibiotics[a]

Parameter	Erythromycin Base	Azithromycin	Clarithromycin	14-Hydroxy-Clarithromycin	Telithromycin
Bioavailability %	25	37	55	35	57
C_{max} (mg/L)	0.3–0.9	0.4	2.1–2.4	0.6	1.9–2.0
t_{max} (h)	3–4	2	2	2–3	1.0
$t_{1/2}$ (h)	2–3	40–68	3–5	4–7	7.16–13
AUC (mg/L × h)	8	3.4	19	5.7	7.9–8.25

Abbreviations: AUC, area under plasma concentration time curve; C_{max}, peak serum concentration; t_{max}, time to peak serum concentration; $t_{1/2}$, serum half-life.
[a] Mean values after a single 500-mg oral dose (800-mg dose for telithromycin).
Data from Zhanel GG, Dueck M, Hoban DJ, et al. Review of macrolides and ketolides: focus on respiratory tract infections. Drugs 2001;61(4):443–98.

Tigecycline is only available in an injectable formulation. The recommended dosage is an initial load of 100 mg, followed by a maintenance dose of 50 mg every 12 hours infused over 30 to 60 minutes. Pooled data from healthy volunteers showed that the C_{max} after a single 100-mg dose was 1.45 mg/L and 0.90 mg/L after 30- and 60-minute infusions, respectively. The C_{max} at steady state was 0.87 mg/L and 0.63 mg/L after 30- and 60-minute infusions, respectively, and the 24-hour AUC was 4.70 mg/L $\times$ h. The serum half-life was 27.1 hours after a single 100-mg dose and increased to 42.2 hours with multiple doses of 50 mg twice daily. The pharmacokinetics of tigecycline are not affected by the presence of food or differences in sex or age.[28–30]

The macrolides and ketolides are lipophilic and are extensively distributed in body fluids and tissues. Mean tissue concentrations are 2- to 20-fold greater than serum concentrations for clarithromycin and are 10- to 100-fold greater than serum concentrations for azithromycin.[31,32] Tissue concentrations do not peak until 48 hours after administration of azithromycin and persist for several days afterwards.[2] Twenty-four hours after the last dose of drug administration, concentrations of clarithromycin and azithromycin in lung epithelial cell lining fluid exceeded serum concentrations by 20-fold.[33] Measurements at this interval also revealed that alveolar macrophage concentrations were 400 times (clarithromycin) and 800 times (azithromycin) greater than their respective serum concentrations. Telithromycin also has excellent penetration into bronchopulmonary tissues. Levels in alveolar macrophages (median concentration 81 mg/L) significantly exceeded plasma levels 8 hours after dosing and maintained elevated levels 24 and 48 hours after dosing (23 mg/L and 2.15 mg/L, respectively).[34] Concentrations of telithromycin in bronchial mucosa and epithelial lining fluid exceeded for 24 hours the mean MIC_{90} of *S pneumoniae, Moraxella catarrhalis,* and *Mycoplasma pneumoniae.*[35] In these studies, 24 hours after the last dose of drug administration, concentrations of telithromycin in lung epithelial cell lining fluid were 12-fold, and in alveolar macrophages the levels were 400-fold greater than their respective serum concentrations.

Tigecycline is also distributed widely in tissues, with a steady-state volume of distribution of 7 to 10 L/kg.[30] At steady-state levels, the tigecycline $AUC_{0–12h}$ in alveolar cells and epithelial lining fluid was 78-fold higher and 32% higher compared with serum.[36] Tissue levels of tigecycline were higher in the gallbladder (38-fold), lung (8.6-fold), and colon (2.1-fold) compared with serum levels 4 hours after a single 100-mg dose. Synovial fluid and bone concentrations, however, were 0.58 and 0.35 lower, respectively, relative to serum.[37] Tissue penetration of tigecycline into skin blister fluid was 74% of serum concentration.[38]

Clarithromycin is metabolized in the liver by the cytochrome P450 3A4 (CYP3A4) enzymes to the active 14-hydroxy form and six additional products. Thirty percent to 40% of an oral dose of clarithromycin is excreted in the urine either unchanged or as the active 14-hydroxy metabolite.[39] The remainder is excreted into the bile. In patients with moderate to severe renal impairment (ie, creatinine clearance <30 mL/min), the dose should be reduced.[39] In patients with moderate to severe hepatic impairment and normal renal function, there is less metabolism of clarithromycin to the 14-hydroxy form, which results in decreased peak plasma concentrations of the metabolite and increased renal excretion of unchanged clarithromycin. Dosing modifications do not seem to be necessary for these patients.[40]

Azithromycin elimination occurs primarily in the feces as the unchanged drug, and urinary excretion is minimal.[41] Unlike clarithromycin, azithromycin does not interact with the cytochrome P450 system.[42] In patients with mild or moderate hepatic impairment, dosing modifications do not seem to be necessary.[42,43]

Telithromycin is eliminated via multiple pathways, including unchanged drug in feces (7%) and urine (13%) and the remainder via hepatic metabolism by the

CYP 3A4 and 1A isoenzymes.[44] Four metabolites of telithromycin do not have appreciable antibacterial activity.[10] Plasma concentrations and AUC were 1.4- and 1.9-fold higher in patients with creatinine clearance less than 30 mL/min. In patients with mild to moderate renal impairment, there was no significant change in the pharmacokinetics of telithromycin.[10] Dosing modifications are not necessary when administering telithromycin to patients with hepatic impairment because pharmacokinetics do not change significantly as the result of a compensatory increase in renal excretion.[45]

Tigecycline is not extensively metabolized and is primarily eliminated unchanged via biliary excretion. In healthy male volunteers who received ^{14}C-tigecycline, 59% of the radioactive dose was recovered in the feces and 33% recovered in the urine.[46] Secondary elimination pathways include renal excretion of unchanged drug and, to a lesser degree, metabolism to glucuronide conjugates and N-acetyl-9-aminominocycline. Dose adjustment is not necessary based on age, sex, renal impairment, or mild to moderate hepatic impairment (Child Pugh class A-B).[28,30] In patients with severe hepatic impairment (Child Pugh class C), the maintenance dose should be reduced by 50%.[47]

SPECTRUM OF ACTIVITY

The Clinical and Laboratory Standards Institute provides guidelines for the interpretation of in vitro MICs for clarithromycin, azithromycin, and telithromycin. The FDA established breakpoints for tigecycline (**Table 2**).[47,48] The breakpoints for azithromycin are based on expected tissue concentrations, whereas the breakpoints for clarithromycin are based on achievable serum concentrations. In vitro susceptibility testing does not account for the antimicrobial activity of the active 14-hydroxy metabolite and may underestimate the activity of clarithromycin.[49] In vitro MIC measurements also do not account for the pharmacodynamic properties of an antimicrobial (eg, tissue penetration, intracellular half-life, postantibiotic effect) and may not predict its relative efficacy at the site of infection.

Comparative in vitro susceptibility data for erythromycin, clarithromycin, azithromycin, and telithromycin are shown in **Table 3**. Compared with erythromycin, clarithromycin demonstrates equal or better in vitro activity against gram-positive organisms, whereas azithromycin is two- to fourfold less active.[53] Azithromycin and clarithromycin are generally inactive against methicillin-resistant staphylococci.

Table 2
Susceptibility test result interpretative criteria

	Clarithromycin		Azithromycin		Telithromycin		Tigecycline	
	S	R	S	R	S	R	S	R
S aureus	≤2	≥8	≤2	≥8	≤1	≥4	≤0.5	N/A
Streptococcus spp, including pneumoniae	≤0.25	≥1	≤0.50	≥2	≤1	≥4	≤0.25	N/A
Enterococcus faecalis	N/A	N/A	N/A	N/A	N/A	N/A	≤0.25	N/A
Haemophilus spp	≤8	≥32	≤4	NA	≤4	≥16	N/A	N/A
Enterobacteriaceae	N/A	N/A	N/A	N/A	N/A	N/A	≤2	≥8
Anaerobes	N/A	N/A	N/A	N/A	N/A	N/A	≤4	≥16

Values expressed as MIC (mg/L).
Data from Tygacil (tigecycline) prescribing information. Revised January, 2011; Clinical and Laboratory Standards Institute. Performance standards for antimicrobial susceptibility Testing; Twenty-First Informational Supplement; 2011.

Table 3
Comparative in vitro activities of macrolide/ketolide antibiotics*

Organism	Erythromycin	Azithromycin	Clarithromycin	Telithromycin
Gram-positive aerobes				
Streptococcus pyogenes				
erythromycin susceptible	0.06–0.12	0.12–0.25	0.06–0.12	0.03
*erm*A resistance	1–32	16–32	2–16	0.015–0.25
*erm*B resistance	>64	>64	>64	>8
*mef*A resistance	8–16	8	8–16	0.25–1
Streptococcus pneumoniae				
erythromycin sensitive	0.03–0.12	0.06–0.25	0.03–0.12	0.08–0.03
erythromycin resistant *erm*B	≥32	≥64	≥64	0.125–0.5
erythromycin resistant *mef*A	8–16	8–16	8	0.25–1
Gram-negative aerobes				
Haemophilus influenzae	8	2–4	4–16	2–4
Moraxella catarrhalis	0.125–0.25	0.06–0.12	0.12–0.25	0.12
Legionella pneumophila	0.12–2	0.25–2	0.06–0.25	0.015–0.06
Neisseria gonorrhoeae	0.5	0.25		0.12
Other pathogens				
Chlamydophila pneumoniae	0.06–0.25	0.125–0.25	0.03–0.06	0.06–0.25
Mycoplasma pneumoniae	≤0.015–0.06	≤0.015	≤0.015–0.03	≤0.015

* Values expressed as MIC 90 (mg/L). Ranges indicate the different values reported in references.
Data from Refs.[3,44,50–52]

Telithromycin is more active in vitro against *S pneumoniae* compared with clarithromycin and azithromycin and maintains activity against strains that are macrolide resistant.[54] In one study, the MIC_{90} for telithromycin against *S pneumoniae* strains with the *mef*A gene was 0.25 mg/L or less, compared with 1 to 4 mg/L for macrolides. Against strains expressing the *erm*B gene, telithromycin had an MIC_{90} of 0.5 mg/L, whereas the macrolides had an MIC_{90} of more than 64 mg/L.[55] Telithromycin MIC_{90} increased from 0.015 mg/L to 0.25 mg/L and 0.5 mg/L for penicillin-intermediate and penicillin-resistant pneumococcal strains, respectively.[56] Telithromycin is also two- to eightfold more active against erythromycin-susceptible strains of *S aureus* compared with clarithromycin and azithromycin. Telithromycin maintains activity against macrolide-resistant strains of *S aureus* that have an inducible MLS_B gene but not against strains in which resistance is constitutively expressed.[57]

The newer macrolides demonstrate enhanced activity against respiratory pathogens. The MIC against *H influenzae* for clarithromycin, combined with its active metabolite, 14-hydroxyclarithromycin, is two- to fourfold lower compared with erythromcyin.[58] Azithromycin and telithromycin are more active against *H influenzae* with an MIC four- to eightfold lower compared with erythromycin.[59] Clarithromycin seems more active in vitro than azithromycin and erythromycin against *Legionella pneumophila* and *Chlamydophila pneumoniae*, whereas azithromycin demonstrates better activity against *M catarrhalis* and *M pneumoniae*.[53,60] Telithromycin has excellent in vitro activity against *Mycoplasma*, *Chlamydia*, and *Legionella* and is more active compared with the macrolides.[44]

Azithromycin has activity against enteric pathogens, including *Escherichia coli*, *Salmonella* spp, *Yersinia enterocolitica*, and *Shigella* spp.[53] Clarithromycin and telithromycin have no in vitro activity against these gram-negative organisms. Azithromycin is more active against *Campylobacter jejuni* than erythromycin or clarithromycin, whereas clarithromycin has greater activity against *H pylori*.[61,62]

Azithromycin and clarithromycin have similar or increased in vitro activity against genital pathogens compared with erythromycin. *Neisseria gonorrhoeae, Haemophilus ducreyi,* and *Ureaplasma urealyticum* are susceptible to both antibiotics, with azithromycin demonstrating lower MICs.[61,62] Clarithromycin is approximately tenfold more active than erythromycin against *Chlamydia trachomatis*, whereas azithromycin's activity is similar to that of erythromycin.[61,62] Only azithromycin demonstrated in vitro activity against *Mycoplasma hominis*.[49]

Tigecycline has a broad spectrum of activity against aerobic and anaerobic gram-positive and -negative pathogens, including micro-organisms that demonstrate resistance to multiple classes of antimicrobials. *P aeruginosa* isolates are intrinsically resistant to tigecycline. Tigecycline also has limited activity against *Proteus* spp and *Providencia* spp.[63]

The Tigecycline Evaluation and Surveillance Trial (TEST) is an ongoing global surveillance study initiated in 2004 to assess the in vitro activity of tigecycline.[64,65] In vitro susceptibility data showed that tigecycline was highly active against most gram-positive organisms, including nearly 100% of the methicillin-resistant *S aureus* isolates tested. Though breakpoints for tigecycline susceptibility and resistance have not been defined for *E fecalis* or *E fecium*, aggregate data demonstrated that tigecycline's MIC 90 against these two bacteria are $\leq$0.25 mg/L and 0.12 mg/L respectively. The MIC 90 was unaffected by the presence of vancomycin reistance. Ninety-five percent of *Enterobacteriaceae* were susceptible to tigecycline at the FDA susceptibility breakpoint of 2 mg/L or less and susceptibility patterns have remained stable since surveillance began in 2004.[66] As mentioned previously, tigecycline has limited activity against *P aeruginosa*. Tigecycline maintained in vitro activity against MDR gram-negative organisms, including *E coli* and *Klebsiella* spp isolates expressing extended-spectrum β-lactamases and carbapenemase-producing strains of *Enterobacteriaceae*.[67] Tigecycline demonstrated excellent activity against *Acinetobacter baumanii* with an MIC 90 results of 1 to 2 mg/L.[68,69] Tigecycline also was active against community-acquired infectious agents such as *S pneumoniae* and *H influenzae* regardless of penicillin susceptibility or β-lactamase production, with MIC 90 values of less than 0.5 mg/L.[70] In a European study, tigecycline had good in vitro activity against both gram-positive (MIC 90 <1 mg/L) and gram-negative (MIC 90 1-2 mg/L) anaerobes. Additionally, tigecycline was found to have the lowest MIC 90 (0.25 mg/L) against *Clostridium difficile*.[71]

CLINICAL USE: MACROLIDES AND KETOLIDES
Respiratory Tract Infections

Upper respiratory tract infections
Clarithromycin, azithromycin, and telithromycin are effective against the most frequently isolated bacterial causes of pharyngitis, otitis media, and sinusitis. A 5-day course of the extended-release formulation of clarithromycin, azithromycin, or telithromycin is equally as effective as a 10-day course of penicillin for the treatment of streptococcal pharyngitis.[2,72,73] In comparative trials, clarithromycin has proved to be equivalent to amoxicillin, amoxicillin-clavulanate, and cefaclor for the treatment of acute otitis media in children.[74,75] Otitis media in children was also treated equally well with azithromycin (3 or 5 days) versus 10 days of amoxicillin/clavulanate or cefaclor or 5 days of cefdinir.[76,77] One study showed greater efficacy with a 10-day course

of high-dose amoxicillin/clavulanate compared with a 5-day course of azithromycin.[78] A single oral dose of azithromycin at 30 mg/kg was as effective as a 10-day course of high-dose amoxicillin.[79]

For the treatment of acute sinusitis, clarithromycin had equivalent efficacy compared with cefuroxime axetil, levofloxacin, or ciprofloxacin.[80–82] Once-daily dosing of the extended-release formulation of clarithromycin was comparable to amoxicillin/clavulanate in the treatment of acute maxillary sinusitis.[83] Studies for acute sinusitis treatment with azithromycin concluded that a 3-day regimen (500 mg daily) was equally efficacious as a 10-day course of amoxicillin-clavulanate, and a single dose of the 2-g azithromycin extended-release microsphere formulation had a similar cure rate as a 10-day course of levofloxacin.[84,85] A 5-day course of telithromycin was equally effective as a 10-day course of high-dose amoxicillin-clavulanate, cefuroxime axetil, or moxifloxacin.[86–88]

Currently, clarithromycin is approved for the treatment of pharyngitis caused by S pyogenes; the recommended dose is 250 mg every 12 hours for 10 days. Dosage for treatment of acute maxillary sinusitis is either 500 mg every 12 hours with the immediate-release tablets for 14 days or 2 × 500 mg every 24 hours with the extended-release tablets for 7 days. For children, the recommended dose is 7.5 mg/kg every 12 hours. Azithromycin is approved as a second-line agent for the treatment of pharyngitis. The recommended adult dose is 500 mg on the first day followed by 250 mg once daily on days 2 through 5. For children, the following azithromycin dosing regimens can be used for the treatment of otitis media: 30 mg/kg as a single dose, 10 mg/kg once daily for 3 days, or 10 mg/kg on the first day followed by 5 mg/kg on days 2 through 5. Azithromycin is also approved for the treatment of acute bacterial sinusitis; the adult dose is either 500 mg daily for 3 days or a single 2-g dose of the extended-release formulation and for children it is 10 mg/kg once daily for 3 days. Telithromycin is not FDA approved for the treatment of upper respiratory tract infections.

Lower respiratory tract infections

Various trials have demonstrated the efficacy of clarithromycin, azithromycin, and telithromycin for treatment of lower respiratory tract infections, including acute bronchitis, acute exacerbation of chronic bronchitis (AECB), and community-acquired pneumonia. Most studies involved patients who were not hospitalized. Studies have shown equal efficacy of clarithromycin compared with ceftibuten, cefaclor, cefuroxime axetil, and cefixime for the treatment of lower respiratory tract infections.[89] Comparable efficacy was also demonstrated between the once-daily dosing of the extended-release formulation of clarithromycin and the twice-daily dosing of the immediate-release formulation for the treatment of lower respiratory tract infections.[90,91] Clinical cure rates for the treatment of AECB were similar between a 10-day course of clarithromycin compared with levofloxacin or cefuroxime axetil and a 5- or 7-day course of extended-release tablets of clarithromycin compared with telithromycin or amoxicillin/clavulanic acid.[92–95] In a comparative trial between 5 days of gemifloxacin and 7 days of clarithromycin, clinical and bacteriologic cures were similar, but significantly more patients in the gemifloxacin group remained free of AECB recurrences.[96] For the outpatient treatment of community-acquired pneumonia, equivalent efficacy has been shown between (1) clarithromycin 500 mg twice daily for 10 days and moxifloxacin or gatifloxacin and (2) clarithromycin extended-release tablets (2 × 500 mg tablets once daily for 7 days) and levofloxacin or trovafloxacin.[97–100]

Azithromycin (500 mg on day 1 followed by 250 mg daily for 4 days) was equivalent to cefaclor in patients with outpatient community-acquired pneumonia.[101] Outcomes for the treatment of community-acquired pneumonia were also similar between a 3-day course of azithromycin (1 g daily) and a 7-day course of amoxicillin-clavulanate.[102] Two comparative trials showed that the efficacy of a single 2-g dose of azithromycin extended-release microsphere formulation was equivalent to a 7-day course of extended-release clarithromycin or levofloxacin for the treatment of mild to moderate community-acquired pneumonia in adults.[103,104]

In an analysis of randomized controlled trials comparing azithromycin with alternative antimicrobials, azithromycin was found to have comparable clinical cure rates for the treatment of acute bronchitis and AECB and superior efficacy in the treatment of community-acquired pneumonia.[105,106] For the treatment of AECB, azithromycin (500 mg daily for 3 days) was as efficacious as clarithromycin (500 mg twice daily for 10 days).[107] Equivalent efficacy was also demonstrated between a 3- or 5-day course of azithromycin with either a 5-day course of moxifloxacin or a 7-day course of levofloxacin for the treatment of AECB[108,109] The clinical efficacy of telithromycin has been demonstrated in the outpatient treatment of community-acquired pneumonia in open-label studies and comparator trials. Telithromycin was equally effective when compared with a 10-day course of high-dose amoxicillin, twice-daily clarithromycin, or a 7- to 10-day course of trovafloxacin.[110–112] Clinical cure rates and bacterial eradication were comparable in patients treated with either a 5- or 7-day course of telithromycin or a 10-day course of clarithromycin.[113] Pooled analysis from clinical trials showed that telithromycin was effective in community-acquired pneumonia caused by erythromycin-resistant *S pneumoniae* infections, including bacteremic patients.[114,115] For the treatment of AECB, a 5-day course of telithromycin was equally effective as a 10-day course with cefuroxime axetil, clarithromycin, or amoxicillin-clavulanate.[116,117] In several studies, however, eradication rates for *H influenzae* were lower for telithromycin (66%) than comparators (88%).[118]

Azithromycin and clarithromycin have been shown to be effective in the treatment of community-acquired pneumonia in patients who require hospitalization. Monotherapy with intravenous azithromycin was equally effective as a respiratory fluoroquinolone or a β-lactam plus macrolide regimen for patients hospitalized with community-acquired pneumonia.[119–121] Recent comparative trials showed equivalent efficacy between respiratory fluoroquinolones and ceftriaxone plus azithromycin or clarithromycin in patients with community-acquired pneumonia who required hospitalization.[122–124] Other studies imply an advantage in dual empiric therapy, including a macrolide, in reducing mortality in patients with community-acquired pneumonia or bacteremic pneumococcal pneumonia.[125–127] Azithromycin monotherapy successfully treated 96% of patients (22/23) hospitalized with legionella pneumonia with a mean total duration of antibiotic therapy (intravenous plus oral) of 7.92 days.[128] To date, limited data have been published on the use of telithromycin with a β-lactam antimicrobial for the treatment of community-acquired pneumonia in hospitalized patients.

Pneumococcal resistance to macrolides is prevalent. Surveillance studies in the United States revealed that 28% to 35% of *S pneumoniae* isolates are macrolide resistant.[129–132] Telithromycin resistance was infrequent in these studies. In the United States, 50-60% of the macrolide-resistant isolates exhibited low-level erythromycin resistance (16 mg/L) via expression of the *mef*(A) gene, and nearly 20–25% expressed the *mef*(A) gene and the *erm*(B) gene, resulting in high-level resistance.[132,133] The prevalence of macrolide resistance among *S pneumoniae* isolates varies greatly among geographic regions, with the highest prevalence of resistance reported from Asia.[134] Telithromycin resistance among *S pneumoniae* isolates has been reported in a small number of case series. One surveillance study of *S pneumoniae* isolates from Taiwan revealed that 2% were resistant to telithromycin and 96% were macrolide resistant.[13,14,135,136]

Despite the high prevalence of macrolide resistance, reported clinical failures have been limited to small case series. In a prospective cohort study of patients who were discharged from emergency departments and prescribed clarithromycin for the treatment of community-acquired pneumonia, macrolide resistance among S pneumoniae isolates did not affect outcomes.[137] A matched-case control study of patients with bacteremic pneumococcal infections investigated whether development of breakthrough bacteremia during macrolide treatment was related to macrolide susceptibility of the isolate.[138] Breakthrough bacteremia with an erythromycin-resistant isolate occurred in 18 (24%) of 76 patients taking a macrolide, compared with none of the 136 matched patients with bacteremia with an erythromycin-susceptible isolate. Given the possibility of treatment failure, most guidelines recommend combining a macrolide with a β-lactam if risk factors are present for drug-resistant S pneumoniae. Telithromycin maintains in vitro activity against macrolide-resistant isolates. Whether this translates into a therapeutic advantage in the empiric treatment of respiratory tract infections, especially when drug-resistant S pneumoniae is of concern, needs to be determined.

Practice guidelines from the Infectious Diseases Society of America (IDSA) and American Thoracic Society (ATS) provide recommendations for the empiric treatment of community-acquired pneumonia based on the clinical setting, presence of comorbidities, severity of disease, and risk for drug-resistant S pneumoniae.[139] Only treatment options that include a macrolide are discussed, and the reader is referred to the guidelines for alternative options. In the outpatient setting, recommended antimicrobial therapy for patients who were previously healthy and have no risk factors for drug-resistant S pneumoniae includes any macrolide (erythromycin, azithromycin, clarithromycin). Recommended outpatient therapy for individuals who have comorbid conditions, have received antibiotics within the previous 3 months, or have other risk factors for drug-resistant S pneumoniae includes a macrolide in combination with a β-lactam. The IDSA/ATS guidelines suggest that in regions in which high-level (MIC $\geq$16 mg/L) macrolide resistance among S pneumoniae exceeds 25%, alternative antimicrobials should be considered in lieu of the macrolides. For patients who require hospitalization, a macrolide combined with a β-lactam is one of the preferred regimens recommended. Azithromycin monotherapy is not endorsed as a routine treatment option. The use of telithromycin is not addressed in the practice guidelines because at the time of publication, telithromycin's safety profile was being re-evaluated by the FDA.

The approved dose of azithromycin for treatment of lower respiratory tract infections is 500 mg the first day followed by 250 mg for days 2 through 5. An alternative regimen for the treatment of AECB is 500 mg daily for 3 days. The recommended treatment of community-acquired pneumonia with the extended-release microsphere formulation of azithromycin is a single 2-g dose. The recommended dose of intravenous azithromycin for the treatment of community-acquired pneumonia is 500 mg daily for at least 2 days followed by oral azithromycin 500 mg daily to complete a 7- to 10-day course. Clarithromycin immediate- and extended-release tablets are approved for treatment of community-acquired pneumonia and AECB. The dose of the immediate-release tablets is 250 mg twice daily for 7 to 14 days. The dose should be increased to 500 mg if H influenzae is being treated. The dose of the extended-release formulation is 2 × 500 mg tablets daily for 7 days. Telithromycin is FDA approved for the treatment of community-acquired pneumonia (including infections caused by multidrug-resistant S pneumoniae) at a dose of 800 mg daily for 7 to 10 days.

Sexually Transmitted Diseases

The use of the advanced macrolides in the treatment of sexually transmitted diseases has focused primarily on azithromycin. The prolonged tissue half-life of azithromycin allows single-dose treatment courses, directly observed therapy, and improved patient compliance. A meta-analysis of randomized clinical trials concluded that a single 1-gram dose of azithromycin was equally efficacious and had similar tolerability as a standard 7-day regimen of doxycycline for the treatment of uncomplicated urethritis or cervicitis caused by C trachomatis.[140] Another meta-analysis for treatment of C trachomatis infection during pregnancy found similar efficacy between a single 1-gram dose of azithromycin compared with erythromycin or amoxicillin.[141] Guidelines published by the US Public Health Service (USPHS) currently recommend either doxycycline, 100 mg twice daily for 7 days, or azithromycin, 1 g as a single dose, for either chlamydial infections or nongonococcal urethritis among adolescents and adults.[142] In a comparative study for the treatment of chronic prostatitis caused by C trachomatis, azithromycin (500 mg daily for 3 days on a weekly basis for 3 weeks) resulted in a significantly higher eradication rate and clinical cure compared with ciprofloxacin (500 mg twice daily for 20 days).[143] Another trial showed equivalent outcomes between azithromycin (1 g weekly for 4 weeks) and doxycycline (100 mg twice daily for 28 days).[144] A single 1-g dose of azithromycin is also one of the recommended treatments for genital ulcer disease caused by H ducreyi (chancroid).[142]

Azithromycin has in vitro activity against N gonorrhoeae, and a single 2-g oral dose was found to be equally efficacious as ceftriaxone, 250 mg intramuscularly, in the treatment of uncomplicated gonorrhea.[145] Gastrointestinal side effects occurred in 35% of patients who received azithromycin. Azithromycin resistance among gonococcal isolates is low in the United States, but 5.2% of isolates in Scotland had reduced susceptibility to azithromycin.[144,145] The concerned about possible emergence of resistance to macrolides, the USPHS recommended limited use of the 2-g azithromycin dose for the treatment of uncomplicated gonorrhea.[142] If chlamydia infection is not ruled out in a patient with uncomplicated gonococcal urethritis or cervicitis, then either a single 1-g dose of azithromycin or 7-day course of doxycycline should be used in addition to the gonorrhea treatment regimen. Azithromycin with or without metronidazole has been shown to have similar clinical response rates to comparative agents (metronidazole + doxycycline + cefoxitin + probenicid or doxycycline + amoxicillin/clavulanate) in the treatment of pelvic inflammatory disease.[146] The USPHS list this as an alternative regimen for the treatment of pelvic inflammatory disease.

The use of azithromycin for the treatment of early syphilis also has been evaluated. A meta-analysis of four randomized controlled trials for the treatment of early syphilis concluded that azithromycin achieved a higher cure rate compared with penicillin G benzathine.[147] A large comparative trial conducted in Tanzania compared the efficacy of a single 2-g dose of azithromycin with an intramuscular injection of 2.4 million U of penicillin G benzathine. Cure rates at 3-, 6-, and 9-months were similar between the two treatment groups.[148] Similar results were also obtained in a study conducted in Madagascar and the United States. Recently, a 23S rRNA gene mutation in Treponema pallidum conferring resistance to azithromycin was identified in 32 of 114 isolates (28%) obtained from four sexually transmitted disease clinics located in either the United States or Ireland.[149] The USPHS recommends the use of azithromycin for the treatment of primary or secondary syphilis in the United States only when treatment with penicillin or doxycycline is not feasible.[142]

Helicobacter Pylori Infections

Antibiotic therapy for H pylori–associated peptic ulcer disease decreases ulcer recurrence and promotes healing. Triple-therapy regimens that consist of clarithromycin, amoxicillin, or metronidazole and an antisecretory agent for 7 to 14 days are preferable for the treatment of H pylori infections.[150,151] These combinations maximize H pylori eradication, minimize the risk of antimicrobial resistance, and allow shorter and simplified treatment courses, which results in improved compliance. Clinical efficacy of different triple-therapy clarithromycin-based regimens for 7 to 14 days had cure rates of 70% to 80% based on intention-to-treat analyses.[152–154] One meta-analysis and a recent randomized trial found that a 14-day course of clarithromycin triple therapy was more effective than a 7-day treatment course.[155,156] Sequential therapy involving a proton pump inhibitor plus amoxicillin for 5 days followed by a proton pump inhibitor, clarithromycin, and tinidazole for 5 days for the treatment of H pylori was evaluated, mainly in Italy. Eradication rates of H pylori with the sequential regimen were 90% or more and were more effective than standard clarithromycin-based triple-therapy regimens.[157,158] A recent meta-analysis concluded that sequential therapy seems to be superior to standard triple therapy, with crude eradication rates of H pylori of 93.4% and 76.9%, respectively.[159]

Clarithromycin resistance rates vary in different regions of the world and, within a region, among different population subgroups.[160] In the United States, the clarithromycin resistance rate among H pylori isolates was reported to be 13%.[161] In a 15-year interval, the frequency of primary clarithromycin resistance in Italy increased from 10.2% (1989–1990) to 21.3% (2004–2005).[162] H pylori resistance to clarithromycin has been shown to be associated with any previous use of macrolides.[163] Pretreatment clarithromycin resistance has a negative impact on treatment efficacy (55% reduction in cure rates) and is associated with failure to eradicate H pylori.[164,165]

In the United States, the American College of Gastroenterology practice guidelines recommend a clarithromycin-based regimen as one of two primary treatment options for H pylori infection. The recommended regimen includes a proton pump inhibitor, clarithromycin (500 mg twice daily), and either amoxicillin (1000 mg twice daily) or metronidazole (500 mg twice daily) given for 14 days. The alternative primary therapy recommended is a non–clarithromycin-based regimen that includes a proton pump inhibitor or ranitidine, bismuth subsalicylate, metronidazole, and tetracycline for 10 to 14 days. Until validation studies are conducted in other countries, the American College of Gastroenterology recommends that the sequential regimen outlined previously be considered as an alternative to the other standard first-line therapy options.[150]

MAC

Clarithromycin and azithromycin have both been shown to be effective in preventing and treating disseminated MAC disease in HIV-infected patients. Azithromycin is effective as prophylaxis against disseminated MAC disease in patients with CD4 counts of less than 100 cells/mm^3. In a comparative trial with rifabutin, the 1-year incidence rate of disseminated MAC disease was 15.3% in the rifabutin group (300 mg/d) compared with 7.6% in the azithromycin group (1200 mg weekly).[166] Combination of azithromycin and rifabutin decreased the 1-year incidence rate of MAC to 2.8%, but 22.7% of patients discontinued therapy because of drug-related toxicity compared with 13.5% of patients who received azithromycin alone. Azithromycin resistance was seen in 11% of isolates obtained from patients who developed breakthrough disease. Similarly, clarithromycin was shown to be effective for MAC prophylaxis. In a comparative trial, clarithromycin (500 mg twice daily) was more effective in preventing MAC bacteremia than rifabutin (300 mg daily), with rates of 9% and 15%, respectively.[167] Clarithromycin resistance was reported in 29% of the patients with breakthrough MAC bacteremia while on clarithromycin prophylaxis. Current USPHS/IDSA guidelines recommend either azithromycin, 1200 mg weekly, or clarithromycin, 500 mg twice daily, as the preferred regimens for MAC prophylaxis in HIV-infected individuals with a CD4 count of less than 50 cells/mm^3.[168]

The effectiveness of clarithromycin in combination with other antibiotics, especially ethambutol, for treatment of disseminated MAC disease in HIV-infected patients has been demonstrated in several randomized trials. A regimen of clarithromycin, rifabutin, and ethambutol was more effective in clearing MAC bacteremia and improving survival than a four-drug regimen of rifampin, ethambutol, clofazamine, and ciprofloxacin.[169] Another trial compared dosing regimens of clarithromycin in combination with ethambutol plus either rifabutin or clofazamine. Mortality was significantly higher at 4.5 months in patients who received clarithromycin at a dose of 1 g twice daily rather than the lower dose of 500 mg twice daily.[170] In another trial that compared clarithromycin with rifabutin, ethambutol, or both, eradication of MAC bacteremia occurred in 40% to 50% of patients at 12 weeks of treatment.[171] Response rates were not statistically different between the various treatment arms at 12 weeks. The relapse rate (24%) was higher in patients treated with clarithromycin and rifabutin than patients who received clarithromycin plus ethambutol (relapse rate 7%) or clarithromycin plus ethambutol plus rifabutin (relapse rate 6%).

Azithromycin, 600 mg daily, was compared with clarithromycin, 500 mg twice daily, for the treatment of disseminated MAC disease.[172] Both were administered with ethambutol 15 mg/kg/d. Two consecutive sterile blood cultures at 24 weeks were obtained in 46% (31/68) of patients in the azithromycin group compared with 56% (32/57) in the clarithromycin group. There was no difference in mortality between the two treatment groups. Another study that used the same regimens found that clarithromycin was significantly better and more rapid in clearance of MAC bacteremia.[173] Current recommendations for the treatment of disseminated MAC disease are to use at least two or more antimycobacterial drugs. Clarithromycin is the preferred first agent. Azithromycin is an alternative when drug interactions or intolerance preclude the use of clarithromycin.[168]

Clarithromycin and azithromycin are also useful in the treatment of pulmonary MAC infections in HIV-negative patients. In noncomparative studies, sputum conversion rates at 6 months were comparable between azithromycin- and clarithromycin-containing regimens (67 vs 74%).[174,175] The development of clarithromycin-resistant isolates was associated with microbiologic relapse. Intermittent treatment regimens also have been studied. Sixty-five percent of patients achieved treatment success with azithromycin-containing treatment regimens administered three times per week.[176] Clarithromycin-containing regimens administered three times weekly resulted in a 78% sputum conversion to acid fast bacilli culture negative.[177] Three times weekly clarithromycin therapy was less effective in patients with MAC infection and cavitary lung disease.[178] The current ATS/IDSA guidelines recommend a three times weekly regimen, including clarithromycin, 1000 mg, or azithromycin, 500 mg, with ethambutol and rifampin for patients with nodular/bronchiectatic MAC lung disease. For patients with fibrocavitary or severe nodular/bronchiectatic MAC lung disease, the recommended regimen is daily dosing of clarithromycin, 500 to 1000 mg, or azithromycin, 250 mg, with ethambutol and rifampin.[179]

CLINICAL USE: TIGECYCLINE

Tigecycline is FDA approved for the treatment of complicated skin and skin structure infections, complicated intra-abdominal infections, or community-acquired bacterial pneumonia. Two double-blind multicenter studies were conducted to evaluate the efficacy and safety of tigecycline monotherapy versus the combination of vancomycin and aztreonam for the treatment of hospitalized adults with complicated skin and skin structure infections.[180–182] Tigecycline monotherapy was demonstrated to be noninferior to the combination of vancomycin and aztreonam; test-of-cure rates in the clinical evaluable population were 86.5% and 88.6%, respectively. Outcomes were similar between the two groups regardless of the type of skin and soft tissue infection present or bacterial species isolated. In another trial that compared tigecycline to vancomycin for the treatment of complicated skin and skin structure infections caused by methicillin-resistant *S aureus*, the clinical cure rates in the microbiologically evaluable population were 86.4% and 86.9% for tigecycline and vancomycin, respectively.[183]

The efficacy of tigecycline was compared with imipenem/cilastatin in patients with complicated intra-abdominal infections in two double-blind randomized multicenter studies.[184–186] In the microbiologically evaluable population, clinical cure rates were similar between tigecycline and imipenem/cilastin (80.2% and 81.5%, respectively). Tigecycline cure rates were 80.6% versus 82.4% for imipenem/cilastatin, a statistically noninferior result. More than 80% of *E coli* and *Klebsiella* spp (the most frequently isolated gram-negative aerobes) were eradicated by tigecycline; 78% of *Streptococcus* spp and 70% of *B fragilis* were also eradicated.

Tigecycline has been evaluated against levofloxacin for the treatment of hospitalized patients with community-acquired pneumonia in two phase III, multicenter, double-blind studies. Pooled clinical cure rates were similar between the two treatment groups (89.7% and 86.3%). There were no significant differences in length of hospital stay, median duration of study antibiotic therapy, or hospital readmissions.[187,188]

Recent studies have evaluated the efficacy of tigecycline for the treatment of infections caused by MDR gram-negative organisms. Twenty-three of 33 patients treated with tigecycline had resolution of their infection caused by either a carbapenem-resistant or extended-spectrum beta lactamase-producing or MDR *Enterobacteriaceae*.[189] An open-label, phase 3, noncomparative, multicenter study assessed tigecycline's efficacy in hospitalized patients with either complicated intra-abdominal infections, complicated skin and skin structure infections, or hospital-acquired pneumonia caused by resistant gram-negative organisms. In the microbiologically evaluable population, the clinical cure rate was 72.2% and the microbiologic eradication rate was 66.7%. The most commonly isolated resistant gram-negative pathogens were *A baumanii* (47%), *E coli* (25%), *K pneumoniae* (16.7%) and *Enterobacter* spp (11%).[190] In a small retrospective review of patients with serious infections caused by MDR gram-negative bacilli, pretherapy MIC values for tigecycline predicted clinical success.[191,192] Despite in vitro activity, the clinical efficacy of tigecycline for treatment of MDR Acinetobacter infections remains uncertain. In a one case series only 8 of 29 patients who received tigecycline for the treatment of acinetobacter infections, only 8 (28%) demonstrated clinical improvement or cure. None of the isolates was fully susceptible to tigecycline (median MIC 4 mg/L).[193] Two other retrospective case series reported more favorable clinical outcomes. Tigecycline therapy (most often in combination with other antimcirobials) resulted in clinical improvement in 32 of 42 patients in one study and 23 of 32 patients in the other. Tigecycline resistance emerged during therapy in four patients within these 2 case series.[194,195]

ADVERSE EFFECTS

Gastrointestinal intolerance is the primary adverse side effect of the newer macrolides and ketolides, but they occur at a significantly reduced rate when compared with erythromycin. The most common adverse effects reported with azithromycin were diarrhea (3.6%), nausea (2.6%), abdominal pain (2.5%), and headache or dizziness (1.3%). Laboratory abnormalities were infrequent and minor, including transient increases in transaminases in 1.5% of patients. Only 0.7% of patients discontinued azithromycin therapy compared with 2.6% of patients who receive comparative medications.[196] Gastrointestinal adverse effects (primarily diarrhea) occurred in 17% of patients treated with the 2-g extended-release microsphere formulation of azithromycin.[83,102] Adverse events related to the intravenous infusion of azithromycin were pain at the injection site (6.5%) and local inflammation (3.1%).[197] The most common adverse reactions reported with clarithromycin were similar (eg, nausea, 3.8%; diarrhea, 3.0%; abdominal pain, 1.9%; and headache, 1.7%).[198] There was no difference in the spectrum and frequency of adverse reactions between the extended-release or immediate-release formulations of clarithromycin.[20] Gastrointestinal adverse events with the extended-release formulation tended to be less severe and resulted in fewer discontinuations of the medication. Laboratory abnormalities were also rare and included abnormal liver function test results and decreased white blood cell counts. Overall, less than 3% of patients receiving clarithromycin withdrew from studies because of adverse effects. Clarithromycin has been associated with teratogenic effects in animal studies and should not be used in pregnant patients.

In phase 3 clinical trials with telithromycin, the most common adverse effects reported were diarrhea (10.8%), nausea (7.9%), headache (5.5%), dizziness (3.7%), and vomiting (2.9%). These adverse effects were generally mild to moderate in severity and the number of patients discontinuing telithromycin (4.4%) was similar to those receiving comparator agents (4.3%).[199] In a large study to assess clinical safety, more than 12,000 subjects with either community-acquired pneumonia or AECB received a course of telithromycin. Diarrhea occurred in 3.5% of study patients and gastrointestinal side effects occurred in 10.6%. Transient blurred vision occurred in 0.6% of telithromycin-treated patients.[10] Clinical trials have shown a small increase (1.5 ms) in the QTc interval with telithromycin. No significant clinical effect on the QT interval in healthy adults was observed.[200] Because of the potential risk of ventricular arrhythmias, however, telithromycin should be avoided in patients with congenital prolongation of the QT interval and patients with ongoing proarrhythmic conditions.[199]

During clinical trials for treatment of community-acquired pneumonia, patients receiving telithromycin had a greater incidence of transient rises in hepatic transaminases compared with patients receiving alternative antibiotics.[3] In the large clinical safety study mentioned previously, no clinically significant hepatic events were reported. An increase in alanine aminotransferase of more than 3 times upper limit of normal occurred in 1% of patients receiving telithromycin compared with 0.8% in patients receiving amoxicillin-clavulanic acid.[10] Site investigations identified serious irregularities in the conduct of the trial, however, which raised concerns about the integrity of the study results.[200,201]

Postmarketing surveillance reports described severe cases of hepatotoxicity in patients who received telithromycin. In a case series of 3 patients who developed acute hepatitis within days of receiving telithromycin therapy, one patient died and one required liver transplantation. Liver histology revealed inflammation consistent with a hypersensitivity reaction.[202] By the end of 2006, telithromycin was implicated in 53 cases of hepatotoxicity, which included some fatalities.[201] Telithromycin also was associated with myasthenia gravis exacerbations, including fatal and life-threatening acute respiratory failure.[197,203] On February 12, 2007, the FDA removed telithromycin's indication for the treatment of acute sinusitis and AECB and limited its approved indication to the treatment of community-acquired pneumonia alone. The FDA also issued a black box warning of the risk of respiratory failure in patients with myasthenia gravis and strengthened the warnings concerning the risk of acute hepatic failure and liver injury, which may be fatal.[204]

The most common side effects associated with tigecycline use in clinical trials were nausea and vomiting, both of which were mild to moderate in intensity and transient.[183,187] Overall, 29.5% of tigecycline recipients experienced nausea and

19.7% experienced vomiting. Diarrhea occurred in 13% of patients. Antimicrobial discontinuation as a result of an adverse event in these trials was similar between tigecycline recipients (5%) and the comparator antimicrobials (4.7%). There have been case reports of acute pancreatitis in patients treated with tigecycline.[205] Because tigecycline is structurally similar to tetracyclines, it may have the same safety concerns.[47] Tigecycline is labeled as a pregnancy category class D drug. Animal studies have shown that it crosses the placenta and is found in fetal tissues. Safety and efficacy of tigecycline in children younger than age 18 has not been established. As with tetracyclines, its use during tooth development may be associated with permanent tooth discoloration. On September 1, 2010, an FDA drug safety communication described an increased mortality risk associated with the use of tigecycline compared with other antimicrobials used to treat serious infections.[206] The increased mortality risk was based on a pooled analysis review of 13 clinical trials which showed overall mortality was 4% in patients treated with tigecycline compared to 3% in patients who received comparator antibiotics. The greatest risk of death was seen in patients who received tigecycline for the treatment of ventilator-associated pneumonia. The reason for the increased mortality risk in these clinical trials is unknown.

DRUG INTERACTIONS

Several reviews have discussed drug interactions between either clarithromycin or azithromycin and other agents.[42,207] Clarithromycin, like erythromycin, is oxidized by the cytochrome P450 system, primarily the CYP3A4 subclass of hepatic enzymes. This converts clarithromycin to a nitrosalkalane metabolite that forms an inactive metabolite/enzyme complex by binding to the iron of the CYP3A4 enzyme. This interaction inhibits the CYP3A4 enzymes and results in decreased clearance of other agents given concurrently that are metabolized by the same enzyme system. Clarithromycin is a less potent inhibitor of the CYP 3A4 enzymes than erythromycin and azithromycin interferes poorly with this system.[42]

Appropriate dose reductions and clinical and therapeutic drug level monitoring are necessary when drugs metabolized by the CYP3A enzymes are given concurrently with clarithromycin. The concurrent use of cisapride, pimozide, terfenadine, and aztemizole with clarithromycin is contraindicated because of the possible cardiotoxic effects of these agents and the occurrence of torsades de pointes. The concomitant administration of clarithromycin with ergotamine or dihydroergotamine is contraindicated because of the risk of acute ergot toxicity. Other medications such as benzodiazepines (eg, triazolam, midazolam, alprazolam), HMG-CoA reductase inhibitors (eg, lovastatin, simvastatin, atorvastatin), class 1A antiarrhythmic agents (eg, quinidine, disopyramide), theophylline, carbamazepine, warfarin, sildenafil, colchicine, and cyclosporine should be used cautiously when given with clarithromycin.[19] These drug-drug interactions are less likely to occur with azithromycin, because it is not a potent inhibitor of the CYP3A enzymes. There are case reports of toxicity related to coadministration of azithromycin and lovastatin, warfarin, cyclosporine, disopyramide and theophylline, however.[42,208] Clarithromycin and azithromycin have been associated with digoxin toxicity presumably due to inhibition of intestinal and renal P-glycoproteins.[209]

The potential for telithromycin to inhibit the cytochrome P450 3A4 pathway is comparable to clarithromycin, although metabolism of telithromycin does not result in the formation of nitrosalkalene metabolite. Telithromycin also competitively inhibits the CYP2D6 system. The concomitant administration of telithromycin with cisapride or pimozide is contraindicated. The use of HMG-CoA reductase inhibitors (simvastatin, lovastatin, or atorvastatin), rifampin, or ergot alkaloid derivatives with telithromycin should be avoided. Caution should be used when administering telithromycin with digoxin, midazolam, metoprolol, oral anticoagulants, or other drugs metabolized by the CYP3A4 enzymes.[198]

Tigecycline does not interact with cytochrome P450 enzymes, making pharmacokinetic drug interactions uncommon. No significant drug interactions were noted during concomitant administration of tigecycline and digoxin or warfarin.[210–213]

SUMMARY

The advanced macrolides (azithromycin and clarithromycin) and ketolides (telithromycin) are structural analogs of erythromycin that have similar mechanisms of action. These antimicrobials have several distinct advantages over erythromycin, including improved oral bioavailability, longer half-life (allowing once- or twice-daily administration), higher tissue concentrations, enhanced antimicrobial activity, and reduced gastrointestinal adverse effects. Clarithromycin and azithromycin have been used extensively for the treatment of upper and lower respiratory tract infections. Despite the increasing prevalence of macrolide resistance among *S pneumoniae*, clinical failures have been reported infrequently. Treatment guidelines have solidified the roles of azithromycin in the treatment of certain sexually transmitted diseases and clarithromycin for the treatment of *H pylori*–associated peptic ulcer disease. Azithromycin and clarithromycin have been used successfully to prevent and treat MAC infections.

Telithromycin has been shown to be clinically effective in the treatment of outpatient respiratory diseases. Because of safety concerns, however, especially the possibility of hepatotoxicity, the approved indication for telithromycin is limited to the treatment of community-acquired pneumonia. Tigecycline, a derivative of minocycline, has a broad spectrum of antimicrobial activity, including activity against many MDR pathogens. Tigecycline, available only as an intravenous preparation, is indicated for the treatment of complicated skin and skin structure and intra-abdominal infections. It is also approved for the treatment of community-acquired pneumonia. The role for tigecycline in the treatment of other types of infections with MDR organisms needs to be further clarified.

REFERENCES

1. Omura S, Tsuzuki K, Sunazuka T, et al. Macrolides with gastrointestinal motor stimulating activity. J Med Chem 1987;30(11):1941–3.
2. Piscitelli SC, Danziger LH, Rodvold KA. Clarithromycin and azithromycin: new macrolide antibiotics. Clin Pharm 1992;11(2):137–52.
3. Shain CS, Amsden GW. Telithromycin: the first of the ketolides. Ann Pharmacother 2002;36(3):452–64.
4. Douthwaite S, Champney WS. Structures of ketolides and macrolides determine their mode of interaction with the ribosomal target site. J Antimicrob Chemother 2001;48(Suppl T1):1–8.
5. Champney WS, Tober CL. Superiority of 11,12 carbonate macrolide antibiotics as inhibitors of translation and 50S ribosomal subunit formation in *Staphylococcus aureus* cells. Curr Microbiol 1999;38(6):342–8.
6. Frampton JE, Curran MP. Tigecycline. Drugs 2005;65(18):2623–35.
7. Sturgill MG, Rapp RP. Clarithromycin: review of a new macrolide antibiotic with improved microbiologic spectrum and favorable pharmacokinetic and adverse effect profiles. Ann Pharmacother 1992;26(9):1099–108.

8. Hansen LH, Mauvais P, Douthwaite S. The macrolide-ketolide antibiotic binding site is formed by structures in domains II and V of 23S ribosomal RNA. Mol Microbiol 1999;31(2):623–31.
9. Tait-Kamradt A, Clancy J, Cronan M, et al. mefE is necessary for the erythromycin-resistant M phenotype in *Streptococcus pneumoniae*. Antimicrob Agents Chemother 1997;41(10):2251–5.
10. Ketek (telithromycin): briefing document for the FDA Anti-Infective Drug Products Advisory Committee Meeting, January 8, 2003. Gaithersburg, MD.
11. Bonnefoy A, Girard AM, Agouridas C, et al. Ketolides lack inducibility properties of MLS(B) resistance phenotype. J Antimicrob Chemother 1997;40(1):85–90.
12. Malhotra-Kumar S, Lammens C, Chapelle S, et al. Macrolide- and telithromycin-resistant *Streptococcus pyogenes*, Belgium, 1999–2003. Emerg Infect Dis 2005; 11(6):939–42.
13. Al-Lahham A, Appelbaum PC, van der Linden M, et al. Telithromycin-nonsusceptible clinical isolates of *Streptococcus pneumoniae* from Europe. Antimicrob Agents Chemother 2006;50(11):3897–900.
14. Wolter N, Smith AM, Farrell DJ, et al. Telithromycin resistance in *Streptococcus pneumoniae* is conferred by a deletion in the leader sequence of erm(B) that increases rRNA methylation. Antimicrob Agents Chemother 2008;52(2):435–40.
15. Bergeron J, Ammirati M, Danley D, et al. Glycylcyclines bind to the high-affinity tetracycline ribosomal binding site and evade Tet(M)- and Tet(O)-mediated ribosomal protection. Antimicrob Agents Chemother 1996;40(9):2226–8.
16. Hirata T, Saito A, Nishino K, et al. Effects of efflux transporter genes on susceptibility of *Escherichia coli* to tigecycline (GAR-936). Antimicrob Agents Chemother 2004;48(6):2179–84.
17. Dean CR, Visalli MA, Projan SJ, et al. Efflux-mediated resistance to tigecycline (GAR-936) in *Pseudomonas aeruginosa* PAO1. Antimicrob Agents Chemother 2003;47(3):972–8.
18. Peleg AY, Adams J, Paterson DL. Tigecycline efflux as a mechanism for nonsusceptibility in *Acinetobacter baumannii*. Antimicrob Agents Chemother 2007;51(6): 2065–9.
19. Abbott Laboratories. Biaxin (Clarithromycin): prescribing information. 2008;2008(12/23). Available at: http://www.rxabbott.com/pdf/biapi.PDF. Accessed August, 2009.
20. Guay DR, Gustavson LE, Devcich KJ, et al. Pharmacokinetics and tolerability of extended-release clarithromycin. Clin Ther 2001;23(4):566–77.
21. Foulds G, Luke DR, Teng R, et al. The absence of an effect of food on the bioavailability of azithromycin administered as tablets, sachet or suspension. J Antimicrob Chemother 1996;37(Suppl C):37–44.
22. Chandra R, Liu P, Breen JD, et al. Clinical pharmacokinetics and gastrointestinal tolerability of a novel extended-release microsphere formulation of azithromycin. Clin Pharmacokinet 2007;46(3):247–59.
23. Perret C, Lenfant B, Weinling E, et al. Pharmacokinetics and absolute oral bioavailability of an 800-mg oral dose of telithromycin in healthy young and elderly volunteers. Chemotherapy 2002;48(5):217–23.
24. Bhargava V, Lenfant B, Perret C, et al. Lack of effect of food on the bioavailability of a new ketolide antibacterial, telithromycin. Scand J Infect Dis 2002;34(11):823–6.
25. Ferrero JL, Bopp BA, Marsh KC, et al. Metabolism and disposition of clarithromycin in man. Drug Metab Dispos 1990;18(4):441–6.
26. Liu P, Allaudeen H, Chandra R, et al. Comparative pharmacokinetics of azithromycin in serum and white blood cells of healthy subjects receiving a single-dose

extended-release regimen versus a 3-day immediate-release regimen. Antimicrob Agents Chemother 2007;51(1):103–9.

27. Namour F, Wessels DH, Pascual MH, et al. Pharmacokinetics of the new ketolide telithromycin (HMR 3647) administered in ascending single and multiple doses. Antimicrob Agents Chemother 2001;45(1):170–5.

28. Muralidharan G, Fruncillo RJ, Micalizzi M, et al. Effects of age and sex on single-dose pharmacokinetics of tigecycline in healthy subjects. Antimicrob Agents Chemother 2005;49(4):1656–9.

29. Muralidharan G, Micalizzi M, Speth J, et al. Pharmacokinetics of tigecycline after single and multiple doses in healthy subjects. Antimicrob Agents Chemother 2005;49(1):220–9.

30. Meagher AK, Ambrose PG, Grasela TH, et al. The pharmacokinetic and pharmacodynamic profile of tigecycline. Clin Infect Dis 2005;41(Suppl 5): S333–40.

31. Foulds G, Shepard RM, Johnson RB. The pharmacokinetics of azithromycin in human serum and tissues. J Antimicrob Chemother 1990;25(Suppl A):73–82.

32. Fraschini F, Scaglione F, Pintucci G, et al. The diffusion of clarithromycin and roxithromycin into nasal mucosa, tonsil and lung in humans. J Antimicrob Chemother 1991;27(Suppl A):61–5.

33. Rodvold KA, Gotfried MH, Danziger LH, et al. Intrapulmonary steady-state concentrations of clarithromycin and azithromycin in healthy adult volunteers. Antimicrob Agents Chemother 1997;41(6):1399–402.

34. Muller-Serieys C, Soler P, Cantalloube C, et al. Bronchopulmonary disposition of the ketolide telithromycin (HMR 3647). Antimicrob Agents Chemother 2001; 45(11):3104–8.

35. Khair OA, Andrews JM, Honeybourne D, et al. Lung concentrations of telithromycin after oral dosing. J Antimicrob Chemother 2001;47(6):837–40.

36. Conte JE Jr, Golden JA, Kelly MG, et al. Steady-state serum and intrapulmonary pharmacokinetics and pharmacodynamics of tigecycline. Int J Antimicrob Agents 2005;25(6):523–9.

37. Rodvold KA, Gotfried MH, Cwik M, et al. Serum, tissue and body fluid concentrations of tigecycline after a single 100 mg dose. J Antimicrob Chemother 2006; 58(6):1221–9.

38. Sun HK, Ong CT, Umer A, et al. Pharmacokinetic profile of tigecycline in serum and skin blister fluid of healthy subjects after multiple intravenous administrations. Antimicrob Agents Chemother 2005;49(4):1629–32.

39. Hardy DJ, Guay DR, Jones RN. Clarithromycin, a unique macrolide: a pharmacokinetic, microbiological, and clinical overview. Diagn Microbiol Infect Dis 1992; 15(1):39–53.

40. Chu SY, Granneman GR, Pichotta PJ, et al. Effect of moderate or severe hepatic impairment on clarithromycin pharmacokinetics. J Clin Pharmacol 1993;33(5): 480–5.

41. Ballow CH, Amsden GW. Azithromycin: the first azalide antibiotic. Ann Pharmacother 1992;26(10):1253–61.

42. Westphal JF. Macrolide -induced clinically relevant drug interactions with cytochrome P-450A (CYP) 3A4: an update focused on clarithromycin, azithromycin and dirithromycin. Br J Clin Pharmacol 2000;50(4):285–95.

43. Mazzei T, Surrenti C, Novelli A, et al. Pharmacokinetics of azithromycin in patients with impaired hepatic function. J Antimicrob Chemother 1993;31(Suppl E):57–63.

44. Zhanel GG, Dueck M, Hoban DJ, et al. Review of macrolides and ketolides: focus on respiratory tract infections. Drugs 2001;61(4):443–98.

45. Cantalloube C, Bhargava V, Sultan E, et al. Pharmacokinetics of the ketolide te-lithromycin after single and repeated doses in patients with hepatic impairment. Int J Antimicrob Agents 2003;22(2):112–21.
46. Hoffmann M, DeMaio W, Jordan RA, et al. Metabolism, excretion, and pharma-cokinetics of [14C]tigecycline, a first-in-class glycylcycline antibiotic, after intra-venous infusion to healthy male subjects. Drug Metab Dispos 2007;35(9): 1543–53.
47. Tygacil (tigecycline) prescribing information. Available at: http://labeling.pfizer.com/showlabeling.aspx?id=491. Accessed January, 2011.
48. Clinical and Laboratory Standards Institute. Performance standards for antimicro-bial susceptibility testing. Eighteenth Informational Supplement. Wayne (PA): Clinical and Laboratory Standards Institute; 2011.
49. Whitman MS, Tunkel AR. Azithromycin and clarithromycin: overview and compar-ison with erythromycin. Infect Control Hosp Epidemiol 1992;13(6):357–68.
50. Goldstein EJ, Citron DM, Merriam CV, et al. In vitro activities of telithromycin and 10 oral agents against aerobic and anaerobic pathogens isolated from antral puncture specimens from patients with sinusitis. Antimicrob Agents Chemother 2003;47(6):1963–7.
51. Nagai K, Davies TA, Ednie LM, et al. Activities of a new fluoroketolide, HMR 3787, and its (des)-fluor derivative RU 64399 compared to those of telithromy-cin, erythromycin A, azithromycin, clarithromycin, and clindamycin against macrolide-susceptible or -resistant *Streptococcus pneumoniae* and *S. pyo-genes*. Antimicrob Agents Chemother 2001;45(11):3242–5.
52. Shortridge VD, Zhong P, Cao Z, et al. Comparison of in vitro activities of ABT-773 and telithromycin against macrolide-susceptible and -resistant streptococci and staphylococci. Antimicrob Agents Chemother 2002;46(3):783–6.
53. Retsema J, Girard A, Schelkly W, et al. Spectrum and mode of action of azithro-mycin (CP-62,993), a new 15-membered-ring macrolide with improved potency against gram-negative organisms. Antimicrob Agents Chemother 1987;31(12): 1939–47.
54. Barry AL, Fuchs PC, Brown SD. Antipneumococcal activities of a ketolide (HMR 3647), a streptogramin (quinupristin-dalfopristin), a macrolide (erythromycin), and a lincosamide (clindamycin). Antimicrob Agents Chemother 1998;42(4):945–6.
55. Ubukata K, Iwata S, Sunakawa K. In vitro activities of new ketolide, telithromycin, and eight other macrolide antibiotics against *Streptococcus pneumoniae* having mefA and ermB genes that mediate macrolide resistance. J Infect Chemother 2003;9(3):221–6.
56. Doern GV, Heilmann KP, Huynh HK, et al. Antimicrobial resistance among clin-ical isolates of *Streptococcus pneumoniae* in the United States during 1999–2000, including a comparison of resistance rates since 1994–1995. Antimicrob Agents Chemother 2001;45(6):1721–9.
57. Clark JP, Langston E. Ketolides: a new class of antibacterial agents for treatment of community-acquired respiratory tract infections in a primary care setting. Mayo Clin Proc 2003;78(9):1113–24.
58. Hardy DJ, Swanson RN, Rode RA, et al. Enhancement of the in vitro and in vivo activities of clarithromycin against *Haemophilus influenzae* by 14-hydroxy-clari-thromycin, its major metabolite in humans. Antimicrob Agents Chemother 1990; 34(7):1407–13.
59. Barry AL, Fuchs PC, Brown SD. In vitro activities of the ketolide HMR 3647 against recent gram-positive clinical isolates and *Haemophilus influenzae*. Anti-microb Agents Chemother 1998;42(8):2138–40.

60. Fernandes PB, Bailer R, Swanson R, et al. In vitro and in vivo evaluation of A-56268 (TE-031), a new macrolide. Antimicrob Agents Chemother 1986; 30(6):865–73.
61. Peters DH, Clissold SP. Clarithromycin: a review of its antimicrobial activity, pharmacokinetic properties and therapeutic potential. Drugs 1992;44(1):117–64.
62. Peters DH, Friedel HA, McTavish D. Azithromycin: a review of its antimicrobial activity, pharmacokinetic properties and clinical efficacy. Drugs 1992;44(5): 750–99.
63. Slover CM, Rodvold KA, Danziger LH. Tigecycline: a novel broad-spectrum antimicrobial. Ann Pharmacother 2007;41(6):965–72.
64. Garrison MW, Mutters R, Dowzicky MJ. In vitro activity of tigecycline and comparator agents against a global collection of Gram-negative and Gram-positive organisms: Tigecycline Evaluation and Surveillance Trial 2004 to 2007. Diagn Microbiol Infect Dis 2009;65(3):288–99.
65. Dowzicky MJ, Park CH. Update on antimicrobial susceptibility rates among Gram-negative and Gram-positive organisms in the United States: results from the Tigecycline Evaluation and Surveillance Trial (TEST) 2005–2007. Clin Ther 2008;30(11):2040–50.
66. Kresken M, Becker K, Siefert, et al. Resistance trends and in vitro activity of tigecycline and 17 other antimicrobial agents against Gram-positive and Gram-negative organisms, including multidrug-resistant pathogens in Germany. Eur J Clin Microbiol Infect Dis 2011. [Epub ahead of print].
67. Castanheira M, Sader HS, Deshpande LM, et al. Antimicrobial activities of tigecycline and other broad-spectrum antimicrobials tested against serine carbapenemase- and metallo-beta-lactamase-producing Enterobacteriaceae: report from the SENTRY Antimicrobial Surveillance Program. Antimicrob Agents Chemother 2008;52(2):570–3.
68. Hoban DJ, Bouchillon SK, Dowzicky MJ. Antimicrobial susceptibility of extended-spectrum beta-lactamase producers and multidrug-resistant *Acinetobacter baumannii* throughout the United States and comparative in vitro activity of tigecycline, a new glycylcycline antimicrobial. Diagn Microbiol Infect Dis 2007;57(4):423–8.
69. Wang YF, Dowzicky MJ. In vitro activity of tigecycline and comparators on *Acinetobacter* spp. isoaltes collected from patients with bacteremia and MIC change during the Tigecycline Evaluation and Surveillance Trial 2004 to 2008. Diagn Microbiol Infect Dis 2010;68(1):73–9.
70. Darabi A, Hocquet D, Dowzicky MJ. Antimicrobial activity against Streptococcus pneumoniae and Haemophilus influenzae collected globally between 2004 and 2008 as part of the tigecycline Evaluation and Surveillance Trial. Diagn Microbiol Infec Dis 2010;67(1):78–86.
71. Nagy E, Dowzicky MJ. In vitro activity of tigecycline and comparators against a European compilation of anaerobes collected as part of the Tigecycline Evaluation and Surveillance Trial (TEST). Scan J Infect Dis 2010;42(1):33–8.
72. Portier H, Filipecki J, Weber P, et al. Five day clarithromycin modified release versus 10 day penicillin V for group A streptococcal pharyngitis: a multi-centre, open-label, randomized study. J Antimicrob Chemother 2002;49(2):337–44.
73. Norrby SR, Quinn J, Rangaraju M, et al. Evaluation of 5-day therapy with telithromycin, a novel ketolide antibacterial, for the treatment of tonsillopharyngitis. Clin Microbiol Infect 2004;10(7):615–23.
74. Quinn J, Ruoff GE, Ziter PS. Efficacy and tolerability of 5-day, once-daily telithromycin compared with 10-day, twice-daily clarithromycin for the treatment of

group A beta-hemolytic streptococcal tonsillitis/pharyngitis: a multicenter, randomized, double-blind, parallel-group study. Clin Ther 2003;25(2):422–43.

75. McCarty JM, Phillips A, Wiisanen R. Comparative safety and efficacy of clarithromycin and amoxicillin/clavulanate in the treatment of acute otitis media in children. Pediatr Infect Dis J 1993;12(12):S122–7.

76. Block SL, Cifaldi M, Gu Y, et al. A comparison of 5 days of therapy with cefdinir or azithromycin in children with acute otitis media: a multicenter, prospective, single-blind study. Clin Ther 2005;27(6):786–94.

77. Ioannidis JP, Contopoulos-Ioannidis DG, Chew P, et al. Meta-analysis of randomized controlled trials on the comparative efficacy and safety of azithromycin against other antibiotics for upper respiratory tract infections. J Antimicrob Chemother 2001;48(5):677–89.

78. Hoberman A, Dagan R, Leibovitz E, et al. Large dosage amoxicillin/clavulanate, compared with azithromycin, for the treatment of bacterial acute otitis media in children. Pediatr Infect Dis J 2005;24(6):525–32.

79. Arguedas A, Emparanza P, Schwartz RH, et al. A randomized, multicenter, double blind, double dummy trial of single dose azithromycin versus high dose amoxicillin for treatment of uncomplicated acute otitis media. Pediatr Infect Dis J 2005;24(2):153–61.

80. Adelglass J, Jones TM, Ruoff G, et al. A multicenter, investigator-blinded, randomized comparison of oral levofloxacin and oral clarithromycin in the treatment of acute bacterial sinusitis. Pharmacotherapy 1998;18(6):1255–63.

81. Clifford K, Huck W, Shan M, et al. Double-blind comparative trial of ciprofloxacin versus clarithromycin in the treatment of acute bacterial sinusitis: Sinusitis Infection Study Group. Ann Otol Rhinol Laryngol 1999;108(4):360–7.

82. Stefansson P, Jacovides A, Jablonicky P, et al. Cefuroxime axetil versus clarithromycin in the treatment of acute maxillary sinusitis. Rhinology 1998;36(4): 173–8.

83. Riffer E, Spiller J, Palmer R, et al. Once daily clarithromycin extended-release vs twice-daily amoxicillin/clavulanate in patients with acute bacterial sinusitis: a randomized, investigator-blinded study. Curr Med Res Opin 2005;21(1): 61–70.

84. Murray JJ, Emparanza P, Lesinskas E, et al. Efficacy and safety of a novel, single-dose azithromycin microsphere formulation versus 10 days of levofloxacin for the treatment of acute bacterial sinusitis in adults. Otolaryngol Head Neck Surg 2005;133(2):194–200.

85. Henry DC, Riffer E, Sokol WN, et al. Randomized double-blind study comparing 3- and 6-day regimens of azithromycin with a 10-day amoxicillin-clavulanate regimen for treatment of acute bacterial sinusitis. Antimicrob Agents Chemother 2003;47(9):2770–4.

86. Desrosiers M, Ferguson B, Klossek JM, et al. Clinical efficacy and time to symptom resolution of 5-day telithromycin versus 10-day amoxicillin-clavulanate in the treatment of acute bacterial sinusitis. Curr Med Res Opin 2008;24(6):1691–702.

87. Roos K, Tellier G, Baz M, et al. Clinical and bacteriological efficacy of 5-day telithromycin in acute maxillary sinusitis: a pooled analysis. J Infect 2005;50(3): 210–20.

88. Ferguson BJ, Guzzetta RV, Spector SL, et al. Efficacy and safety of oral telithromycin once daily for 5 days versus moxifloxacin once daily for 10 days in the treatment of acute bacterial rhinosinusitis. Otolaryngol Head Neck Surg 2004; 131(3):207–14.

89. Langtry HD, Brogden RN. Clarithromycin. A review of its efficacy in the treatment of respiratory tract infections in immunocompetent patients. Drugs 1997; 53(6):973–1004.

90. Weiss K, Vanjaka A. An open-label, randomized, multicenter, comparative study of the efficacy and safety of 7 days of treatment with clarithromycin extended-release tablets versus clarithromycin immediate-release tablets for the treatment of patients with acute bacterial exacerbation of chronic bronchitis. Clin Ther 2002;24(12):2105–22.

91. Adler JL, Jannetti W, Schneider D, et al. Phase III, randomized, double-blind study of clarithromycin extended-release and immediate-release formulations in the treatment of patients with acute exacerbation of chronic bronchitis. Clin Ther 2000;22(12):1410–20.

92. Martinot JB, Carr WD, Cullen S, et al. A comparative study of clarithromycin modified release and amoxicillin/clavulanic acid in the treatment of acute exacerbation of chronic bronchitis. Adv Ther 2001;18(1):1–11.

93. Anzueto A, Fisher CL Jr, Busman T, et al. Comparison of the efficacy of extended-release clarithromycin tablets and amoxicillin/clavulanate tablets in the treatment of acute exacerbation of chronic bronchitis. Clin Ther 2001; 23(1):72–86.

94. Gotfried M, Busman TA, Norris S, et al. Role for 5-day, once-daily extended-release clarithromycin in acute bacterial exacerbation of chronic bronchitis. Curr Med Res Opin 2007;23(2):459–66.

95. Weiss LR. Open-label, randomized comparison of the efficacy and tolerability of clarithromycin, levofloxacin, and cefuroxime axetil in the treatment of adults with acute bacterial exacerbations of chronic bronchitis. Clin Ther 2002;24(9):1414–25.

96. Wilson R, Schentag JJ, Ball P, et al. A comparison of gemifloxacin and clarithromycin in acute exacerbations of chronic bronchitis and long-term clinical outcomes. Clin Ther 2002;24(4):639–52.

97. Hoeffken G, Meyer HP, Winter J, et al. The efficacy and safety of two oral moxifloxacin regimens compared to oral clarithromycin in the treatment of community-acquired pneumonia. Respir Med 2001;95(7):553–64.

98. Gotfried MH, Dattani D, Riffer E, et al. A controlled, double-blind, multicenter study comparing clarithromycin extended-release tablets and levofloxacin tablets in the treatment of community-acquired pneumonia. Clin Ther 2002;24(5):736–51.

99. Sokol WN Jr, Sullivan JG, Acampora MD, et al. A prospective, double-blind, multicenter study comparing clarithromycin extended-release with trovafloxacin in patients with community-acquired pneumonia. Clin Ther 2002;24(4):605–15.

100. Lode H, Aronkyto T, Chuchalin AG, et al. A randomised, double-blind, double-dummy comparative study of gatifloxacin with clarithromycin in the treatment of community-acquired pneumonia. Clin Microbiol Infect 2004;10(5):403–8.

101. Kinasewitz G, Wood RG. Azithromycin versus cefaclor in the treatment of acute bacterial pneumonia. Eur J Clin Microbiol Infect Dis 1991;10(10):872–7.

102. Paris R, Confalonieri M, Dal Negro R, et al. Efficacy and safety of azithromycin 1 g once daily for 3 days in the treatment of community-acquired pneumonia: an open-label randomised comparison with amoxicillin-clavulanate 875/125 mg twice daily for 7 days. J Chemother 2008;20(1):77–86.

103. Drehobl MA, De Salvo MC, Lewis DE, et al. Single-dose azithromycin microspheres vs clarithromycin extended release for the treatment of mild-to-moderate community-acquired pneumonia in adults. Chest 2005;128(4):2230–7.

104. D'Ignazio J, Camere MA, Lewis DE, et al. Novel, single-dose microsphere formulation of azithromycin versus 7-day levofloxacin therapy for treatment of

mild to moderate community-acquired pneumonia in adults. Antimicrob Agents Chemother 2005;49(10):4035–41.

105. Contopoulos-Ioannidis DG, Ioannidis JP, Chew P, et al. Meta-analysis of randomized controlled trials on the comparative efficacy and safety of azithromycin against other antibiotics for lower respiratory tract infections. J Antimicrob Chemother 2001;48(5):691–703.

106. Panpanich R, Lerttrakarnnon P, Laopaiboon M. Azithromycin for acute lower respiratory tract infections. Cochrane Database Syst Rev 2008;1:CD001954.

107. Swanson RN, Lainez-Ventosilla A, De Salvo MC, et al. Once-daily azithromycin for 3 days compared with clarithromycin for 10 days for acute exacerbation of chronic bronchitis: a multicenter, double-blind, randomized study. Treat Respir Med 2005;4(1):31–9.

108. Amsden GW, Baird IM, Simon S, et al. Efficacy and safety of azithromycin vs levofloxacin in the outpatient treatment of acute bacterial exacerbations of chronic bronchitis. Chest 2003;123(3):772–7.

109. Zervos M, Martinez FJ, Amsden GW, et al. Efficacy and safety of 3-day azithromycin versus 5-day moxifloxacin for the treatment of acute bacterial exacerbations of chronic bronchitis. Int J Antimicrob Agents 2007;29(1):56–61.

110. Hagberg L, Carbon C, van Rensburg DJ, et al. Telithromycin in the treatment of community-acquired pneumonia: a pooled analysis. Respir Med 2003;97(6): 625–33.

111. Pullman J, Champlin J, Vrooman PS Jr. Efficacy and tolerability of once-daily oral therapy with telithromycin compared with trovafloxacin for the treatment of community-acquired pneumonia in adults. Int J Clin Pract 2003;57(5):377–84.

112. Mathers Dunbar L, Hassman J, Tellier G. Efficacy and tolerability of once-daily oral telithromycin compared with clarithromycin for the treatment of community-acquired pneumonia in adults. Clin Ther 2004;26(1):48–62.

113. Tellier G, Niederman MS, Nusrat R, et al. Clinical and bacteriological efficacy and safety of 5 and 7 day regimens of telithromycin once daily compared with a 10 day regimen of clarithromycin twice daily in patients with mild to moderate community-acquired pneumonia. J Antimicrob Chemother 2004;54(2):515–23.

114. van Rensburg DJ, Fogarty C, Kohno S, et al. Efficacy of telithromycin in community-acquired pneumonia caused by pneumococci with reduced susceptibility to penicillin and/or erythromycin. Chemotherapy 2005;51(4): 186–92.

115. Carbon C, van Rensburg D, Hagberg L, et al. Clinical and bacteriologic efficacy of telithromycin in patients with bacteremic community-acquired pneumonia. Respir Med 2006;100(4):577–85.

116. Fogarty C, de Wet R, Mandell L, et al. Five-day telithromycin once daily is as effective as 10-day clarithromycin twice daily for the treatment of acute exacerbations of chronic bronchitis and is associated with reduced health-care resource utilization. Chest 2005;128(4):1980–8.

117. Aubier M, Aldons PM, Leak A, et al. Telithromycin is as effective as amoxicillin/clavulanate in acute exacerbations of chronic bronchitis. Respir Med 2002; 96(11):862–71.

118. Carbon C. A pooled analysis of telithromycin in the treatment of community-acquired respiratory tract infections in adults. Infection 2003;31(5):308–17.

119. Vergis EN, Indorf A, File TM Jr, et al. Azithromycin vs cefuroxime plus erythromycin for empirical treatment of community-acquired pneumonia in hospitalized patients: a prospective, randomized, multicenter trial. Arch Intern Med 2000; 160(9):1294–300.

120. Plouffe J, Schwartz DB, Kolokathis A, et al. Clinical efficacy of intravenous followed by oral azithromycin monotherapy in hospitalized patients with community-acquired pneumonia: the Azithromycin Intravenous Clinical Trials Group. Antimicrob Agents Chemother 2000;44(7):1796–802.

121. Feldman RB, Rhew DC, Wong JY, et al. Azithromycin monotherapy for patients hospitalized with community-acquired pneumonia: a 31/2-year experience from a veterans affairs hospital. Arch Intern Med 2003;163(14):1718–26.

122. Zervos M, Mandell LA, Vrooman PS, et al. Comparative efficacies and tolerabilities of intravenous azithromycin plus ceftriaxone and intravenous levofloxacin with step-down oral therapy for hospitalized patients with moderate to severe community-acquired pneumonia. Treat Respir Med 2004;3(5):329–36.

123. Frank E, Liu J, Kinasewitz G, et al. A multicenter, open-label, randomized comparison of levofloxacin and azithromycin plus ceftriaxone in hospitalized adults with moderate to severe community-acquired pneumonia. Clin Ther 2002;24(8):1292–308.

124. Correa JC, Badaro R, Bumroongkit C, et al. Randomized, open-label, parallel-group, multicenter study of the efficacy and tolerability of IV gatifloxacin with the option for oral stepdown gatifloxacin versus IV ceftriaxone (with or without erythromycin or clarithromycin) with the option for oral stepdown clarithromycin for treatment of patients with mild to moderate community-acquired pneumonia requiring hospitalization. Clin Ther 2003;25(5):1453–68.

125. Weiss K, Low DE, Cortes L, et al. Clinical characteristics at initial presentation and impact of dual therapy on the outcome of bacteremic Streptococcus pneumoniae pneumonia in adults. Can Respir J 2004;11(8):589–93.

126. Garcia Vazquez E, Mensa J, Martinez JA, et al. Lower mortality among patients with community-acquired pneumonia treated with a macrolide plus a beta-lactam agent versus a beta-lactam agent alone. Eur J Clin Microbiol Infect Dis 2005;24(3):190–5.

127. Martinez JA, Horcajada JP, Almela M, et al. Addition of a macrolide to a beta-lactam-based empirical antibiotic regimen is associated with lower in-hospital mortality for patients with bacteremic pneumococcal pneumonia. Clin Infect Dis 2003;36(4):389–95.

128. Plouffe JF, Breiman RF, Fields BS, et al. Azithromycin in the treatment of Legionella pneumonia requiring hospitalization. Clin Infect Dis 2003;37(11):1475–80.

129. Sahm DF, Brown NP, Draghi DC, et al. Tracking resistance among bacterial respiratory tract pathogens: summary of findings of the TRUST Surveillance Initiative, 2001–2005. Postgrad Med 2008;120(3 Suppl 1):8–15.

130. Jenkins SG, Brown SD, Farrell DJ. Trends in antibacterial resistance among Streptococcus pneumoniae isolated in the USA: update from PROTEKT US Years 1–4. Ann Clin Microbiol Antimicrob 2008;7:1.

131. Critchley IA, Brown SD, Traczewski MM, et al. National and regional assessment of antimicrobial resistance among community-acquired respiratory tract pathogens identified in a 2005–2006 U.S. Faropenem surveillance study. Antimicrob Agents Chemother 2007;51(12):4382–9.

132. Jenkins SG, Farrell DJ. Increase in pneumococcus macrolide resistance, United States. Emerg Infect Dis 2009;15(8):1260–4.

133. Farrell DJ, File TM, Jenkins SG. Prevalence and antibacterial susceptibility of mef(A)-positive macrolide-resistant Streptococcus pneumoniae over 4 years (2000 to 2004) of the PROTEKT US Study. J Clin Microbiol 2007;45(2):290–3.

134. Sahm DF, Brown NP, Thornsberry C, et al. Antimicrobial susceptibility profiles among common respiratory tract pathogens: a GLOBAL perspective. Postgrad Med 2008;120(3 Suppl 1):16–24.

135. Rantala M, Haanpera-Heikkinen M, Lindgren M, et al. *Streptococcus pneumoniae* isolates resistant to telithromycin. Antimicrob Agents Chemother 2006;50(5):1855–8.
136. Lau YJ, Hsueh PR, Liu YC, et al. Comparison of in vitro activities of tigecycline with other antimicrobial agents against *Streptococcus pneumoniae, Haemophilus influenzae,* and *Moraxella catarrhalis* in Taiwan. Microb Drug Resist 2006;12(2):130–5.
137. Rowe BH, Campbell SG, Boudreaux ED, et al. Community-acquired pneumonia in North American emergency departments: drug resistance and treatment success with clarithromycin. Acad Emerg Med 2007;14(7):607–15.
138. Lonks JR, Garau J, Gomez L, et al. Failure of macrolide antibiotic treatment in patients with bacteremia due to erythromycin-resistant *Streptococcus pneumoniae*. Clin Infect Dis 2002;35(5):556–64.
139. Mandell LA, Wunderink RG, Anzueto A, et al. Infectious Diseases Society of America/American Thoracic Society consensus guidelines on the management of community-acquired pneumonia in adults. Clin Infect Dis 2007;44(Suppl 2): S27–72.
140. Lau CY, Qureshi AK. Azithromycin versus doxycycline for genital chlamydial infections: a meta-analysis of randomized clinical trials. Sex Transm Dis 2002; 29(9):497–502.
141. Pitsouni E, Iavazzo C, Athanasiou S, et al. Single-dose azithromycin versus erythromycin or amoxicillin for *Chlamydia trachomatis* infection during pregnancy: a meta-analysis of randomised controlled trials. Int J Antimicrob Agents 2007;30(3):213–21.
142. Workowski KA, Berman SM. Centers for Disease Control and Prevention. Sexually transmitted diseases treatment guidelines, 2010. MMWR Recomm Rep 2010;59(RR-12):1–110.
143. Skerk V, Schonwald S, Krhen I, et al. Comparative analysis of azithromycin and ciprofloxacin in the treatment of chronic prostatitis caused by *Chlamydia trachomatis*. Int J Antimicrob Agents 2003;21(5):457–62.
144. Skerk V, Krhen I, Lisic M, et al. Comparative randomized pilot study of azithromycin and doxycycline efficacy in the treatment of prostate infection caused by *Chlamydia trachomatis*. Int J Antimicrob Agents 2004;24(2):188–91.
145. Handsfield HH, Dalu ZA, Martin DH, et al. Multicenter trial of single-dose azithromycin vs. ceftriaxone in the treatment of uncomplicated gonorrhea: Azithromycin Gonorrhea Study Group. Sex Transm Dis 1994;21(2):107–11.
146. Bevan CD, Ridgway GL, Rothermel CD. Efficacy and safety of azithromycin as monotherapy or combined with metronidazole compared with two standard multidrug regimens for the treatment of acute pelvic inflammatory disease. J Int Med Res 2003;31(1):45–54.
147. Bai ZG, Yang KH, Liu YL, et al. Azithromycin vs. benzathine penicillin G for early syphilis: a meta-analysis of randomized clinical trials. Int J STD AIDS 2008; 19(4):217–21.
148. Riedner G, Rusizoka M, Todd J, et al. Single-dose azithromycin versus penicillin G benzathine for the treatment of early syphilis. N Engl J Med 2005;353(12): 1236–44.
149. Hook EW 3rd, Behets F, Van Damme K, et al. A phase III equivalence trial of azithromycin versus benzathine penicillin for treatment of early syphilis. J Infect Dis 2010;201(11):1729–35.
150. Su JR, Hook E, Kenney K, et al. Prevalence of the 23S rRNA point mutation in *Treponema pallidum* in the United States and Associated Factors, 2006–2008. 18th International Society for Sexually Transmitted Diseases Research, #OS1.11.03. London, England: June 2009.

151. Chey WD, Wong BC, Practice Parameters Committee of the American College of Gastroenterology. American College of Gastroenterology guideline on the management of *Helicobacter pylori* infection. Am J Gastroenterol 2007;102(8):1808–25.

152. Suerbaum S, Michetti P. *Helicobacter pylori* infection. N Engl J Med 2002;347(15):1175–86.

153. Vergara M, Vallve M, Gisbert JP, et al. Meta-analysis: comparative efficacy of different proton-pump inhibitors in triple therapy for *Helicobacter pylori* eradication. Aliment Pharmacol Ther 2003;18(6):647–54.

154. Gene E, Calvet X, Azagra R, et al. Triple vs. quadruple therapy for treating *Helicobacter pylori* infection: a meta-analysis. Aliment Pharmacol Ther 2003;17(9):1137–43.

155. Laheij RJ, Rossum LG, Jansen JB, et al. Evaluation of treatment regimens to cure *Helicobacter pylori* infection: a meta-analysis. Aliment Pharmacol Ther 1999;13(7):857–64.

156. Calvet X, Garcia N, Lopez T, et al. A meta-analysis of short versus long therapy with a proton pump inhibitor, clarithromycin and either metronidazole or amoxycillin for treating *Helicobacter pylori* infection. Aliment Pharmacol Ther 2000;14(5):603–9.

157. Paoluzi P, Iacopini F, Crispino P, et al. 2-week triple therapy for *Helicobacter pylori* infection is better than 1-week in clinical practice: a large prospective single-center randomized study. Helicobacter 2006;11(6):562–8.

158. Vaira D, Zullo A, Vakil N, et al. Sequential therapy versus standard triple-drug therapy for *Helicobacter pylori* eradication: a randomized trial. Ann Intern Med 2007;146(8):556–63.

159. Zullo A, De Francesco V, Hassan C, et al. The sequential therapy regimen for *Helicobacter pylori* eradication: a pooled-data analysis. Gut 2007;56(10):1353–7.

160. Jafri NS, Hornung CA, Howden CW. Meta-analysis: sequential therapy appears superior to standard therapy for *Helicobacter pylori* infection in patients naive to treatment. Ann Intern Med 2008;148(12):923–31.

161. Meyer JM, Silliman NP, Wang W, et al. Risk factors for *Helicobacter pylori* resistance in the United States: the surveillance of *H. pylori* antimicrobial resistance partnership (SHARP) study, 1993–1999. Ann Intern Med 2002;136(1):13–24.

162. Duck WM, Sobel J, Pruckler JM, et al. Antimicrobial resistance incidence and risk factors among *Helicobacter pylori*-infected persons, United States. Emerg Infect Dis 2004;10(6):1088–94.

163. De Francesco V, Margiotta M, Zullo A, et al. Prevalence of primary clarithromycin resistance in *Helicobacter pylori* strains over a 15 year period in Italy. J Antimicrob Chemother 2007;59(4):783–5.

164. McMahon BJ, Hennessy TW, Bensler JM, et al. The relationship among previous antimicrobial use, antimicrobial resistance, and treatment outcomes for *Helicobacter pylori* infections. Ann Intern Med 2003;139(6):463–9.

165. Lee JH, Shin JH, Roe IH, et al. Impact of clarithromycin resistance on eradication of *Helicobacter pylori* in infected adults. Antimicrob Agents Chemother 2005;49(4):1600–3.

166. Dore MP, Leandro G, Realdi G, et al. Effect of pretreatment antibiotic resistance to metronidazole and clarithromycin on outcome of *Helicobacter pylori* therapy: a meta-analytical approach. Dig Dis Sci 2000;45(1):68–76.

167. Havlir DV, Dube MP, Sattler FR, et al. Prophylaxis against disseminated *Mycobacterium avium* complex with weekly azithromycin, daily rifabutin, or both: California Collaborative Treatment Group. N Engl J Med 1996;335(6):392–8.

168. Benson CA, Williams PL, Cohn DL, et al. Clarithromycin or rifabutin alone or in combination for primary prophylaxis of *Mycobacterium avium* complex disease in patients with AIDS: a randomized, double-blind, placebo-controlled trial. The AIDS Clinical Trials Group 196/Terry Beirn Community Programs for Clinical Research on AIDS 009 Protocol Team. J Infect Dis 2000;181(4):1289–97.

169. Kaplan JE, Benson C, Holmes KK, et al. Guidelines for the prevention and treatment of opportunistic infections among HIV-Exposed and HIV-Infected Children—Recommendations from CDC, the National Institutes of Health, the HIV Medicine Association of the Infectious Diseases Society of America, the Pediatric Infectious Diseases Society, and the American Academy of Pediatrics. MMWR Recomm Rep 2009;58(RR-11):1–166.

170. Shafran SD, Singer J, Zarowny DP, et al. A comparison of two regimens for the treatment of *Mycobacterium avium* complex bacteremia in AIDS: rifabutin, ethambutol, and clarithromycin versus rifampin, ethambutol, clofazimine, and ciprofloxacin. Canadian HIV Trials Network Protocol 010 Study Group. N Engl J Med 1996;335(6):377–83.

171. Cohn DL, Fisher EJ, Peng GT, et al. A prospective randomized trial of four three-drug regimens in the treatment of disseminated *Mycobacterium avium* complex disease in AIDS patients: excess mortality associated with high-dose clarithromycin. Terry Beirn Community Programs for Clinical Research on AIDS. Clin Infect Dis 1999;29(1):125–33.

172. Benson CA, Williams PL, Currier JS, et al. A prospective, randomized trial examining the efficacy and safety of clarithromycin in combination with ethambutol, rifabutin, or both for the treatment of disseminated *Mycobacterium avium* complex disease in persons with acquired immunodeficiency syndrome. Clin Infect Dis 2003;37(9):1234–43.

173. Dunne M, Fessel J, Kumar P, et al. A randomized, double-blind trial comparing azithromycin and clarithromycin in the treatment of disseminated *Mycobacterium avium* infection in patients with human immunodeficiency virus. Clin Infect Dis 2000;31(5):1245–52.

174. Ward TT, Rimland D, Kauffman C, et al. Randomized, open-label trial of azithromycin plus ethambutol vs. clarithromycin plus ethambutol as therapy for *Mycobacterium avium* complex bacteremia in patients with human immunodeficiency virus infection. Veterans Affairs HIV Research Consortium. Clin Infect Dis 1998; 27(5):1278–85.

175. Wallace RJ Jr, Brown BA, Griffith DE, et al. Initial clarithromycin monotherapy for Mycobacterium avium-intracellulare complex lung disease. Am J Respir Crit Care Med 1994;149(5):1335–41.

176. Griffith DE, Brown BA, Girard WM, et al. Azithromycin activity against *Mycobacterium avium* complex lung disease in patients who were not infected with human immunodeficiency virus. Clin Infect Dis 1996;23(5):983–9.

177. Griffith DE, Brown BA, Murphy DT, et al. Initial (6-month) results of three-times-weekly azithromycin in treatment regimens for *Mycobacterium avium* complex lung disease in human immunodeficiency virus-negative patients. J Infect Dis 1998;178(1):121–6.

178. Griffith DE, Brown BA, Cegielski P, et al. Early results (at 6 months) with intermittent clarithromycin-including regimens for lung disease due to *Mycobacterium avium* complex. Clin Infect Dis 2000;30(2):288–92.

179. Lam PK, Griffith DE, Aksamit TR, et al. Factors related to response to intermittent treatment of *Mycobacterium avium* complex lung disease. Am J Respir Crit Care Med 2006;173(11):1283–9.

180. Griffith DE, Aksamit T, Brown-Elliott BA, et al. An official ATS/IDSA statement: diagnosis, treatment, and prevention of nontuberculous mycobacterial diseases. Am J Respir Crit Care Med 2007;175(4):367–416.
181. Sacchidanand S, Penn RL, Embil JM, et al. Efficacy and safety of tigecycline monotherapy compared with vancomycin plus aztreonam in patients with complicated skin and skin structure infections: results from a phase 3, randomized, double-blind trial. Int J Infect Dis 2005;9(5):251–61.
182. Breedt J, Teras J, Gardovskis J, et al. Safety and efficacy of tigecycline in treatment of skin and skin structure infections: results of a double-blind phase 3 comparison study with vancomycin-aztreonam. Antimicrob Agents Chemother 2005;49(11):4658–66.
183. Ellis-Grosse EJ, Babinchak T, Dartois N, et al. The efficacy and safety of tigecycline in the treatment of skin and skin-structure infections: results of 2 double-blind phase 3 comparison studies with vancomycin-aztreonam. Clin Infect Dis 2005;41(Suppl 5):S341–53.
184. Florescu I, Beuran M, Dimov R, et al. Efficacy and safety of tigecycline compared with vancomycin or linezolid for treatment of serious infections with methicillin-resistant *Staphylococcus aureus* or vancomycin-resistant enterococci: a phase 3, multicentre, double-blind, randomized study. J Antimicrob Chemother 2008;62(Suppl 1):i17–28.
185. Fomin P, Beuran M, Gradauskas A, et al. Tigecycline is efficacious in the treatment of complicated intra-abdominal infections. Int J Surg 2005;3(1):35–47.
186. Oliva ME, Rekha A, Yellin A, et al. A multicenter trial of the efficacy and safety of tigecycline versus imipenem/cilastatin in patients with complicated intra-abdominal infections [Study ID Numbers: 3074A1-301-WW; ClinicalTrials.gov Identifier: NCT00081744]. BMC Infect Dis 2005;5:88.
187. Babinchak T, Ellis-Grosse E, Dartois N, et al. The efficacy and safety of tigecycline for the treatment of complicated intra-abdominal infections: analysis of pooled clinical trial data. Clin Infect Dis 2005;41(Suppl 5):S354–67.
188. Bergallo C, Jasovich A, Teglia O, et al. Safety and efficacy of intravenous tigecycline in treatment of community-acquired pneumonia: results from a double-blind randomized phase 3 comparison study with levofloxacin. Diagn Microbiol Infect Dis 2009;63(1):52–61.
189. Tanaseanu C, Bergallo C, Teglia O, et al. Integrated results of 2 phase 3 studies comparing tigecycline and levofloxacin in community-acquired pneumonia. Diagn Microbiol Infect Dis 2008;61(3):329–38.
190. Kelesidis T, Karageorgopoulos DE, Kelesidis I, et al. Tigecycline for the treatment of multidrug-resistant Enterobacteriaceae: a systematic review of the evidence from microbiological and clinical studies. J Antimicrob Chemother 2008;62(5):895–904.
191. Vasilev K, Reshedko G, Orasan R, et al. A phase 3, open-label, non-comparative study of tigecycline in the treatment of patients with selected serious infections due to resistant Gram-negative organisms including *Enterobacter* species, *Acinetobacter baumannii* and *Klebsiella pneumoniae*. J Antimicrob Chemother 2008;62(Suppl 1):i29–40.
192. Gallagher JC, Rouse HM. Tigecycline for the treatment of *Acinetobacter* infections: a case series. Ann Pharmacother 2008;42(9):1188–94.
193. Karageorgopoulos DE, Kelesidis T, Kelesidis I, et al. Tigecycline for the treatment of multidrug-resistant (including carbapenem-resistant) Acinetobacter infections: a review of the scientific evidence. J Antimicrob Chemother 2008;62(1):45–55.

194. Gordon NC, Wareham DW. A review of clinical and microbiological outcomes following treatment of infections involving multidrug-resistant Acinetobacter baumannii with tigecycline. J Antimicrob Chemother 2009;63(4):775–80.

195. Nieman RB, Sharma K, Edelberg H, et al. Telithromycin and myasthenia gravis. Clin Infect Dis 2003;37(11):1579.

196. Anthony KB, Fishman NO, Linkin DR, et al. Clinical and microbiological outcomes of serious infections with multidrug-resistant gram-negative organisms treated with tigecycline. Clin Infect Dis 2008;46(4):567–70.

197. Hopkins S. Clinical toleration and safety of azithromycin. Am J Med 1991;91(3): 40S–5S.

198. Garey KW, Amsden GW. Intravenous azithromycin. Ann Pharmacother 1999; 33(2):218–28.

199. Guay DR, Patterson DR, Seipman N, et al. Overview of the tolerability profile of clarithromycin in preclinical and clinical trials. Drug Saf 1993;8(5):350–64.

200. Ketek (telithromycin) tablets: prescribing information. 2007;2008(November, 28).

201. Demolis JL, Vacheron F, Cardus S, et al. Effect of single and repeated oral doses of telithromycin on cardiac QT interval in healthy subjects. Clin Pharmacol Ther 2003;73(3):242–52.

202. Ross DB. The FDA and the case of Ketek. N Engl J Med 2007;356(16):1601–4.

203. Brinker AD, Wassel RT, Lyndly J, et al. Telithromycin-associated hepatotoxicity: Clinical spectrum and causality assessment of 42 cases. Hepatology 2009;49: 250–7.

204. Clay KD, Hanson JS, Pope SD, et al. Brief communication: severe hepatotoxicity of telithromycin: three case reports and literature review. Ann Intern Med 2006; 144(6):415–20.

205. Perrot X, Bernard N, Vial C, et al. Myasthenia gravis exacerbation or unmasking associated with telithromycin treatment. Neurology 2006;67(12):2256–8.

206. U.S. Food and Drug Administration. Telithromycin (marketed as Ketek) Information. 2007;2008(12/22).

207. Gilson M, Moachon L, Jeanne L, et al. Acute pancreatitis related to tigecycline: case report and review of the literature. Scand J Infect Dis 2008;40(3):1–3.

208. Rubinstein E. Comparative safety of the different macrolides. Int J Antimicrob Agents 2001;18(Suppl 1):S71–6.

209. Amsden GW. Macrolides versus azalides: a drug interaction update. Ann Pharmacother 1995;29(9):906–17.

210. Gomes T, Mamdani MM, Juurlink DN. Macrolide-induced digoxin toxicity: a population-based study. Clin Pharmacol Ther 2009;86(4):383–6.

211. Zimmerman JJ, Harper DM, Matschke K, et al. Absence of an interaction between tigecycline and digoxin in healthy men. Pharmacotherapy 2007; 27(6):835–44.

212. Zimmerman JJ, Raible DG, Harper DM, et al. Evaluation of a potential tigecycline-warfarin drug interaction. Pharmacotherapy 2008;28(7):895–905.

213. FDA. FDA Drug Safety Communication: increased risk of death with Tygacil (tigecycline) compared to other antibiotics used to treat similar infections. Available at: http://www.fda.gov/Drugs/DrugSafety/ucm224370.htm. Accessed March 23, 2011.

The Newer Fluoroquinolones

Maureen K. Bolon, MD, MS

KEYWORDS

- Fluoroquinolones • Antiinfective agents • Pharmacology
- Pharmacokinetics • Microbial drug resistance
- Therapeutic use

Quinolones are unusual among antimicrobials in that they were not isolated from living organisms, but rather synthesized by chemists. The first quinolone, nalidixic acid, was derived from the antimalarial drug chloroquine.[1] Subsequent agents were derived through side chain and nuclear manipulation.[2] The development of the fluoroquinolone class may be described in generational terms, with each generation sharing similar features or antimicrobial spectra (**Table 1**).[1–3] First-generation agents possess activity against aerobic gram-negative bacteria, but little activity against aerobic gram-positive bacteria or anaerobes. Second-generation agents are the original fluoroquinolones, named for the addition of a fluorine atom at position C-6 (**Fig. 1**). These agents offer improved coverage against gram-negative bacteria and moderately improved gram-positive coverage. Third-generation agents achieve greater potency against gram-positive bacteria, particularly pneumococci, in combination with good activity against anaerobes. Fourth-generation fluoroquinolones have superior coverage against pneumococci and anaerobes. This article focuses on the fluoroquinolone agents most commonly used in clinical practice: ciprofloxacin, levofloxacin, and moxifloxacin.

CHEMISTRY
Basic Antimicrobial Activity

Fluoroquinolones interfere with bacterial cell replication, transcription, and DNA repair by disabling two bacterial enzymes crucial to these processes, DNA gyrase (formerly topoisomerase II) and topoisomerase IV. These enzymes are necessary for bacteria to manage the topological challenge of containing their genetic material. Using *Escherichia coli* as an example, a bacterial cell that is 1 to 3 μm long must accommodate a chromosome that is a double-stranded DNA circle longer than 1000 μm. Chromosomal volume is reduced via tertiary folding and compaction. These processes

A version of this article appeared in the 23:4 issue of the *Infectious Disease Clinics of North America*.

Division of Infectious Diseases, Department of Medicine, Northwestern University Feinberg School of Medicine, 645 North Michigan Avenue, Suite 900, Chicago, IL 60611, USA

E-mail address: m-bolon@northwestern.edu

Med Clin N Am 95 (2011) 793–817

doi:10.1016/j.mcna.2011.03.006

medical.theclinics.com

Table 1
Evolution of the fluoroquinolone class of antimicrobials

Generation	Agent	Comment
First generation	Nalidixic acid	Generic form available
	Cinoxacin	Discontinued
Second generation	Norfloxacin	Available as Noroxin
	Ciprofloxacin	Available as Cipro and generic form
	Lomefloxacin	Discontinued
	Ofloxacin	Available as Floxin and generic form
	Levofloxacin	Available as Levaquin and generic form
Third generation	Sparfloxacin	Discontinued
	Gatifloxacin	Discontinued
	Grepafloxacin	Discontinued
Fourth generation	Trovafloxacin	Discontinued
	Moxifloxacin	Available as Avelox
	Gemifloxacin	Available as Factive
	Garenoxacin	Not approved

Data from Andriole VT. The quinolones: past, present, and future. Clinical Infectious Diseases 2005;41(Suppl 2):S113–9; Ball P. Adverse drug reactions: Implications for the development of fluoroquinolones. Journal of Antimicrobial Chemotherapy 2003;51(Suppl 1):21–7; and Drugs@FDA page. Available at: http://www.accessdata.fda.gov/scripts/cder/drugsatfda/index.cfm. Accessed April 18, 2011.

must be reversed in order for bacterial replication to occur; DNA topoisomerases facilitate this.[4]

DNA gyrase is a tetramer of two A and two B subunits, encoded by *gyrA* and *gyrB*.[4] DNA gyrase introduces negative DNA supercoils, removes positive and negative supercoils, and catenates and decatenates (links and unlinks) chromosomal material.[5] Topoisomerase IV is a homologue of DNA gyrase and possesses two C and two E subunits, encoded by *parC* and *parE*.[4] It too can remove positive and negative supercoils, but is primarily involved in the separation of the daughter chromosome.[5,6]

Fluoroquinolones bind to the enzyme–DNA complex, causing a conformational change in the enzyme. This leads to DNA cleavage by the enzyme while the continued presence of the fluoroquinolone prevents ligation of broken DNA strands. The fluoroquinolone traps the enzyme on the DNA as a fluoroquinolone–enzyme–DNA complex, inhibiting further DNA replication. The process of complex-formation inhibits bacterial cell growth and is thus believed to be bacteriostatic in nature. The bactericidal action of fluoroquinolones is attributed to DNA cleavage.[4,5]

Structure–activity Relationships

Decades of fluoroquinolone development provide considerable insight into the effects of structural modification upon the antimicrobial activity and pharmacologic properties

Fig. 1. The core quinolone nucleus.

of these agents. **Fig. 1** depicts the core quinolone nucleus. Position 1 affects drug potency, pharmacokinetics, and the potential for interaction with theophylline. Positions 2, 3, and 4 determine antibacterial activity by influencing the affinity for bacterial enzymes. Additionally, positions 3 and 4 are involved in metal chelation and the resulting interaction with di- and trivalent cations. The presence of a methoxy side chain at position 5 enhances gram-positive activity and phototoxicity. The addition of a fluorine atom to position 6 transforms a quinolone into a fluoroquinolone, enhancing drug penetration into the bacterial cell and activity against gram-negative bacteria. Position 7, like position 1, is instrumental in drug potency, pharmacokinetics, and the interaction with theophylline. This position is also implicated in the central nervous system toxicity of some fluoroquinolones owing to their proclivity to bind to gamma-aminobutyric acid (GABA). The addition of a piperazine moiety at position 7 augments activity against *Pseudomonas aeruginosa*, whereas a pyrrolidine group improves gram-positive activity. The presence of any halogen at position 8 can increase a drug's half-life, absorption, and antianaerobic activity; however, the resulting phototoxicity of di-halogenated compounds renders them unacceptable for clinical use. In contrast, superior pneumococcal activity is achieved by the addition of a methoxy group at position 8 without attendant phototoxicity.[6,7]

Pharmacologic Considerations

Fluoroquinolones have favorable pharmacokinetic properties that have encouraged their widespread use (**Table 2**). They are well absorbed and have good tissue penetration, which facilitates their use for many clinical syndromes.[6,8] While ciprofloxacin must be dosed more frequently, the longer half-lives of the later generation fluoroquinolones allow them to be dosed daily. Most fluoroquinolones are eliminated via the kidney. Moxifloxacin, which is eliminated via the hepatic route, is unusual among fluoroquinolones in lacking efficacy for the treatment of genitourinary infections.

In general, because fluoroquinolones are not highly protein-bound and inhibition of the cytochrome P450 system is limited to the CYP1A2 enzyme, concerns for drug–drug interactions are somewhat minimized.[6,8,9] Fluoroquinolones are known to interact with xanthines, including theophylline and caffeine; however, this is primarily a concern for the older agents.[10] Concomitant use of fluoroquinolones and warfarin can result in supratherapeutic anticoagulation.[11] Perhaps the most common fluoroquinolone interaction involves di- and trivalent cations. Coadministration with antacids may result in subtherapeutic levels of fluoroquinolone agents and, potentially, clinical failure. This issue may be particularly relevant in the inpatient setting given the prevalent use of both fluoroquinolones and antacids; coadministration of fluoroquinolones

Agent	Dose (mg)	Bioavailability (%)	Protein Binding (%)	Half-life (Hours)	Elimination	Formulation
Ciprofloxacin	500	60–80	20–40	3–5	Renal/other	IV and PO
Gemifloxacin	320	71	60	7	Renal/other	PO only
Levofloxacin	500	99	40	7	Renal	IV and PO
Moxifloxacin	400	90	50	13	Hepatic	IV and PO

Table 2
Pharmacokinetic properties of fluoroquinolones

Abbreviations: IV, intravenous; PO, by mouth.
Data from Ball P. The quinolones: history and overview. In: Andriole VT, editor. The quinolones, Third edition. San Diego: Academic Press; 2000. p. 1–33; and O'Donnell JA, Gelone SP. The newer fluoroquinolones. Infect Disease Clinics of North America 2004;18(3):691–716.

and antacids has been implicated by some authors in the emergence of resistance to fluoroquinolones.[12,13]

Pharmacodynamics

Decisions regarding the choice and dosing of an agent are greatly enhanced by considering the pharmacokinetic and pharmacodynamic properties of that agent. Using the minimal inhibitory concentration (MIC) of a bacterial isolate as the sole criterion for choosing an agent fails to take into account the likely concentration of the agent at the site of the infection, individual variation in drug metabolism and clearance, and the mechanism of antimicrobial killing. The pharmacodynamic parameters typically used to predict antimicrobial efficacy are: the time over MIC (T>MIC), the ratio of peak concentration to the MIC (C_{max}/MIC), and the ratio of the area under the concentration-versus-time curve to the MIC (AUC/MIC).[14] Consistent with the characterization of fluoroquinolones as concentration-dependent killers, the parameters regarded as most useful for predicting fluoroquinolone efficacy are C_{max}/MIC and AUC/MIC. These parameters may also be useful to guide therapy in order to prevent the development of resistance to fluoroquinolone agents.

One of the earliest studies to correlate pharmacodynamic parameters with bacteriologic and clinical outcomes evaluated several regimens of intravenous ciprofloxacin administered to acutely ill subjects.[15] Although subjects were treated for a variety of infectious syndromes, the majority were receiving therapy for gram-negative pneumonia. An AUC/MIC ratio greater than 125 was associated with a superior likelihood of clinical and microbiologic cure. Additionally, the time to bacterial eradication was significantly shorter if the AUC/MIC exceeded 125. Subsequent studies have not validated the AUC/MIC threshold value of 125 for all infectious processes, but rather suggest that this value varies by disease state and target pathogen.[16,17] As an example, an AUC/MIC ratio of greater than 33.7 was necessary for a superior microbiologic response when treating pneumococcal pneumonia using levofloxacin or gatifloxacin.[18] Another study in subjects who had nosocomial pneumonia determined that an AUC/MIC threshold of 87 was required for bacterial eradication when treating with levofloxacin.[19] The usefulness of the C_{max}/MIC parameter was established by modeling the pharmacodynamic data from phase 3 trials for levofloxacin.[20] Favorable clinical and microbiologic outcomes were associated with a C_{max}/MIC ratio of at least 12.2. In this particular study, the C_{max}/MIC was highly correlated with the AUC/MIC.

One of the earliest studies to examine whether pharmacodynamic parameters correlate with the emergence of resistance analyzed retrospective data from four nosocomial pneumonia trials.[21] The AUC/MIC ratio was a significant predictor of resistance: resistance was significantly more likely to occur when the AUC/MIC was below 100. Although dosing antimicrobials aggressively in order to achieve adequate pharmacodynamic parameters is fairly well accepted, subsequent studies have not conclusively established that this approach prevents the emergence of resistance. Falagas and colleagues[22] reviewed 12 studies that compared different dosing regimens of fluoroquinolones and reported the development of resistance. Only five of the studies identified fluoroquinolone-resistant isolates following treatment. There was no statistical difference in the emergence of resistance between the high- and low-dose arms, highlighting the need for more studies in this area.

Given trends of worsening antimicrobial resistance, the feasibility of achieving desirable pharmacodynamic thresholds has become an issue of great concern. Pharmacodynamic modeling using antimicrobial susceptibility data from gram-negative organisms collected in the United States for the 2004 Meropenem Yearly Susceptibility Test Information Collection (MYSTIC) surveillance program substantiates this concern.[23] Ciprofloxacin and levofloxacin could be anticipated to be active against only 78% of *E coli*, 40.4%–65.5% of *P aeruginosa* and 43.6%–48.2% of *Acinetobacter baumannii*. These are findings that call into question whether these agents can continue to be used empirically for nonfermenters and Enterobacteriaceae. Finally, altered pharmacokinetics may impact the likelihood of achieving desirable pharmaco-dynamic thresholds on an individual level. Target AUC/MIC ratios for ciprofloxacin in critically ill individuals are attainable for organisms with the lowest levels of resistance.[24] However, standard doses of ciprofloxacin do not achieve AUC/MIC ratios above 125 for organisms with higher MICs in this population. Higher doses of ciprofloxacin should be considered in critically ill patients to accommodate the MICs of bacteria likely to be encountered.

MECHANISMS OF RESISTANCE

Resistance to fluoroquinolones was traditionally believed to be caused by one of two possible mechanisms: mutation of the target enzymes or reduction of intracellular drug concentrations by way of efflux pumps or alterations in porin channels. The discovery of transferable resistance due to plasmids has uncovered additional mechanisms.[5] A complete understanding of resistance mechanisms continues to evolve—one contemporary appraisal in *E coli* estimated that 50–70% of resistance was explained by known mechanisms.[25]

Target Mutations

Mutations in DNA gyrase or topoisomerase IV are due to amino acid substitutions in the corresponding genes (*gyrA* or *gyrB* for DNA gyrase and *parC* or *parE* for topoiso-merase IV) at a site known as the quinolone resistance determining region (QRDR). This location corresponds to a region on the DNA-binding surface of the enzyme and influences drug affinity at the DNA–enzyme complex.[5] Resistance to fluoroquino-lones occurs in a stepwise fashion, with accumulation of additional mutations resulting in a greater degree of resistance. The primary target enzyme for an organism is gener-ally the first affected by mutation. Thus, *gyrA* mutations are the first to occur in *E coli*, because DNA gyrase is the primary target of fluoroquinolones in gram-negative organisms.[4,26] Additional mutations in *gyrA* and *parC* lead to higher levels of resis-tance in gram-negative organisms.[27] The fact that relatively more mutations are required for high-level resistance in *E coli* may account for the superior activity of flu-oroquinolones in *E coli* compared to that of other gram-negatives with intrinsic resis-tance to fluoroquinolones.[28,29]

Topoisomerase IV is believed to be the primary target of fluoroquinolones in the gram-positive organisms. Typically, *parC* mutations are the first to occur in *Staphylococcus aureus* or *Streptococcus pneumoniae* and are associated with low-level resistance. Progressive resistance in gram-positives also occurs in a stepwise fashion, with accumu-lation of subsequent mutations in *gyrA* leading to higher levels of fluoroquinolone resistance.[30,31] Many of the older studies in the gram-positives were performed using older agents, such as ciprofloxacin. Studies of the newer generations of fluoroquinolones demonstrate some divergence from the previously held understanding. For instance, gatifloxacin and moxifloxacin bind strongly to both DNA gyrase and topoisomerase IV.[32] Thus, the primary mutations leading to resistance to these agents occur in *gyrA*, rather than *parC*.[33,34] This feature may explain the preserved activity of later generation fluoroquinolones against *S pneumoniae* strains that are resistant to ciprofloxacin.

One continuing challenge for clinicians is the failure of standard susceptibility testing methods to identify isolates with low-level resistance caused by single-step mutations. These isolates may develop high-level resistance upon exposure to fluoro-quinolone therapy. Studies indicate a high prevalence of single-step mutants exists among pneumococcal isolates.[35] The clinical relevance of this issue has been under-scored by a report of treatment failure and death due to the emergence of high-level resistance in a single-step mutant following levofloxacin therapy.[36] This phenomenon has led to calls advocating for use of a more sensitive screening test for single-step mutants, similar to what is done for *Salmonella* isolates.[37]

Efflux Pumps

Efflux pumps are intrinsic components of the bacterial cell membrane that expel waste and other harmful substances from cells. In general, efflux pumps are responsible for lower levels of resistance to fluoroquinolones than target enzyme mutations.[38] However, by allowing short-term survival of the organism in the presence of the drug, efflux pumps encourage the development of mutations in the QRDR.[16]

The efflux transport mechanism is seen in wild-type *E coli*[39] and may explain the intrinsic fluoroquinolone resistance among *P aeruginosa*.[40] This mechanism has also been described in gram-positive organisms, including *S aureus* and *S pneumoniae*,[38,41] although agents with a bulky side chain at position 7 such as moxi-floxacin are less susceptible to efflux pumps.[32] Because efflux pumps may expel multiple classes of antimicrobial agents, the phenomenon of efflux pump overexpres-sion may contribute to the selection of multidrug-resistant organisms.[42]

Plasmid-mediated Resistance Mechanisms

Transferable fluoroquinolone resistance was conclusively established by the inadver-tent discovery of a plasmid from *Klebsiella pneumoniae* that conferred resistance to ciprofloxacin.[43] The plasmid-mediated locus was initially termed *qnr*. Although the impact upon the MIC for ciprofloxacin was fairly minimal in wild-type strains, clinically significant resistance was achieved in strains with deficient porin channels. It was theorized that the low levels of resistance conferred by this mechanism could facilitate the development of secondary mutations that would produce greater resistance. The implication of this discovery was the understanding that Enterobacteriaceae were vulnerable to the rapid development and dissemination of fluoroquinolone and multi-drug resistance.

Since the initial discovery of plasmid-mediated fluoroquinolone resistance, several additional plasmid-mediated resistance determinants have been described. Qnr-type determinants, which are now thought to produce proteins that protect DNA gyrase and topoisomerase IV from fluoroquinolone inhibition, are geographically widespread and have been identified in many species of Enterobacteriaceae.[44,45] Another plasmid-mediated resistance determinant is an aminoglycoside acetyltransferase, AAC(6')-Ib-cr, which acts in Enterobacteriaceae by acetylating the piperazinyl substit-uent of ciprofloxacin and norfloxacin and is frequently found in association with extended-spectrum β-lactamases.[44,45] Yet another plasmid-mediated fluoroquino-lone resistance determinant is QepA, an efflux pump that has been identified in *E coli* isolates.[44,45]

EPIDEMIOLOGY OF RESISTANCE
Surveillance Studies

Large surveillance studies report fluoroquinolone resistance rates among a variety of pathogens (**Table 3**).[46–56] Data for gram-negative pathogens predominantly come from intensive care units, where one would expect to see the highest rates of resistance. Indeed, the rates of ciprofloxacin resistance are quite high for *P aeruginosa* and other nosocomial pathogens. Notably, fluoroquinolone resistance among Entero-bacteriaceae approaches that of nonfermenters in some settings. Data from the National Nosocomial Infections Surveillance (NNIS) system demonstrate that resis-tance to ciprofloxacin is also being observed in the outpatient setting.[46]

Emerging fluoroquinolone resistance in *S pneumoniae* has been monitored very closely following a report of very high rates of levofloxacin resistance in Hong Kong (13.3% and 27.3% among penicillin-susceptible and penicillin-resistant pneumo-cocci, respectively).[57] As of this writing, pneumococcal resistance to the newer fluo-roquinolone agents does not appear to be prevalent outside of Asia.

Correlation with Use

Fluoroquinolone use has been correlated with the development of resistance in gram-negative organisms on an individual level and on an ecologic level.[58–60] These studies are consistent with the understanding that fluoroquinolone use encourages resistance in gram-negatives by selecting organisms whose survival is favored because of target enzyme mutations or other resistance determinants. The association of fluoroquino-lone use with methicillin-resistanct *S aureus* (MRSA) is also fairly well established,[61–64] but the explanation for this association is not akin to that for gram-negative organisms. De novo resistance to methicillin in *S aureus* is not believed to explain the development of MRSA colonization or infection. Rather, MRSA strains are acquired from contact with colonized individuals or the environment. Fluoroquinolones may increase the like-lihood of acquisition of MRSA colonization or amplify the resistant population following colonization.[63]

Clostridium difficile Infection

The association between fluoroquinolone use and the epidemic of *Clostridium difficile* infection (CDI) noted in Quebec and other regions of North America deserves mention. The responsible strain of *C difficile*, referred to as BI/NAP/027, is a fluoroquinolone-resistant, binary toxin-producing strain that also produces high levels of toxins A and B.[65,66] Numerous studies have demonstrated a relationship between fluoroquino-lone use and this epidemic strain of *C difficile*.[65,67,68] Some investigators have proposed that the risk for CDI may be higher in association with the newer generations of respiratory fluoroquinolones, possibly because of their greater anaerobic activity.[69] Other investigators have failed to correlate a differential risk among individual fluoro-quinolone agents.[7,70]

Resistance in Gonococcal Infections

Although ciprofloxacin received an indication from the US Food and Drug Administra-tion (FDA) for treatment of gonococcal infections, the utility of this drug has been steadily decreasing secondary to the advance of resistance among vulnerable popu-lations. Resistance in *Neisseria gonorrhoeae* is tracked by the Gonococcal Isolate Surveillance Project (GISP), a surveillance program sponsored by the Centers for Disease Control and Prevention (CDC).[71] In 2007, the CDC recommended that fluoro-quinolones no longer be used in the United States to treat gonococcal infections and associated conditions. This was based on GISP data that demonstrated that 8.6% of *N gonorrhoeae* isolates outside of Hawaii and California were fluoroquinolone resis-tant. Of 26 GISP sites, fluoroquinolone resistance was identified in 25.

Table 3
Summary data of fluoroquinolone resistance from selected large surveillance studies

Author or Name of Study	Patient Population	Details of Microbiologic Isolate Collection	Time Period of Study	Summary of Findings
Gram-negative pathogens				
Meropenem Yearly Susceptibility Test Information Collection (MYSTIC) Program[53]	15 United States medical centers	Up to 200 consecutive clinical isolates submitted by each center; 2894 total isolates	2007	Ciprofloxacin resistance in 18.3% of Enterobacteriaceae Ciprofloxacin resistance in 3.4% of *Citrobacter* spp Ciprofloxacin resistance in 8.8% of *Enterobacter* spp Ciprofloxacin resistance in 29% of *E coli* Ciprofloxacin resistance in 20.8% of *Klebsiella* spp Ciprofloxacin resistance in 20.3% of *P mirabilis* Ciprofloxacin resistance in 4.3% of *Serratia* spp Ciprofloxacin resistance in 19.6% of *P aeruginosa* Ciprofloxacin resistance in 60.9% of *Acinetobacter* spp
International Nosocomial Infection Control Consortium (INICC) surveillance study[55]	ICU patients from 98 ICUs in Latin America, Asia, Africa, and Europe	Bacterial susceptibilities provided from patients with device-associated infections	2002–2007	Ciprofloxacin or ofloxacin resistance in 52.4% of *P aeruginosa* Ciprofloxacin or ofloxacin resistance in 42.9% of *E coli*

Lockhart et al[54]	ICU patients from multiple US hospitals	74,000 gram-negative clinical isolates	1993–2004	Ciprofloxacin resistance in *Acinetobacter* spp increased from 38.5% to 64.8%
				Ciprofloxacin resistance in *P aeruginosa* increased from 16.8% to 33.7%
				Ciprofloxacin resistance in *E coli* increased from 1.1% to 17.5%
				Ciprofloxacin resistance in *C freundii* increased from 12% to 26.1%
				Ciprofloxacin resistance in *P mirabilis* increased from 3.6% to 17.1%
				Ciprofloxacin resistance in *E cloacae* increased from 6.5% to 14.1%
				Ciprofloxacin resistance in *K pneumoniae* increased from 11% to 18.2%
				Multidrug resistance (resistance to one or more of extended-spectrum cephalosporins, one aminoglycoside and ciprofloxacin) increased fourfold in *Acinetobacter* spp and more than fivefold in *P aeruginosa*.
National Nosocomial Infections Surveillance (NNIS) system[46]	United States patients in ICU, non-ICU inpatient areas, and outpatient areas	Bacterial susceptibilities reported by participating centers	1992–2004	In the ICU: ciprofloxacin or ofloxacin resistance in 34.8% of *P aeruginosa*
				In the ICU: ciprofloxacin or ofloxacin resistance in 7.3% of *E coli*
				In non-ICU inpatient areas: ciprofloxacin or ofloxacin resistance in 27.7% of *P aeruginosa*
				In non-ICU inpatient areas: ciprofloxacin or ofloxacin resistance in 8.2% of *E coli*
				In outpatient areas: ciprofloxacin or ofloxacin resistance in 23.4% of *P aeruginosa*
				In outpatient areas: ciprofloxacin or ofloxacin resistance in 3.6% of *E coli*

(continued on next page)

Table 3
(*continued*)

S pneumoniae and other respiratory pathogens

Author or Name of Study	Patient Population	Details of Microbiologic Isolate Collection	Time Period of Study	Summary of Findings
MOXIAKTIV Study[51]	Patients admitted to one of 29 hospitals in Germany	Laboratories submitted respiratory or bloodstream isolates: 426 *S pneumoniae* isolates; 398 *H influenzae* isolates; 112 *M catarrhalis* isolates	Not specified	Moxifloxacin resistance in 0.7% of *S pneumoniae* isolates Moxifloxacin resistance in 0.8% of *H influenzae* isolates Moxifloxacin resistance in 0.9% of *M catarrhalis* isolates
Ip et al[50]	Patients admitted to a 1350-bed teaching hospital in Hong Kong	1388 nonduplicate *S pneumoniae* isolates from respiratory tract or blood	2000–2005	Ciprofloxacin resistance in 10.5% Levofloxacin resistance in 1.6% In penicillin-nonsusceptible isolates, ciprofloxacin resistance was 11.2% In penicillin nonsusceptible isolates, levofloxacin resistance was 2.2%
Prospective Resistant Organism Tracking and Epidemiology for the Ketolide Telithromycin (PROTEKT)[48]	151 centers from 40 countries worldwide	20,142 respiratory tract isolates of *S pneumoniae* from outpatients with community-acquired respiratory tract infections and from hospitalized patients within 48 hours of admission	2001–2004	Levofloxacin resistance in 0.8% to 1.1%
SENTRY Antimicrobial Surveillance Program[52]	Medical centers in North America, Latin America, and Europe	2379 strains of *S pneumoniae* from patients diagnosed with community-acquired respiratory tract infections	1999–2003	Ciprofloxacin resistance in 4.9%–8.0% Levofloxacin resistance in 0–1.1% Gatifloxacin resistance in 0–1%

Prospective Resistant Organism Tracking and Epidemiology for the Ketolide Telithromycin (PROTEKT)[49]	Six centers from Japan, two centers from South Korea, and one center from Hong Kong	515 isolates of S pneumoniae, 373 isolates of H influenzae, 165 isolates of M catarrhalis from blood and respiratory samples	1999–2000	Levofloxacin resistance in 4.7% of S pneumoniae Moxifloxacin resistance in 3.3% of S pneumoniae In Hong Kong, 14% of S pneumoniae isolates were resistant to fluoroquinolones No fluoroquinolone resistance in H influenzae or M catarrhalis isolates
Other organisms				
Canadian National Intensive Care Unit (CAN-ICU)[56]	19 medical centers from all regions of Canada	Consecutive isolates from clinical specimens: 687 MSSA isolates, 197 MRSA isolates	2005–2006	Ciprofloxacin resistance in 9.2% of MSSA Levofloxacin resistance in 7.5% of MSSA Moxifloxacin resistance in 7.3% of MSSA Ciprofloxacin resistance in 91.8% of MRSA Levofloxacin resistance in 91.8% of MRSA Moxifloxacin resistance in 91.1% of MRSA
Bozeman et al[47]	United States and Canadian patients enrolled in Tuberculosis Trials Consortium (TBTC) Isolates from state health departments submitted to the CDC microbiology lab for additional testing	1373 M tuberculosis isolates from the TBTC studies	1995–2001	Ciprofloxacin resistance in 0.15%
		1852 M tuberculosis isolates referred to CDC	1996–2000	Ciprofloxacin resistance in 1.8% 75.8% of ciprofloxacin-resistant isolates were multidrug resistant

Abbreviations: CDC, Centers for Disease Control and Prevention; ICU, intensive care unit; MRSA, methicillin-resistant Staphylococcus aureus.

TOXICITY

Although generally considered safe and well tolerated, a number of fluoroquinolones have been removed from the United States market for reasons of toxicity. Reported toxicities may be class-wide or limited to single agents or to agents that share a particular structural characteristic. The discussion below is divided into a general account of adverse effects, followed by mention of toxicities that are fairly unique to the fluoroquinolone class, and concludes with a description of the idiosyncratic and typically most severe toxicities that have been associated with individual agents.

Adverse Effects

As with many other antimicrobials, patients may experience gastrointestinal distress when taking fluoroquinolones. In clinical trials, nausea and diarrhea were the most commonly reported adverse effects.[7] There is no particular structural component of fluoroquinolones known to correlate with gastrointestinal toxicity.[72]

A range of adverse effects of the central nervous system can accompany fluoroquinolone administration. Symptoms can range from relatively mild, such as headache or drowsiness, to more severe, such as dizziness or confusion. Seizures have been reported, but are quite rare and are most likely to occur in patients who have a predisposition.[2,72] As mentioned above, fluoroquinolones with certain substituents at position 7 can cause CNS stimulation through one of several hypothesized mechanisms: displacement of GABA, competition with GABA at the receptor site, or interaction with glutamate receptors.[7]

Rash due to fluoroquinolones is fairly uncommon and should be distinguished from phototoxicity, which is specific to certain agents and is discussed in more detail below. Gemifloxacin had an increased rate of rash in clinical trials that appeared to be associated with prolonged use (longer than 5 days) and with use in younger women.[72,73]

Apart from the severe, immune-mediated idiosyncratic reactions leading to hepatitis and renal failure that are discussed below, hepatotoxicity and nephrotoxicity are uncommon following administration of available fluoroquinolones. Liver enzyme abnormalities are reported in 2% to 3% of patients.[74] These have generally been limited to mild, reversible elevations in serum transaminases and alkaline phosphatase.

Anaphylactoid reactions and anaphylaxis can occur following fluoroquinolone administration, but are fairly infrequent, occurring in 0.46 to1.2 cases per 100,000.[74] Unfortunately, there is substantial cross reactivity among the fluoroquinolones, and skin testing is believed to be unreliable due to the frequency of false-positive results.[72]

Class-wide Toxicities

Arthropathy

Tendinopathy was reported in association with the earliest quinolones, and subsequent study established it as a class-wide effect. In 2008, the FDA added a "black box" warning to all fluoroquinolone agents cautioning of the risk of tendonitis and tendon rupture that may be increased in certain populations.[75–79] Although the Achilles tendon is most frequently involved, other tendons of weight-bearing joints may also be affected. Patients typically complain of pain, stiffness, and joint swelling within the first few days of therapy.[80] Symptoms typically resolve within several weeks after discontinuation, although recovery can be prolonged. Achilles tendon rupture may occur in up to half of those with involvement at this site.[80] Fluoroquinolones should be discontinued in patients who have symptoms of tendonitis and exercise should be avoided until recovery.

The mechanism for fluoroquinolone-induced tendinopathy has not been fully elucidated. Fluoroquinolones may be directly toxic to collagen fibers or may cause defective proteoglycan and procollagen synthesis.[7,72] Yet another possibility is that magnesium deficiency caused by fluoroquinolone chelation of ions alters the functionality of chondrocyte surface integrin receptors.[72,81]

QT prolongation

QT interval prolongation is a potentially serious class effect of fluoroquinolones that may provoke torsades de pointes or other ventricular arrhythmias. Grepafloxacin and sparfloxacin were removed from the market for increased risk of arrhythmia.[7] There are certain patient populations who are at increased risk for developing arrhythmia in association with fluoroquinolone use. Fluoroquinolones should be used cautiously in elderly female patients, those who have electrolyte abnormalities (particularly hypokalemia or hypomagnesemia), those who have significant cardiac disease or pre-existing arrhythmia or QTc prolongation, and those receiving coadministration of other drugs likely to prolong the QT interval (particularly class Ia or class III antiarrhythmics).[2,7] The package inserts for levofloxacin, moxifloxacin, and gemifloxacin recommend that these drugs be avoided in patients who have known QTc interval prolongation, uncorrected hypokalemia, and in patients receiving class Ia or class III antiarrhythmics.[7]

The structural moiety responsible for QT interval prolongation by fluoroquinolones has not been identified. The mechanism, however, is known to be blockade of the delayed rectifier potassium current, which regulates the outward flow of potassium ions from the myocyte.[82] The resultant accumulation of intracellular potassium ions within the myocyte delays ventricular repolarization. Because the magnitude of the effect upon repolarization is influenced by fluoroquinolone concentration, factors that increase drug concentration or reduce clearance increase the risk for arrhythmia.[82]

QT interval prolongation should be considered to be a possibility for all available fluoroquinolone agents, although there is some variation in the reported risk. A review of case reports of torsades de pointes from 1996 to 2001 demonstrated an extremely low risk for ciprofloxacin and moxifloxacin, whereas that for levofloxacin and gatifloxacin was 10- to 100-fold higher, respectively.[83] However, no case reports of torsades de pointes caused by moxifloxacin existed at the time of this review. Data that were submitted to the FDA confirm that moxifloxacin may prolong the QT interval.[7] Several case reports documenting torsades de pointes following moxifloxacin administration have since been published.[84,85] Although there is certainly more accumulated clinical experience with ciprofloxacin, it is difficult to compare older and new agents for the risk of torsades de pointes. Agents that have been approved since 2002 undergo much more rigorous testing for QT interval prolongation as directed by the FDA's International Conference on Harmonization S7B document.[72]

Dysglycemia

Fluoroquinolones may cause both hypoglycemia and hyperglycemia. Although a number of fluoroquinolones may have this effect, there is clearly a greater risk associated with gatifloxacin, which was consequently removed from the market in 2006.[7] Development of the agent clinafloxacin was also halted for this reason. Park-Wyllie and colleagues'[86] influential study established that gatifloxacin administration was associated with an increased risk of both hypoglycemia and hyperglycemia. Levofloxacin use was noted to slightly increase the risk for hypoglycemia.

The structural moiety responsible for dysglycemia is not known at this time. Fluoro-quinolones are believed to increase pancreatic insulin secretion by inhibiting adeno-sine triphosphate–sensitive potassium channels in the beta cells.[7] The mechanism of hyperglycemia is unknown, but, according to one theory, gatifloxacin may reduce insulin levels by triggering the vacuolation of pancreatic beta cells.[86]

Phototoxicity

Fluoroquinolone-induced phototoxicity typically manifests as an intense sunburn that occurs within hours of exposure to UV light.[72] Reactions can be severe, however, particularly in association with multifluorinated agents or agents with halogen atoms at position 8, such as clinafloxacin and sitafloxacin, which are no longer available.[2] Patients should be cautioned to avoid excessive UV exposure during fluoroquinolone administration.[7] Phototoxicity following fluoroquinolone use is believed to be secondary to the generation of reactive oxygen species and free radicals following exposure of these agents to UV light.[7]

Idiosyncratic Toxicities

Several fluoroquinolone agents are known to cause severe, idiosyncratic reactions that are believed to be immune-mediated. Two such agents, temofloxacin and trova-floxacin, are both trifluorinated compounds and possess a 1-2,4-difluorophenyl substituent.[2,72] Temafloxacin was withdrawn from the market after reports of an asso-ciation with immune hemolytic anemia. The original report by the FDA detailed 95 cases of fevers, rigors, and jaundice that developed within a week of therapy and was associated with hemolysis, hepatitis, and new renal insufficiency.[87] Trovafloxacin was also removed from the market following reports of the development of severe hepatotoxicity, in some cases progressing to hepatic failure, liver transplant, and death.[2]

INDICATIONS
FDA-approved Indications

Table 4 lists complete details regarding indications for the most commonly prescribed fluoroquinolone agents: ciprofloxacin, gemifloxacin, levofloxacin, and moxifloxacin.[76–79]

Ciprofloxacin is the only fluoroquinolone agent approved for gram-negative bone and joint infections. It is also the primary fluoroquinolone approved for gastrointestinal infections, including infectious diarrhea (when therapy is warranted) and typhoid fever. Ciprofloxacin is approved for treatment of uncomplicated and complicated urinary tract infections and chronic bacterial prostatitis. It is also approved for treatment of urethral and cervical gonococcal infections, although it should be noted that the CDC no longer recommends fluoroquinolones for this indication.[71] Ciprofloxacin may be used to treat a range of respiratory tract infections, but is not the agent of choice for *S pneumoniae*. The intravenous formulation of ciprofloxacin may be used for nosocomial pneumonia. Ciprofloxacin is approved for the management of skin and skin structure infections. Ciprofloxacin is approved for postexposure prophylaxis following anthrax exposure. It is the only fluoroquinolone approved for empiric therapy for neutropenic fever, although combination with piperacillin–sodium is recommen-ded. Finally, ciprofloxacin has approval for two pediatric indications: complicated urinary tract infections and pyelonephritis due to *E coli* and postexposure prophylaxis to anthrax.

Gemifloxacin is approved only for respiratory indications: acute bacterial exacerba-tion of chronic bronchitis and community-acquired pneumonia, including that caused by known or suspected multidrug resistant strains of *S pneumoniae*.

Levofloxacin is approved for uncomplicated and complicated urinary tract infections and prostatitis. It is unique in that it has an indication for short-course regimens (5 days) for complicated urinary tract infections and pyelonephritis. Levofloxacin is approved for the treatment of respiratory tract infections, including community-acquired pneumonia caused by multidrug resistant strains of S pneumoniae. A short-course regimen of 5 days may be used to treat community-acquired pneumonia due to sensitive strains of S pneumoniae. Levofloxacin is the only fluoroquinolone agent specifically approved for treatment of Legionella pneumophila using the longer course of therapy (7–14 days). Levofloxacin may be used for the treatment of nosocomial pneumonia; it is suggested that combination therapy with an antipseudomonal β-lactam be used for P aeruginosa. Levofloxacin is approved for the treatment of uncomplicated and complicated skin and skin structure infections due to gram-positive organisms. Lastly, levofloxacin is approved in both adult and pediatric patients for postexposure prophylaxis for inhalation anthrax.

Moxifloxacin is approved for the treatment of complicated intra-abdominal infections, including polymicrobial infections and abscesses. Moxifloxacin is approved for respiratory tract infections, including community-acquired pneumonia caused by multidrug resistant strains of S pneumoniae. Finally, moxifloxacin is approved for the treatment of uncomplicated and complicated skin and skin structure infections caused by gram-positive organisms.

Special Indications

There are several special uses for fluoroquinolones that do not specifically have FDA approval, but nonetheless deserve mention.

Tuberculosis

There are a number of arguments for including a fluoroquinolone agent in a treatment regimen for Mycobacterium tuberculosis (MTB). These agents act by a mechanism that is unique among antituberculous agents, achieve good penetration into many tissues, and their good safety profile and convenient dosing schedule is likely to improve adherence to therapy. However, these agents are not without toxicity and may interact with other antituberculous and antiretroviral agents. A Cochrane review of 11 trials assessed the use of fluoroquinolones as additional or substitute components in antituberculous regimens for both sensitive and resistant strains.[88] There were no significant differences observed in trials substituting ciprofloxacin, ofloxacin, or moxifloxacin for first-line drugs in relation to cure, treatment failure, or clinical or radiologic improvement. However, substituting ciprofloxacin into first-line regimens for cases of drug-sensitive MTB led to a higher incidence of relapse and longer time to sputum culture conversion for HIV-positive subjects. Adding or substituting levofloxacin to basic regimens in drug-resistant areas did not result in adverse outcomes. The sole conclusion of the review was that ciprofloxacin should not be used to treat MTB.

Legionella

Although levofloxacin does have FDA approval for the treatment of pneumonia due to L pneumophila, all agents in the class have become workhorses for lower respiratory tract infections. Thus, it is instructive to examine the evidence supporting the use of fluoroquinolones for this indication. Although fluoroquinolones have been shown to have superior efficacy compared with macrolides in animal and in vitro models, clinical evidence favoring fluoroquinolone use primarily comes from observational studies.[89] It should be noted that no prospective studies or randomized trials have directly

Table 4
FDA-approved indications for the most commonly prescribed fluoroquinolone agents[a]

Type and/or Severity of Infection	Agent	Target Organisms	Dose, Frequency, Route	Duration
Bone and joint infections				
Mild/moderate	Ciprofloxacin	E cloacae, S marcescens, P aeruginosa	500 mg q 12 h PO or 400 mg q 12 h IV	≥4–6 wk
Severe/complicated	Ciprofloxacin	See mild/moderate infections above	750 mg q 12 h PO or 400 mg q 8 h IV	≥4–6 wk
Gastrointestinal infections				
Complicated intra-abdominal infections	Ciprofloxacin[b]	E coli, P aeruginosa, P mirabilis, K pneumoniae, B fragilis	500 mg q 12 h PO or 400 mg q 12 h IV	7–14 d
	Moxifloxacin	E coli, B fragilis, S anginosus, S constellatus, E faecalis, P mirabilis, C perfringens, B thetaiotamicron, Peptostreptococcus spp	400 mg q 24 h PO or 400 mg q 24 h IV	5–14 d
Infectious diarrhea, mild/moderate/severe	Ciprofloxacin	E coli (enterotoxigenic strains), C jejuni, S boydii, S dysenteriae, S flexneri, S sonnei	500 mg q 12 h PO	5–7 d
Typhoid fever, mild/moderate	Ciprofloxacin[c]	S typhi	500 mg q 12 h PO	10 d
Genitourinary Infections				
Urinary tract infection, acute/uncomplicated	Ciprofloxacin	E coli, K pneumoniae, E cloacae, S marcescens, P mirabilis, P rettgeri, M morganii, C diversus, C freundii, P aeruginosa, methicillin-susceptible S epidermidis, S saprophyticus, E faecalis	250 mg q 12 h PO	3 d
	Levofloxacin	E coli, K pneumoniae, S saprophyticus	250 mg q 24 h PO or 250 mg q 24 h IV	3 d
Urinary tract infection, mild/moderate	Ciprofloxacin	See acute/uncomplicated infections above	250 mg q 12 h PO or 200 mg q 12 h IV	7–14 d
Urinary tract infection, severe/complicated	Ciprofloxacin	See acute/uncomplicated infections above	500 mg q 12 h PO or 400 mg q 12 IV	7–14 d

Indication	Drug	Organisms	Dose	Duration
Complicated urinary tract infection	Levofloxacin	E coli, K pneumoniae, P mirabilis	750 mg q 24 h PO	5 d
		E faecalis, E cloacae, E coli, K pneumoniae, P mirabilis, P aeruginosa	250 mg q 24 h PO or 250 mg q 24 h IV	10 d
Acute pyelonephritis	Levofloxacin	E coli	750 mg q 24 h PO	5 d
			250 mg q 24 h PO or 250 mg q 24 h IV	10 d
Chronic bacterial prostatitis	Ciprofloxacin	E coli, P mirabilis	500 mg q 12 h PO or 400 mg q 12 IV	28 d
	Levofloxacin	E coli, E faecalis, methicillin-susceptible S epidermidis	500 mg q 24 h PO	28 d
Urethral and cervical gonococcal infections[d]	Ciprofloxacin	N gonorrhoeae	250 mg PO	Single dose
Respiratory infections				
Acute bacterial sinusitis	Ciprofloxacin	H influenzae, penicillin-susceptible S pneumoniae, M catarrhalis	500 mg q 12 h PO or 400 mg q 12 h IV	10 d
	Levofloxacin	S pneumoniae, H influenzae, M catarrhalis	750 mg q 24 h PO	5 d
			500 mg q 24 h PO or 500 mg q 24 h IV	10–14 d
	Moxifloxacin	S pneumoniae, H influenzae, M catarrhalis	400 mg q 24 h PO or 400 mg q 24 h IV	10 d
Lower respiratory tract, mild/moderate	Ciprofloxacin	E coli, K pneumoniae, E cloacae, P mirabilis, P aeruginosa, H influenzae, H parainfluenzae, penicillin-susceptible S pneumoniae,[e] M catarrhalis[f]	500 mg q 12 h PO or 400 mg q 12 h IV	7–14 d
Lower respiratory tract, severe/complicated	Ciprofloxacin	See mild/moderate infections above	750 mg q 12 h PO or 400 mg q 8 h IV	7–14 d
Acute bacterial exacerbation of chronic bronchitis	Gemifloxacin	S pneumoniae, H influenzae, H parainfluenzae, M catarrhalis	320 mg q 24 h PO	5 d
	Levofloxacin	MSSA, S pneumoniae, H influenzae, H parainfluenzae, M catarrhalis	500 mg q 24 h PO or 500 mg q 24 h IV	7 d
	Moxifloxacin	S pneumoniae, H influenzae, H parainfluenzae, K pneumoniae, MSSA, M catarrhalis	400 mg q 24 h PO or 400 mg q 24 h IV	5 d

(continued on next page)

Table 4
(continued)

Type and/or Severity of Infection	Agent	Target Organisms	Dose, Frequency, Route	Duration
Community-acquired pneumonia	Gemifloxacin	S pneumoniae, H influenzae, M pneumoniae, C pneumoniae	320 mg q 24 h PO	5 d
	Gemifloxacin	Known or suspected multidrug resistant strains of S pneumoniae, K pneumoniae, or M catarrhalis	320 mg q 24 h PO	7 d
	Levofloxacin	S pneumoniae (not multidrug resistant strains), H influenzae, H parainfluenzae, M pneumoniae, C pneumoniae	750 mg q 24 h PO	5 d
	Levofloxacin	MSSA, S pneumoniae (including multidrug resistant strains), H influenzae, H parainfluenzae, K pneumoniae, M catarrhalis, C pneumoniae, L pneumophila, M pneumoniae	500 mg q 24 h PO or 500 mg q 24 h IV	7–14 d
	Moxifloxacin	S pneumoniae (including multidrug resistant strains), H influenzae, M catarrhalis, MSSA, K pneumoniae, M pneumoniae, C pneumoniae	400 mg q 24 h PO or 400 mg q 24 h IV	7–14 d
Nosocomial pneumonia	Ciprofloxacin	H influenzae, K pneumoniae	400 mg q 8 h IV	10–14 d
	Levofloxacin	MSSA, P aeruginosa,[9] S marcescens, E coli, K pneumoniae, H influenzae, S pneumoniae	750 mg q 24 h PO	7–14 d
Skin and skin structure infections				
Mild/moderate	Ciprofloxacin	E coli, K pneumoniae, E cloacae, P mirabilis, P vulgaris, P stuartii, M morganni, C freundii, P aeruginosa, MSSA, methicillin-susceptible S epidermidis, S pyogenes	500 mg q 12 h PO or 400 mg q 12 h IV	7–14 d
Uncomplicated	Levofloxacin	MSSA, S pyogenes	500 mg q 24 h PO or 500 mg q 24 h IV	7–10 d
	Moxifloxacin	MSSA, S pyogenes	400 mg q 24 h PO or 400 mg q 24 h IV	7 d
Severe/complicated	Ciprofloxacin	See mild/moderate infections above	750 mg q 12 h PO or 400 mg q 8 h IV	7–14 d
Complicated	Levofloxacin	MSSA, E faecalis, S pyogenes, P mirabilis	750 mg q 24 h PO	7–14 d
	Moxifloxacin	MSSA, E coli, K pneumoniae, E cloacae	400 mg q 24 h PO or 400 mg q 24 h IV	7–21 d
Other				
Inhalation anthrax (postexposure)	Ciprofloxacin	B anthracis	500 mg q 12 h PO or 400 mg q 12 h IV	60 d
	Levofloxacin	B anthracis	500 mg q 24 h PO	60 d

Indication	Drug	Organism	Dosing	Duration
Empirical therapy in febrile neutropenia	Ciprofloxacin[h]		400 mg q 8 h IV	7–14 d
Indications approved for use in pediatric patients (1–17 years of age)				
Complicated urinary tract infections and pyelonephritis	Ciprofloxacin	E coli	10–20 mg/kg q 12 h PO (not to exceed 750 mg dose) or 6–10 mg/kg q 8 h IV (not to exceed 400 mg dose)	10–21 d
Inhalation anthrax (postexposure)	Ciprofloxacin	B anthracis	15 mg/kg q 12 h PO (not to exceed 500 mg dose) or 10 mg/kg q 12 h IV (not to exceed 400 mg dose)	60 d
	Levofloxacin	B anthracis	For patients <50 kg: 8 mg/kg q 12 h PO (not to exceed 250 mg dose) For patients >50 kg: 500 mg q 24 h PO	60 d

Abbreviations: PO, by mouth; IV, intravenous; MSSA, methicillin-susceptible Staphylococcus aureus.

[a] Please note that the indications, target organisms, dosing, and durations listed below are based on FDA labeling information, but are not consistent with best practices in all cases.

[b] Use in combination with metronidazole.

[c] The efficacy of ciprofloxacin in eradication of the chronic typhoid carrier state has not been demonstrated.

[d] Fluoroquinolones no longer recommended by the CDC for treatment of gonococcal infections.

[e] Ciprofloxacin is not a drug of first choice in the treatment of presumed or confirmed pneumonia secondary to S pneumonia.

[f] For acute exacerbations of chronic bronchitis.

[g] Combination therapy with an antipseudomonal β-lactam is recommended.

[h] Use in combination with piperacillin–sodium.

Data from Cipro labeling information, October 2008. Available at: http://www.fda.gov/cder/foi/label/2008/019537s68,19847s42,19857s49,20780s26,21473s24lbl.pdf; Factive labeling information, October 2008. Available at: http://www.fda.gov/cder/foi/label/2008/021158s012lbl.pdf; Levaquin labeling information, October 2008. Available at: http://www.fda.gov/cder/foi/label/2008/021721s020_02063s557_02063s557_02063452_lbl.pdf; Avelox labeling information, October 2008. Available at: http://www.fda.gov/cder/foi/label/2008/021085s040,021277s034lbl.pdf. All accessed on November 14, 2008.

compared the clinical efficacy of fluoroquinolones with that of newer macrolides such as azithromycin.

Antibacterial prophylaxis after chemotherapy

Clinical trials have evaluated the practice of administering fluoroquinolone prophylaxis during periods of chemotherapy-induced neutropenia. Two studies of note, one of which included subjects who had solid tumors and lymphoma[90] and another that enrolled subjects who had solid tumors, lymphoma, and acute leukemia,[91] found a benefit of levofloxacin compared to placebo for the outcomes of fever and documented infection. The study in subjects who had solid tumors and lymphoma also demonstrated a reduction in hospitalization for infection following levofloxacin prophylaxis. Neither study demonstrated a reduction in mortality attributable to the prophylaxis. A follow-up meta-analysis of randomized, blinded, placebo-controlled trials of fluoroquinolone prophylaxis for neutropenic subjects similarly failed to establish a significant reduction in mortality associated with prophylaxis.[92]

Prevention of meningococcal infections following exposure

Ciprofloxacin may be used for the prevention of meningococcal disease following exposure to an infected individual. A Cochrane review has examined the outcomes associated with the common antimicrobial agents used for this indication.[93] Because no meningococcal disease occurred among secondary contacts in any of the trials, the efficacy of different agents for the prevention of future disease could not be assessed. Ciprofloxacin proved effective at eradicating pharyngeal carriage of *Neisseria meningitidis* for up to 2 weeks following treatment in healthy carriers. The authors concluded that ciprofloxacin could be considered as an alternative to rifampin.

SUMMARY

Fluoroquinolones have gained widespread use owing to their favorable pharmacokinetics and broad antimicrobial spectra. Although a number of agents have been withdrawn from the market for serious safety concerns, the remaining agents have proved quite safe. Worrisome levels of fluoroquinolone resistance have developed as a consequence of heavy use. Resistance in gram-negative organisms, in particular, threatens to jeopardize the continued empiric use of fluoroquinolones. However, recent advances in fluoroquinolone development have primarily resulted in improved pneumococcal coverage, with the consequence that the treatment of respiratory tract infections may become the main use for this class. Appropriate choice of agent and dose while keeping pharmacodynamic principles in mind will, we hope, preserve these very useful agents.

REFERENCES

1. Andriole VT. The quinolones: past, present, and future. Clin Infect Dis 2005; 41(Suppl 2):S113–9.
2. Ball P. Adverse drug reactions: implications for the development of fluoroquinolones. J Antimicrob Chemother 2003;51(Suppl 1):21–7.
3. Drugs@FDA page. Available at: http://www.accessdata.fda.gov/scripts/cder/drugsatfda/index.cfm. Accessed April 18, 2011.
4. Hawkey PM. Mechanisms of quinolone action and microbial response. J Antimicrob Chemother 2003;51(Suppl 1):29–35.
5. Jacoby GA. Mechanisms of resistance to quinolones. Clin Infect Dis 2005; 41(Suppl 2):S120–6.

6. O'Donnell JA, Gelone SP. The newer fluoroquinolones. Infect Dis Clin North Am 2004;18(3):691–716, x.
7. Mehlhorn AJ, Brown DA. Safety concerns with fluoroquinolones. Ann Pharmacother 2007;41(11):1859–66.
8. Ball P. The quinolones: history and overview. In: Andriole VT, editor. The quinolones. 3rd edition. San Diego (CA): Academic Press; 2000. p. 1–33.
9. Stahlman R, Lode H. Safety overview: toxicity, adverse effects, and drug interactions. In: Andriole VT, editor. The quinolones. 3rd edition. San Diego (CA): Academic Press; 2000. p. 397–453.
10. Niki Y, Hashiguchi K, Okimoto N, et al. Quinolone antimicrobial agents and theophylline [letter]. Chest 1992;101(3):881.
11. Carroll DN, Carroll DG. Interactions between warfarin and three commonly prescribed fluoroquinolones. Ann Pharmacother 2008;42(5):680–5.
12. Barton TD, Fishman NO, Weiner MG, et al. High rate of coadministration of di- or trivalent cation-containing compounds with oral fluoroquinolones: risk factors and potential implications. Infect Control Hosp Epidemiol 2005;26(1):93–9.
13. Cohen KA, Lautenbach E, Weiner MG, et al. Coadministration of oral levofloxacin with agents that impair absorption: impact on antibiotic resistance. Infect Control Hosp Epidemiol 2008;29(10):975–7.
14. Rybak MJ. Pharmacodynamics: relation to antimicrobial resistance. Am J Med 2006;119(6 Suppl 1):S37–44 [discussion: S62–70].
15. Forrest A, Nix DE, Ballow CH, et al. Pharmacodynamics of intravenous ciprofloxacin in seriously ill patients. Antimicrob Agents Chemother 1993;37(5):1073–81.
16. Dalhoff A, Schmitz FJ. In vitro antibacterial activity and pharmacodynamics of new quinolones. Eur J Clin Microbiol Infect Dis 2003;22(4):203–21.
17. Wispelwey B. Clinical implications of pharmacokinetics and pharmacodynamics of fluoroquinolones. Clin Infect Dis 2005;41(Suppl 2):S127–35.
18. Ambrose PG, Grasela DM, Grasela TH, et al. Pharmacodynamics of fluoroquinolones against *Streptococcus pneumoniae* in patients with community-acquired respiratory tract infections. Antimicrob Agents Chemother 2001;45(10):2793–7.
19. Drusano GL, Preston SL, Fowler C, et al. Relationship between fluoroquinolone area under the curve: minimum inhibitory concentration ratio and the probability of eradication of the infecting pathogen, in patients with nosocomial pneumonia. J Infect Dis 2004;189(9):1590–7.
20. Preston SL, Drusano GL, Berman AL, et al. Pharmacodynamics of levofloxacin: a new paradigm for early clinical trials. JAMA 1998;279(2):125–9.
21. Thomas JK, Forrest A, Bhavnani SM, et al. Pharmacodynamic evaluation of factors associated with the development of bacterial resistance in acutely ill patients during therapy. Antimicrob Agents Chemother 1998;42(3):521–7.
22. Falagas ME, Bliziotis IA, Rafailidis PI. Do high doses of quinolones decrease the emergence of antibacterial resistance? A systematic review of data from comparative clinical trials. J Infect 2007;55(2):97–105.
23. DeRyke CA, Kuti JL, Nicolau DP. Pharmacodynamic target attainment of six beta-lactams and two fluoroquinolones against *Pseudomonas aeruginosa, Acinetobacter baumannii, Escherichia coli*, and *Klebsiella* species collected from United States intensive care units in 2004. Pharmacotherapy 2007;27(3):333–42.
24. van Zanten AR, Polderman KH, van Geijlswijk IM, et al. Ciprofloxacin pharmacokinetics in critically ill patients: a prospective cohort study. J Crit Care 2008;23(3):422–30.

25. Morgan-Linnell SK, Becnel Boyd L, Steffen D, et al. Mechanisms accounting for fluoroquinolone resistance in *Escherichia coli* clinical isolates. Antimicrob Agents Chemother 2009;53(1):235–41.

26. Oram M, Fisher LM. 4-quinolone resistance mutations in the DNA gyrase of *Escherichia coli* clinical isolates identified by using the polymerase chain reaction. Antimicrob Agents Chemother 1991;35(2):387–9.

27. Khodursky AB, Zechiedrich EL, Cozzarelli NR. Topoisomerase IV is a target of quinolones in *Escherichia coli*. Proc Natl Acad Sci U S A 1995;92(25):11801–5.

28. Vila J, Ruiz J, Goni P, et al. Detection of mutations in *parC* in quinolone-resistant clinical isolates of *Escherichia coli*. Antimicrob Agents Chemother 1996;40(2): 491–3.

29. Vila J, Ruiz J, Goni P, et al. Quinolone-resistance mutations in the topoisomerase IV *parC* gene of *Acinetobacter baumannii*. J Antimicrob Chemother 1997;39(6): 757–62.

30. Ferrero L, Cameron B, Crouzet J. Analysis of *gyrA* and *grlA* mutations in stepwise-selected ciprofloxacin-resistant mutants of *Staphylococcus aureus*. Antimicrob Agents Chemother 1995;39(7):1554–8.

31. Pan XS, Ambler J, Mehtar S, et al. Involvement of topoisomerase IV and DNA gyrase as ciprofloxacin targets in *Streptococcus pneumoniae*. Antimicrob Agents Chemother 1996;40(10):2321–6.

32. Scheld WM. Maintaining fluoroquinolone class efficacy: review of influencing factors. Emerg Infect Dis 2003;9(1):1–9.

33. Fukuda H, Hiramatsu K. Primary targets of fluoroquinolones in *Streptococcus pneumoniae*. Antimicrob Agents Chemother 1999;43(2):410–2.

34. Pestova E, Millichap JJ, Noskin GA, et al. Intracellular targets of moxifloxacin: a comparison with other fluoroquinolones. J Antimicrob Chemother 2000;45(5): 583–90.

35. Pletz MW, Shergill AP, McGee L, et al. Prevalence of first-step mutants among levofloxacin-susceptible invasive isolates of *Streptococcus pneumoniae* in the United States. Antimicrob Agents Chemother 2006;50(4):1561–3.

36. de Cueto M, Rodriguez JM, Soriano MJ, et al. Fatal levofloxacin failure in treatment of a bacteremic patient infected with *Streptococcus pneumoniae* with a preexisting *parC* mutation. J Clin Microbiol 2008;46(4):1558–60.

37. Hakanen A, Kotilainen P, Jalava J, et al. Detection of decreased fluoroquinolone susceptibility in *Salmonella*s and validation of nalidixic acid screening test. J Clin Microbiol 1999;37(11):3572–7.

38. Kaatz GW, Seo SM, Ruble CA. Efflux-mediated fluoroquinolone resistance in *Staphylococcus aureus*. Antimicrob Agents Chemother 1993;37(5):1086–94.

39. Cohen SP, Hooper DC, Wolfson JS, et al. Endogenous active efflux of norfloxacin in susceptible *Escherichia coli*. Antimicrob Agents Chemother 1988;32(8): 1187–91.

40. Li XZ, Livermore DM, Nikaido H. Role of efflux pump(s) in intrinsic resistance of *Pseudomonas aeruginosa*: resistance to tetracycline, chloramphenicol, and norfloxacin. Antimicrob Agents Chemother 1994;38(8):1732–41.

41. Brenwald NP, Gill MJ, Wise R. Prevalence of a putative efflux mechanism among fluoroquinolone-resistant clinical isolates of *Streptococcus pneumoniae*. Antimicrob Agents Chemother 1998;42(8):2032–5.

42. Kriengkauykiat J, Porter E, Lomovskaya O, et al. Use of an efflux pump inhibitor to determine the prevalence of efflux pump-mediated fluoroquinolone resistance and multidrug resistance in *Pseudomonas aeruginosa*. Antimicrob Agents Chemother 2005;49(2):565–70.

43. Martinez-Martinez L, Pascual A, Jacoby GA. Quinolone resistance from a transferable plasmid. Lancet 1998;351(9105):797–9.
44. Poirel L, Cattoir V, Nordmann P. Is plasmid-mediated quinolone resistance a clinically significant problem? Clin Microbiol Infect 2008;14(4):295–7.
45. Yamane K, Wachino J, Suzuki S, et al. New plasmid-mediated fluoroquinolone efflux pump, QepA, found in an *Escherichia coli* clinical isolate. Antimicrob Agents Chemother 2007;51(9):3354–60.
46. National Nosocomial Infections Surveillance System. National nosocomial infections surveillance (NNIS) system report, data summary from January 1992 through June 2004, issued October 2004. Am J Infect Control 2004;32(8):470–85.
47. Bozeman L, Burman W, Metchock B, et al. Fluoroquinolone susceptibility among *Mycobacterium tuberculosis* isolates from the United States and Canada. Clin Infect Dis 2005;40(3):386–91.
48. Felmingham D, Canton R, Jenkins SG. Regional trends in beta-lactam, macrolide, fluoroquinolone and telithromycin resistance among *Streptococcus pneumoniae* isolates 2001–2004. J Infect 2007;55(2):111–8.
49. Inoue M, Lee NY, Hong SW, et al. Protekt 1999–2000: a multicentre study of the antibiotic susceptibility of respiratory tract pathogens in Hong Kong, Japan and South Korea. Int J Antimicrob Agents 2004;23(1):44–51.
50. Ip M, Chau SS, Chi F, et al. Longitudinally tracking fluoroquinolone resistance and its determinants in penicillin-susceptible and -nonsusceptible *Streptococcus pneumoniae* isolates in Hong Kong, 2000 to 2005. Antimicrob Agents Chemother 2007;51(6):2192–4.
51. Jacobs E, Dalhoff A, Korfmann G. Susceptibility patterns of bacterial isolates from hospitalised patients with respiratory tract infections (MOXIAKTIV study). Int J Antimicrob Agents 2009;33(1):52–7.
52. Johnson DM, Stilwell MG, Fritsche TR, et al. Emergence of multidrug-resistant *Streptococcus pneumoniae*: report from the SENTRY antimicrobial surveillance program (1999–2003). Diagn Microbiol Infect Dis 2006;56(1):69–74.
53. Jones RN, Kirby JT, Rhomberg PR. Comparative activity of meropenem in US medical centers (2007): initiating the 2nd decade of MYSTIC program surveillance. Diagn Microbiol Infect Dis 2008;61(2):203–13.
54. Lockhart SR, Abramson MA, Beekmann SE, et al. Antimicrobial resistance among gram-negative bacilli causing infections in intensive care unit patients in the United States between 1993 and 2004. J Clin Microbiol 2007;45(10):3352–9.
55. Rosenthal VD, Maki DG, Mehta A, et al. International nosocomial infection control consortium report, data summary for 2002–2007, issued January 2008. Am J Infect Control 2008;36(9):627–37.
56. Zhanel GG, DeCorby M, Laing N, et al. Antimicrobial-resistant pathogens in intensive care units in Canada: results of the Canadian National Intensive Care Unit (CAN-ICU) study, 2005–2006. Antimicrob Agents Chemother 2008;52(4):1430–7.
57. Ho PL, Yung RW, Tsang DN, et al. Increasing resistance of *Streptococcus pneumoniae* to fluoroquinolones: results of a Hong Kong multicentre study in 2000. J Antimicrob Chemother 2001;48(5):659–65.
58. Gagliotti C, Nobilio L, Moro ML. Emergence of ciprofloxacin resistance in *Escherichia coli* isolates from outpatient urine samples. Clin Microbiol Infect 2007;13(3):328–31.
59. Kaye KS, Kanafani ZA, Dodds AE, et al. Differential effects of levofloxacin and ciprofloxacin on the risk for isolation of quinolone-resistant *Pseudomonas aeruginosa*. Antimicrob Agents Chemother 2006;50(6):2192–6.

60. Ray GT, Baxter R, DeLorenze GN. Hospital-level rates of fluoroquinolone use and the risk of hospital-acquired infection with ciprofloxacin-nonsusceptible *Pseudomonas aeruginosa*. Clin Infect Dis 2005;41(4):441–9.

61. Weber SG, Gold HS, Hooper DC, et al. Fluoroquinolones and the risk for methicillin-resistant *Staphylococcus aureus* in hospitalized patients. Emerg Infect Dis 2003;9(11):1415–22.

62. LeBlanc L, Pepin J, Toulouse K, et al. Fluoroquinolones and risk for methicillin-resistant *Staphylococcus aureus*, Canada. Emerg Infect Dis 2006;12(9):1398–405.

63. MacDougall C, Harpe SE, Powell JP, et al. *Pseudomonas aeruginosa, Staphylococcus aureus*, and fluoroquinolone use. Emerg Infect Dis 2005;11(8):1197–204.

64. MacDougall C, Powell JP, Johnson CK, et al. Hospital and community fluoroquinolone use and resistance in *Staphylococcus aureus* and *Escherichia coli* in 17 US hospitals. Clin Infect Dis 2005;41(4):435–40.

65. Labbe AC, Poirier L, Maccannell D, et al. *Clostridium difficile* infections in a Canadian tertiary care hospital before and during a regional epidemic associated with the bi/nap1/027 strain. Antimicrob Agents Chemother 2008;52(9):3180–7.

66. Razavi B, Apisarnthanarak A, Mundy LM. *Clostridium difficile*: emergence of hypervirulence and fluoroquinolone resistance. Infection 2007;35(5):300–7.

67. Pepin J, Saheb N, Coulombe MA, et al. Emergence of fluoroquinolones as the predominant risk factor for *Clostridium difficile*-associated diarrhea: a cohort study during an epidemic in Quebec. Clin Infect Dis 2005;41(9):1254–60.

68. Loo VG, Poirier L, Miller MA, et al. A predominantly clonal multi-institutional outbreak of *Clostridium difficile*-associated diarrhea with high morbidity and mortality. N Engl J Med 2005;353(23):2442–9.

69. Gaynes R, Rimland D, Killum E, et al. Outbreak of *Clostridium difficile* infection in a long-term care facility: association with gatifloxacin use. Clin Infect Dis 2004; 38(5):640–5.

70. McFarland LV, Clarridge JE, Beneda HW, et al. Fluoroquinolone use and risk factors for *Clostridium difficile*-associated disease within a Veterans Administration health care system. Clin Infect Dis 2007;45(9):1141–51.

71. del Rio C, Hall G, Hook EW, et al. Update to CDC's sexually transmitted diseases treatment guidelines, 2006: Fluoroquinolones no longer recommended for treatment of gonococcal infections. MMWR Morb Mortal Wkly Rep 2007;56(14):332–6.

72. Owens RC Jr, Ambrose PG. Antimicrobial safety: focus on fluoroquinolones. Clin Infect Dis 2005;41(Suppl 2):S144–57.

73. Iannini P, Mandell L, Patou G, et al. Cutaneous adverse events and gemifloxacin: observations from the clinical trial program. J Chemother 2006;18(1):3–11.

74. Lipsky BA, Baker CA. Fluoroquinolone toxicity profiles: a review focusing on newer agents. Clin Infect Dis 1999;28(2):352–64.

75. Tanne JH. FDA adds "black box" warning label to fluoroquinolone antibiotics [comment]. BMJ 2008;337:a816.

76. Cipro [label information October 2008]. Available at: http://www.fda.gov/cder/foi/label/2008/019537s68. 19847s42, 19857s49, 20780s26, 21473s24lbl.pdf. Accessed November 14, 2008.

77. Factive [label information October 2008]. Available at: http://www.fda.gov/cder/foi/label/2008/021158s012lbl.pdf. Accessed November 14, 2008.

78. Levaquin [label information October 2008]. Available at: http://www.fda.gov/cder/foi/label/2008/021721s020_020635s57_020634s52_lbl.pdf. Accessed November 14, 2008.

79. Avelox [label information October 2008]. Available at: http://www.fda.gov/cder/foi/label/2008/021085s040. 021277s034lbl.pdf. Accessed November 14, 2008.

80. Khaliq Y, Zhanel GG. Fluoroquinolone-associated tendinopathy: a critical review of the literature. Clin Infect Dis 2003;36(11):1404–10.
81. Stahlmann R, Forster C, Shakibaei M, et al. Magnesium deficiency induces joint cartilage lesions in juvenile rats which are identical to quinolone-induced arthropathy. Antimicrob Agents Chemother 1995;39(9):2013–8.
82. Owens RC Jr, Nolin TD. Antimicrobial-associated QT interval prolongation: pointes of interest. Clin Infect Dis 2006;43(12):1603–11.
83. Frothingham R. Rates of torsades de pointes associated with ciprofloxacin, ofloxacin, levofloxacin, gatifloxacin, and moxifloxacin. Pharmacotherapy 2001;21(12): 1468–72.
84. Dale KM, Lertsburapa K, Kluger J, et al. Moxifloxacin and torsades de pointes. Ann Pharmacother 2007;41(2):336–40.
85. Altin T, Ozcan O, Turhan S, et al. Torsades de pointes associated with moxifloxacin: a rare but potentially fatal adverse event. Can J Cardiol 2007;23(11):907–8.
86. Park-Wyllie LY, Juurlink DN, Kopp A, et al. Outpatient gatifloxacin therapy and dysglycemia in older adults. N Engl J Med 2006;354(13):1352–61.
87. Blum MD, Graham DJ, McCloskey CA. Temafloxacin syndrome: review of 95 cases. Clin Infect Dis 1994;18(6):946–50.
88. Ziganshina LE, Squire SB. Fluoroquinolones for treating tuberculosis. Cochrane Database Syst Rev 2008;1:CD004795.
89. Pedro-Botet L, Yu VL. Legionella: macrolides or quinolones? Clin Microbiol Infect 2006;12(Suppl 3):25–30.
90. Cullen M, Steven N, Billingham L, et al. Antibacterial prophylaxis after chemotherapy for solid tumors and lymphomas. N Engl J Med 2005;353(10):988–98.
91. Bucaneve G, Micozzi A, Menichetti F, et al. Levofloxacin to prevent bacterial infection in patients with cancer and neutropenia. N Engl J Med 2005;353(10): 977–87.
92. Imran H, Tleyjeh IM, Arndt CA, et al. Fluoroquinolone prophylaxis in patients with neutropenia: a meta-analysis of randomized placebo-controlled trials. Eur J Clin Microbiol Infect Dis 2008;27(1):53–63.
93. Fraser A, Gafter-Gvili A, Paul M, et al. Antibiotics for preventing meningococcal infections. Cochrane Database Syst Rev 2006;4:CD004785.

Current Use for Old Antibacterial Agents: Polymyxins, Rifamycins, and Aminoglycosides

Luke F. Chen, MBBS (Hons), MPH, CIC, FRACP[a],*, Donald Kaye, MD[b,c]

KEYWORDS

- Rifaximin • Pharmacokinetics • Pharmacodynamics • Toxicity
- Polymyxins • Aminoglycoside • Rifampin

The polymyxins, rifamycins, and the aminoglycosides may be considered special use antibacterial agents. They are all old agents and are rarely considered the drugs of choice for common bacterial infections.

The polymyxins are increasingly important because of the continued emergence of multidrug resistant (MDR) gram-negative organisms, such as strains of *Pseudomonas aeruginosa* or carbapenemase-producing Enterobacteriaceae that are susceptible to few remaining drugs. Rifampin is only considered in the context of nonmycobacterial infections where its role is limited and sometimes controversial. Rifaximin is a new enteric rifamycin that is increasingly used for gastrointestinal infections such as traveler's diarrhea and *Clostridium difficile* infections (CDIs). This article will also review the current role of aminoglycosides in nonmycobacterial systemic infections, with an emphasis on the use of single daily administration.

POLYMYXINS

The polymyxins were discovered in 1947. Although there are five known polymyxin molecules, sequentially named polymyxin A through polymyxin E, only two polymyxins are available for therapeutic use: polymyxin B and polymyxin E (colistin) (**Table 1**). Both polymyxin B and polymyxin E are large cyclic cationic polypeptide detergents

A version of this article appeared in the 23:4 issue of the *Infectious Disease Clinics of North America*.

[a] Division of Infectious Diseases and International Health, Department of Medicine, Duke University Medical Center, Box 102359, Hanes House, Durham, NC 27710, USA
[b] Department of Medicine, Drexel University College of Medicine, Philadelphia, PA 19102, USA
[c] 1535 Sweet Briar Road, Gladwyne, PA 19035, USA
* Corresponding author.
E-mail address: luke.chen@duke.edu

Med Clin N Am 95 (2011) 819–842
doi:10.1016/j.mcna.2011.03.007
0025-7125/11/$ – see front matter © 2011 Elsevier Inc. All rights reserved.

Table 1
Routes of administration of different forms of polymyxins

	Alternate Name	Available Preparations	Routes of Administration
Polymyxin B	—	Polymyxin B	Parenteral/topical intrathecal/intraventricular
Polymyxin E	Colistin	Colistin sulfate Colistimethate sodium (Colistin methanesulfonate)	Oral Parenteral/nebulization intrathecal/intraventricular

with molecular weights of 1000 or more. Polymyxin B was initially isolated from *Bacillus polymyxa*, and colistin was isolated from *Bacillus colistinus*. There are two preparations of colistin: colistin sulfate and colistimethate sodium. Colistimethate sodium is inactive until hydrolyzed and such hydrolysis occurs in both in vivo and in vitro testing systems. Notably, colistimethate sodium is the least active polymyxin in vitro (as much as fourfold to eightfold less active)[1] but also is the least nephrotoxic compound compared with polymyxin B and colistin sulfate.[2,3]

The polymyxins were used to treat serious infections caused by gram-negative bacilli in the early 1960s until aminoglycosides active against *P aeruginosa* (eg, gentamicin) came into common use. The polymyxins fell into further disuse by 1980 because of their nephrotoxicity and subsequently they became mainly reserved for topical and oral administration.[4,5] The recent emergence of *P aeruginosa*, *Acinetobacter baumannii*, and MDR gram-negative bacilli resistant to all other antimicrobial agents has resulted in the increasing need for an injectable polymyxin.[6,7]

In recent years, colistimethate sodium has been the most commonly used form of polymyxin for parenteral therapy. Colistimethate has also been used for nebulization therapy in patients with cystic fibrosis and for intrathecal and intraventricular injection. Colistin, on the other hand, has been available as colistin sulfate for use topically and orally, except in the United States, where only colistimethate and polymyxin B are available commercially.

Polymyxin B sulfate can be given intramuscularly and intravenously and is available for topical use. Polymyxin B has also been used intrathecally and intraventricularly for central nervous system infections.

Mechanism of Action and Antimicrobial Activity

The polymyxins act on the cell wall of gram-negative bacteria by way of three known mechanisms of action. (1) Polymyxins are cationic molecules that electrostatically disrupt bacterial surface membranes by displacing Ca^{2+} and Mg^{2+} ions that stabilize lipopolysaccharide (LPS) molecules. (2) Polymyxins are surface-active amphipathic agents containing both lipophilic and lipophobic groups. They penetrate into cell membranes and interact with phospholipids in the membranes, leading to permeability changes that quickly disrupt cell membranes leading to cell death.[8] (3) Polymyxins also bind to the lipid A portion of endotoxin or LPS molecules and, in animal studies, block many of the biologic effects of endotoxins.[9]

The polymyxins are active against commonly isolated gram-negative aerobic bacilli with the exception of *Proteus* spp, which are generally very resistant to the polymyxins. In addition, the polymyxins have poor activity against *Serratia*, *Providencia*, *Burkholderia*, *Vibrio*, *Brucella*, *Helicobacter*, *Moraxella*, *Aeromonas*, *Morganella*, and *Edwardsiella*.[5,10] Fortunately, the polymyxins have retained activity against many drug-resistant gram-negative bacilli, such as *P aeruginosa* and *A baumannii*. When tested against colistin sulfate, most gram-negative bacilli are inhibited by 1.0 μg/mL; *P aeruginosa* strains are more resistant, but most strains are inhibited by 2.0 μg/mL.[10] *Pseudomonas* strains with a minimal inhibitory concentration (MIC) greater than 4.0 μg/mL and *Acinetobacter* strains with a colistin MIC of greater than 2 mcg/ml are defined as resistant.[11]

Polymyxins are not active against gram-positive organisms and most anaerobes. Fortunately, resistance of gram-negative bacteria to the polymyxins remains uncommon[12–14]; however, heteroresistance has been reported in isolates of *Acinetobacter*.[15,16] When resistance is present however, there is complete cross-resistance between the polymyxins.[17] Such resistance of gram-negative bacteria to the polymyxins is usually related to changes in the architecture of LPS molecules in the cell wall that interfere with the interaction between peptides of the polymyxin (which are positively charged) and the LPS molecules (which are negatively charged).[5] The PmrA-PmrB and PhoP-PhoQ systems regulate the charge of Lipid A and LPS in gram-negative bacteria and appear to have important roles in this mechanism of resistance.[18,19] Studies have shown less common mechanisms of resistance to polymyxins. For example, one study of colistin-resistant *Pseudomonas* isolates revealed alterations in bacterial cell membrane, including reduced density of LPS molecules, and reduced concentration of Ca^{2+} and Mg^{2+} ions.[1] Interestingly, the emergence of polymyxin-resistant *P aeruginosa* has been linked to the use of nebulized colistimethate in patients who have cystic fibrosis.[2,20] Another recent report showed that efflux pump/potassium channels may mediate resistance in isolates of polymyxin-resistant *Yersinia* spp.[21] The activity of the polymyxins is diminished in the presence of high concentrations of divalent cations such as calcium and magnesium.[1]

Pharmacokinetics

The basic and clinical evaluation of the polymyxins took place many years ago, and reliable pharmacokinetic data are lacking. Furthermore, review articles often do not differentiate forms of polymyxin and often have internally inconsistent data concerning pharmacokinetics, especially blood levels.[22]

When administered orally, none of the polymyxins are absorbed. According to old literature, following intramuscular injection of 2–4 mg/kg polymyxin B, peak serum levels of 1–8 μg/mL were achieved. There is little reliable data on serum levels after IV administration of polymyxin B. A very recent study using 0.5–1.25 mg/kg polymyxin B, given by IV infusions over an hour to critically ill subjects, reported peak plasma concentrations of 2.4–14 μg/mL drawn after at least 2 days of therapy. Serum protein binding was 79%–92%.[23]

When colistimethate was given intramuscularly to adults at a dose of 2.5 mg/kg, a peak serum level of 5–7 μg/mL was achieved. In old reports, the peak serum level following intravenous administration of colistimethate was about 20 μg/mL. The package insert for colistimethate shows peak levels of about 8 μg/mL and 20 μg/mL, respectively, following intramuscular and intravenous administration of 150 mg.

In very limited studies, however, following 2 to 3 mg/kg intravenous administration of colistimethate, the peak level of colistin, the active metabolite was only about 2 μg/ml (which is much lower than the peak of colistimethate).[24] Because serum protein binding of colistin is about 50%, the peak antibacterial activity in serum of active colistin following administration of recommended doses is borderline at best.[24] Finally, in a recent pharmacokinetic analysis, steady state concentrations of 2.3 mcg/mL were achievable when colistimethate was administered at 240 mg every 8 hours.[25]

According to past literature, the excretion of polymyxin B and colistin is primarily by glomerular filtration. After the initial dose of polymyxin B (but not colistimethate) there is a 12- to 24-hour lag before significant amounts of drug are found in the urine. After administration of subsequent doses, the urine levels of both polymyxin B and colistimethate exceed 15 µg/mL for at least 6 hours. In a recent study, less than 1% of infused polymyxin B was recovered unchanged in the urine.[23]

The half-life of polymyxin B in serum is about 4.5 to 6 hours.[26] There is relatively little information available on the serum half-life of colistin (the active antibiotic) following injection of colistimethate. In subjects who have cystic fibrosis, the serum half-lives of colistimethate and colistin were 2 hours and 4 hours, respectively.[24] Half-lives of these agents are prolonged when given to patients who have renal insufficiency or are critically ill.[27] Distribution to the cerebrospinal fluid (CSF), biliary tract, pleural fluid, and joint fluid is poor.[28] However, in one report, the peak CSF levels following the intravenous administration of colistimethate were 25% of the peak serum levels.[29]

Serum levels of the polymyxins are very low following inhalation therapy.[30] The polymyxins are poorly dialyzed and there is minimal hepatic metabolism or biliary excretion.

Pharmacodynamics

Polymyxin B and colistin have rapid bactericidal effect in vitro in a concentration-dependent manner. There is well-described postantibiotic effect (PAE) for *P aeruginosa* with delayed regrowth, as compared with rapid regrowth of MDR *A baumannii* with no PAE because of heteroresistance.[5,31] Because of the potential lack of PAE, three times a day dosing has been suggested by in vitro studies.[32] It has also been suggested that the polymyxins be used in combination with another active drug if there is one. Studies of in vitro synergy have been limited to relatively few organisms. Using colistin-susceptible strains of MDR bacteria, synergism has been demonstrated between a polymyxin and ceftazidime, rifampin, trimethoprim-sulfametho:azole, imipenem, cefepime, tigecycline, and azithromycin.[33-40]

Toxicity

Dose-related nephrotoxicity is the most common and the most important adverse effect associated with polymyxins.[41] The nephrotoxicity is attributed to direct damage of the cells in the distal convoluted tubules,[42] and is usually reversible after the drug is discontinued.[22,43] Early literature suggested that 10%–30% of subjects who received polymyxins developed reversible renal impairment. However, more recent reports indicate that the nephrotoxicity with polymyxins may be less than aminoglycosides.[15] In addition, studies that adjusted for severity of illness and pre-existing renal impairment have found that subjects receiving colistimethate experienced similar rates of nephrotoxicity compared with cohorts receiving carbapenems and other agents for infections caused by *P aeruginosa* and *A baumanii*.[7,44,45] Nephrotoxic effects are enhanced, however, when the polymyxins are used in subjects receiving other nephrotoxic agents.[46]

Dose-related neurotoxicity occurs in approximately 5% of subjects receiving polymyxins, according to more recent literature. There are several manifestations of neurotoxicity: (1) Neuromuscular blockade, which can involve the respiratory musculature and cause apnea and can be potentiated by aminoglycosides[4,22]; (2) Sensory disturbance with perioral paresthesias, parethesias of the tongue, and parethesias of the extremities; and (3) Polyneuropathy, including cranial nerve palsies (diplopia, nystagmus).

Neuromuscular blockade is most likely to occur when the drug is used in excessive doses in patients who have renal failure, or in those who are receiving curariform drugs. When respiratory paralysis occurs, it is necessary to support respiratory function until the effects of the drug wear off. Intravenous calcium may help reverse the respiratory paralysis. Aminoglycosides may potentiate the neurotoxic effects. Other neurotoxic side effects, such as perioral paresthesias, parathesias of the tongue and extremities, and peripheral neuropathy are not uncommon.[4] Toxicity is less likely to occur with colistimethate than with polymyxin B.

Hypersensitivity to polymyxins is unusual, but up to 2% of patients receiving parenteral polymyxins can develop allergic manifestations, including fever, eosinophilia, and rashes.

In general, toxicity is less likely to occur with colistimethate than with polymyxin B. Intraventricular and intrathecal administration of the polymyxins are generally well tolerated.[46,47] Nebulization may result in bronchoconstriction. A warning has been issued by the FDA against premixing colistimethate too far in advance of nebulization because of one possible drug-related death.[48]

Clinical Indications

In the United States, polymyxin B and colistimethate are approved only for use intravenously (which is preferred) and intramuscularly. However, aerosols and the intrathecal and intraventricular routes have become relatively common.[29,47,49–52]

Polymyxin B is very painful when given intramuscularly, and this route of administration should be avoided. The dosage of polymyxins below are expressed in terms of the polymyxin base. If IM injection is necessary, the usual IM dose is 2.5–3 mg/kg/day in divided doses every 4 to 6 hours. The IV dose is 1.5–2.5 mg/kg/day by continuous IV infusion or in divided doses every 12 hours over a period of 60 to 90 minutes.

For treatment of gram-negative bacillary central nervous system infection, the Infectious Diseases Society of America guidelines recommend a daily dose of 5 mg polymyxin B intraventricularly.[53] Polymyxin B has been given intrathecally in doses of 5–10 mg/day for the initial 3 days of therapy and then every other day until cultures are negative.

The recommended dosage of colistimethate in adults who have normal renal function is 2.5–5 mg/kg (depending on the severity of infection) each day intramuscularly or intravenously in two to four divided doses. The dose should be based on ideal body weight and should not exceed 300 mg/day. Doses must be decreased in patients who have impaired renal function to avoid drug accumulation and toxicity. When given intravenously, colistimethate is administered over 3 to 5 minutes. Administration of doses as high as 8 mg/kg/day has been reported recently.[54] The question has been raised about the use of colistimethate as a single daily dose to theoretically lower the risk of toxicity, but clinical validation is lacking and, for reasons stated above, is not a good idea.

For treatment of central nervous system infection, the Infectious Diseases Society of America guidelines suggest an intraventricular dose of 10 mg of colistimethate.[53] The same dose would presumably be used intrathecally.

Colistin sulfate has been used orally for intestinal decontamination. The oral preparation is not available in the United States.

Inhalation therapy with aerosolized colistimethate has been used with varying success to treat colonization or infection of the bronchial system, especially with MDR *P aeruginosa*, in patients who have cystic fibrosis.[52] Systemic blood levels are not achieved with inhalation therapy. The usual dose in adults is 80 mg every 12 hours. Up to 160 mg every 8 hours has been used.

Most of the literature on the use of the polymyxins for parenteral therapy is old. In recent years, colistimethate has been used parenterally to treat systemic infections caused by MDR gram-negative bacilli, mainly ventilator-associated pneumonia.[1,5,22,29,43,44,47–52,54,55] In contrast with past experience, recent reports claim little in the way of nephrotoxicity or neurotoxicity.[1,4,5,22,29,43,44,47–52,54,55] However, more modern-day experience is necessary before colistimethate can be considered a relatively nontoxic systemic agent. Reports of use of polymyxin B in modern medicine have been sparse.

Recent observations have indicated that emergence of polymyxin resistance in *P aeruginosa, K pneumoniae*, and *A baumannii* is associated with the use of this class of agents.[2,20,56]

Until more clinical data become available, parenteral polymyxin B and colistimethate should be reserved for use only when no other less toxic or potentially more effective drug can be used.

RIFAMPIN AND RIFAXIMIN

Rifamycins are a group of broad-spectrum antibiotics that interfere with bacterial DNA-dependent RNA polymerase and are active against mycobacteria and various gram-positive and gram-negative organisms. This section focuses on the use of rifampin against nonmycobacterial organisms, and is followed by a discussion of rifaximin, a novel rifamycin derivative that is increasingly used as an enteric antibiotic against traveler's diarrhea[57] and is being evaluated for *Clostridium difficile* infections (CDIs).

Rifampin

Rifampin, or rifampicin, the prototypical rifamycin, was first synthesized in 1965 from a fermentation product of *Streptomyces mediterranei*. It kills proliferating extracellular organisms, intracellular mycobacteria, and semidormant subpopulations of mycobacteria that reside in tissues.[58]

Although rifampin is best known for its antimycobacterial activity, the drug is highly active against both coagulase-positive and -negative staphylococci and other gram-positive cocci, such as *S pyogenes* and *S pneumoniae*. Enterococci are only moderately susceptible. Among gram-negative organisms, *N meningitidis, N gonorrhoeae*, and *Hemophilus influenzae* are the most susceptible.

In addition to its broad spectrum of activity, rifampin has interesting pharmacokinetic properties and has the unusual ability to enter cells and mediate antibacterial activity at intracellular sites.[59]

Mechanism of action and antimicrobial activity

Rifampin acts by inhibiting DNA-dependent RNA polymerase after binding to the beta subunit of the enzyme.[60] This interaction interferes with protein synthesis by preventing chain initiation. Rifampin is usually bactericidal, but may be bacteriostatic depending on the organism and the drug concentration. Hence, rifampin demonstrates concentration-dependent killing and has a very long PAE.[61] Those organisms inhibited by 1.0 µg/mL or less are considered to be susceptible to rifampin, those inhibited by 2.0 µg/mL are intermediate, and those with a MIC of 4.0 µg/mL or more are resistant.[10]

Most gram-positive cocci (staphylococci and streptococci) are highly susceptible to rifampin (MICs <1 µg/mL); enterococci, which are only moderately sensitive, are an important exception.[62,63]

Meningococci, gonococci, and *H influenzae* are susceptible to rifampin. In contrast, most gram-negative bacilli are intrinsically resistant to rifampin.

Acquired resistance to rifampin occurs rapidly when it is inappropriately used as monotherapy and often develops by mutations in the gene (*rpoB*) encoding the beta subunit of DNA-dependent RNA polymerase. Additionally, resistance can be mediated by alterations in membrane permeability.[64]

The effects of combining rifampin with other antibiotics remain a confusing area due to conflicting in vitro and in vivo data. When rifampin is added to other bactericidal agents, the effect may be synergistic, additive, indifferent, or antagonistic depending on the drugs, their concentrations, the organisms being studied, and the model. Examples of some of the results follow.

Addition of rifampin to penicillinase-resistant penicillins in vitro inhibited the bactericidal activity of the penicillins against *S aureus*.[65] In a rabbit model of *S aureus* endocarditis, the combination of a penicillinase-resistant penicillin and rifampin was synergistic for some strains and indifferent or antagonistic for other strains.[66] The addition of rifampin to vancomycin or to vancomycin-plus-gentamicin improved the effectiveness of therapy in a rabbit model of *Staphylococcus epidermidis* endocarditis.[67] Similarly, substantial improvements in cure rates for *S epidermidis* prosthetic valve endocarditis were achieved by adding rifampin, gentamicin, or both, to vancomycin.[68]

Experimental meningitis studies with limited number of strains of pneumococci have demonstrated that addition of rifampin to vancomycin or ceftriaxone may have differing effects on the rate of killing of pneumococci in CSF. One study showed a beneficial effect.[69] In contrast, another study demonstrated no increase in killing rate against pneumococci when rifampin was added to vancomycin.[70] Interestingly, an in vitro study showed that the addition of rifampin to ceftriaxone resulted in a marked decrease in killing rates of ceftriaxone-susceptible pneumococci, compared with ceftriaxone alone.[71]

Synergism has been demonstrated between colistin and rifampin in vitro and in vivo against certain MDR strains of bacteria.[34,36,38,72]

Pharmacokinetics

Rifampin is well absorbed when given orally with peak serum concentrations of 7 to 10 µg/mL following a dose of 600 mg. Food interferes with enteric absorption and rifampin should therefore be administered on an empty stomach. An intravenous preparation is available when the oral route cannot be used. Dosing is identical for the oral and intravenous preparations.

Rifampin is widely distributed into tissues and different compartments despite being 80% protein-bound. It penetrates well into body fluids, achieving therapeutic levels in saliva, bile, bone, pleural fluid, prostate, and CSF. Moreover, rifampin readily enters phagocytic cells and can kill microorganisms in the cells.

Rifampin undergoes a multistep process of elimination. It is first de-acetylated in the liver and then cleared by hepatic metabolism and biliary excretion. The half-life of rifampin is 2 to 5 hours, which can be prolonged by hepatic disease and shortened by repeated dosing due to rifampin's propensity to induce its own metabolism by way of the P450 enzymes. Rifampin does not need dose-adjustment in the setting of renal insufficiency.

Toxicity

With administration of rifampin, urine and sweat often develop an orange tinge and soft contact lenses may be stained. This adverse effect of discoloring body fluids is almost universal and may be used as a surrogate marker of adherence. A flulike syndrome can occur in up to 5% of patients who have had prolonged intermittent use of rifampin. Rash and gastrointestinal adverse effects (eg, nausea, vomiting, diarrhea, heartburn) may occur in up to 5% of patients. Abnormal liver function tests are common but frank hepatitis is uncommon (<1%), especially with short courses used for nonmycobacterial infections.

The potential for rifampin to induce hepatic microsomal enzymes can cause multiple drug–drug interactions[73]; such interactions can occur with oral contraceptives, cyclosporine, digoxin, fluconazole, sulfonylureas, theophylline, thyroxine, warfarin, antipsychotics[74] and antiretroviral agents.[75]

Clinical indications

Rifampin should always be coupled with another bacterioactive agent and should never be used as monotherapy, except when used for chemoprophylaxis of meningococcal and H influenzae infections.[76,77] The course of chemoprophylaxis is always short and is designed to eradicate the organism from the nasopharynx. Furthermore, rifampin is now seldom used to prevent H influenzae infections because of decreased rates of the infection due to widespread use of the H influenzae vaccine.

Rifampin is administered in a dose of 10 mg/kg (not to exceed 600 mg) in patients at least 1 month of age, twice a day for 2 days for prevention of meningococcal disease; this generally has had an efficacy of more than 90%. However, rifampin has several shortcomings, including nasopharyngeal eradication rates of only about 70%–80% in some studies, adverse effects, and the necessity for multiple doses over 2 days. Moreover, resistance to rifampin in isolates of N meningitidis in the United States is increasingly detected (up to 10%–27% of N meningitidis isolates).[78,79] Ciprofloxacin may be more effective in eradicating meningococci.[80] To protect children under 4 years of age who have been incompletely immunized against H influenzae type B, all household contacts who have been in contact with a case of severe infection should receive rifampin prophylaxis. The dose in adults is 600 mg twice daily for 2 days.

Rifampin has been used in combination with other nonmycobacterial agents in some limited situations, including (1) Staphylococcal infections, especially on foreign bodies (eg, prosthetic valve endocarditis)[81]; (2) Pneumococcal meningitis in which corticosteroids are being given in addition to vancomycin and a third generation cephalosporin; and (3) As combination therapy for certain zoonoses, such as Brucellosis, Q fever, Bartonellosis and Rhodococcus infections.[82]

Staphylococcal infection In an attempt to achieve higher rates of cure, rifampin has been increasingly used by some in combination with standard antistaphylococcal therapy for severe infections caused by staphylococci. Rifampin has several properties that are theoretically advantageous in the treatment of complicated staphylococcal infections: (1) Rifampin is bactericidal against S aureus, (2) Rifampin achieves high intracellular levels, and (3) Rifampin can penetrate biofilms.[83]

Even though rifampin has these desirable characteristics, data to support the practice of combining rifampin and another antistaphylococcal agent are limited and are typically based on small clinical studies or animal and in vitro investigations. A recent meta-analysis concluded that many animal studies showed a microbiologic benefit of adjunctive rifampin use, particularly in osteomyelitis and infected foreign body infection models.[81] Few human studies have adequately addressed the role of adjunctive rifampin therapy. Adjunctive therapy seems most promising for the treatment of osteomyelitis and prosthetic device-related infections, although studies typically have been underpowered and benefits were not always seen.[81]

A substantial improvement in cure rates for S epidermidis prosthetic valve endocarditis was reported in a noncontrolled study by adding rifampin, gentamicin, or both, to vancomycin.[68] As a result of this study and in vitro and animal studies, the American Heart Association recommends the addition of 300 mg rifampin orally every 8 hours for treatment of *S epidermidis* prosthetic valve endocarditis.[84]

Because of the excellent penetration of rifampin into tissues and organ spaces, there is a general enthusiasm for including rifampin in regimens when treating staphylococcal infections in the presence of abscesses or foreign bodies.

Despite the benefit of adding rifampin to the regimen in animal models of *S aureus* osteomyelitis,[85] clinical studies have not been convincing.[86] However, in the presence of a foreign body, it is reasonable to add rifampin.

Rifampin alone or in combination with another drug (eg, trimethoprim-sulfamethoxazole) has been used to eradicate nasal carriage of *S aureus*, including methicillin-resistant strains (MRSA).[87,88] These combinations have also been used for oral treatment of non–life-threatening MRSA infections.

Pneumococcal meningitis Despite high in vitro susceptibility against *S pneumoniae*, rifampin should never be used alone to treat pneumococcal meningitis. When the infecting organism is highly resistant to ceftriaxone and cefotaxime but is rifampin-susceptible, combination therapy with vancomycin plus ceftriaxone plus rifampin might be effective.[69] In these circumstances, vancomycin concentrations should be maximized to ensure adequate CNS penetration. Steroid therapy can reduce antimicrobial penetration into CSF by decreasing inflammation; in animal models, steroid therapy has been associated with failure of cephalosporin or vancomycin monotherapy, although this has not been observed in all experimental studies. For these reasons the Infectious Disease Society of America recommends addition of rifampin to the vancomycin, third generation cephalosporin, and dexamethasone regimen used for pneumococcal meningitis.[53]

Despite these recommendations, there are no reliable clinical data concerning results of the addition of rifampin to vancomycin and/or a third-generation cephalosporin in subjects who have pneumococcal meningitis. Because there are conflicting results of the benefits of rifampin in animal model and in vitro studies, it has been suggested that rifampin be used for patients in whom the pneumococcal isolate is sensitive to rifampin in vitro and who are not responding appropriately to standard therapy.

Brucellosis Rifampin in combination with doxycycline plus and minus an aminoglycoside has been shown to have better cure rates for brucellosis than other antibiotic combinations in recent meta-analyses.[89,90]

Rifaximin

Rifaximin is a new enteric antibiotic that is only available as an oral preparation. Like other rifamycins, rifaximin binds the beta subunit of the DNA-dependent RNA polymerase, and inhibits RNA synthesis.[91] Unlike rifampicin, however, rifaximin acts exclusively in the gastrointestinal tract and is poorly absorbed due to the presence of a pyridoimidazole moiety.

Spectrum of activity

Rifaximin is active against most gram-positive organisms, including *C difficile* and essentially all enteric gram-negative pathogens, including *E coli, H pylori, Y enterocolitica,* and *Shigella* spp.[92]

Despite its broad antibiotic spectrum, rifaximin appears to have little impact on normal gastrointestinal flora.[93] In one study, there was an initial decrease in the gastrointestinal flora following rifaximin administration, followed by rapid normalization of enteric flora within the month.[94] Development of resistance to rifaximin appears to occur with low frequency.[95,96]

Adverse effects

Rifaximin is generally well tolerated, with similar rates of adverse effects in subjects receiving comparator drugs and placebos.[97–99] Headache was more common in one study. Rifaximin is not expected to have drug–drug interactions via the CYP 450 system because it is not systemically absorbed.[100]

Clinical indications

Rifaximin is currently approved for the treatment of traveler's diarrhea caused by noninvasive strains of *E coli*. Three studies showed rifaximin to be effective in shortening the duration of diarrhea. The approved dosage is 200 mg three times per day for 3 days.

Rifaximin is also being considered in the therapy for *C difficile* infections.[101,102] One study in the hamster model showed oral rifaximin to be as effective, if not more effective, than oral vancomycin for two standard strains of *C difficile*.[103] Several treatment strategies with rifaximin have shown positive outcomes in refractory *C difficile* infections, including combination therapy of vancomycin and rifaximin,[104] drug-cycling regimen of vancomycin and rifaximin,and even a strategy of sequential monotherapy of vancomycin and rifaximin.[105]

In one small case series, eight subjects who had recurrent symptoms of *C difficile* infection received sequential therapy of oral vancomycin and then rifaximin.[105] At the end of the study, all but one subject remained symptom free. Unfortunately, the study also reported that the rifaximin MIC for *C difficile* isolates recovered after therapy (>256 μg/mL) was much higher than the MIC for isolates recovered before therapy (0.0078 μg/mL). The use of rifaximin for *C difficile* infections remains off-label and caution should be exercised because drug resistance was clearly demonstrated after rifaximin use in the study.

AMINOGLYCOSIDES

The aminoglycosides are a class of bactericidal antibiotics characterized by the presence of a six-carbon aminocyclitol ring, covalently bonded to multiple amino sugar groups. Aminoglycosides were once widely used as primary agents in the therapy of gram-negative bacillary infections. However, because of their toxicity and the availability of newer effective agents, systemic aminoglycosides have been primarily relegated to a role as companion drugs either to broaden coverage against gram-negative aerobic bacilli or to provide synergistic killing against gram-positive cocci or certain gram-negative bacilli. Now, because of the emergence of MDR gram-negative bacilli, the aminoglycosides, along with the polymyxins, may become antibiotics of last resort.[106]

The major change in the use of aminoglycosides has been a trend toward single daily dosage, even though this is not an FDA-approved dosing regimen. Gentamicin, the most widely administered and the most studied of the aminoglycosides, is the prototype for our discussion.

Mechanism of Action and Antimicrobial Activity

The aminoglycosides act in part by impairing bacterial protein synthesis through irreversible binding to the 30S subunit of the bacterial ribosome. They are rapidly bactericidal against a broad range of aerobic gram-negative bacilli (including *P aeruginosa*), but lack activity against anaerobes. Although there is activity against some gram-positive aerobic cocci, it is unreliable. The aminoglycosides are generally used against gram-positive cocci such as enterococci and staphylococci in combination with beta-lactam antibiotics and vancomycin to achieve synergistic bactericidal activity.

This clinical application of drug synergy is based primarily on in vitro and animal studies because there are no comparative trials showing better cure rates with addition of an aminoglycoside.[107] Synergy is lacking or variable when aminoglycosides are combined with newer drugs such as daptomycin, quinupristin-dalfopristin, or linezolid.[108]

Acquired resistance to the aminoglycosides is usually mediated by bacterial elaboration of aminoglycoside-inactivating enzymes. These enzymes are widely distributed in both gram-positive and gram-negative bacteria, and usually are plasmid-mediated.[109] Amikacin is the most likely of all aminoglycosides to be effective against MDR gram-negative bacilli because amikacin only has one locus that is susceptible to aminoglycoside-inactivating enzymes compared with six susceptible loci on gentamicin and tobramycin.[110,111]

Among gram-positive cocci, the most clinically significant resistance occurs in enterococci, where the synergistic killing activity of aminoglycosides is required for a high cure rate of endocarditis. Although all enterococci are intrinsically resistant to low concentrations of aminoglycosides, the clinical problem arises with high level gentamicin resistant (HLGR) enterococci.[84] HLGR enterococci are resistant to all other aminoglycosides in clinical use in the United States, with the possible exception of streptomycin, and do not demonstrate synergistic killing of enterococci when aminoglycosides are combined with penicillin or vancomycin.[84] Detection of HLGR requires either special susceptibility wells or screening plates with high concentrations of gentamicin or streptomycin (eg, $\geq$500 µg/mL gentamicin; $\geq$1000µg/ml streptomycin).

The synergistic killing effect of beta-lactam antibiotics and aminoglycosides has been demonstrated with multiple aerobic gram-negative bacilli and gram-positive cocci and in multiple animal models. In uncontrolled clinical studies, synergistic activity has been demonstrated to be important in the treatment of native valve endocarditis caused by enterococci and in prosthetic valve endocarditis due to S epidermidis.[84] There is a lack of clinical studies to clearly demonstrate benefits of drug synergy with aminoglycosides in serious P aeruginosa infections, and in infections caused by gram-negative bacilli in neutropenic patients. The aminoglycosides remain among the most active antibiotics against P aeruginosa.[109]

Pharmacokinetics

Aminoglycosides are poorly absorbed orally. After intravenous infusion of 1.7 mg/kg gentamicin (every 8 hour dosage), peak serum levels (C_{max}) are 4 to10 µg/mL. After infusion of 5 mg/kg (once daily dosage), peak levels are about 20 µg/mL serum. The half-life of all of the aminoglycosides is about 2 to 3 hours. Protein binding is low (<10%) and, because the agents are water soluble, they are distributed in the intravascular space and into interstitial fluid. The drugs diffuse into synovial, pleural, and peritoneal fluids, but penetration into CSF and bile is poor.

In general, in the absence of large effusions and edema, the volume of distribution is low. Increases in the volume of distribution tend to decrease the C_{max} and area under the serum-concentration-time curve (AUC), and increases in clearance tend to decrease the AUC. For example, the volume of distribution tends to be elevated and peak serum levels decreased in patients who have large effusions, fever, burns, or congestive heart failure and in critically ill patients.[112] Excretion of aminoglycosides is primarily by glomerular filtration; clearance is decreased with renal insufficiency and increased in children, in pregnancy and in patients who have cystic fibrosis.

Pharmacodynamics

The aminoglycosides show the following well-studied pharmacodynamic properties: (1) Concentration-dependent killing, (2) PAE, and (3) Postantibiotic leucocyte enhancement.

Concentration-dependent killing

Bacterial killing by aminoglycosides in vitro is concentration-dependent.[109] In vivo, higher doses of the drug not only increase the rate of reduction of bacteria, but also the length of time of drug exposure to bactericidal concentrations as measured by the AUC. In animal studies, aminoglycoside efficacy is correlated with the ratio of C_{max} to MIC of the infecting organism and also with the AUC. In animal studies, effective dosing regimens for concentration-dependent antibiotics require that either the 24-hour AUC/MIC be 80 to100 against gram-negative bacilli or the C_{max}/MIC of the causative pathogen be 8 to10.[113]

Some clinical studies have demonstrated a relationship between peak aminoglycoside concentrations and response to therapy. For concentration-dependent drugs, such as aminoglycosides, giving the total daily dose once every 24 hours rather than smaller divided doses would maximize the C_{max} and possibly allow for comparable or better efficacy at greater convenience and lower cost. A C_{max}/MIC of 10 to 12 appears to be the optimal ratio to ensure clinical response.[109] To achieve this ratio with single daily dose gentamicin, the MIC must be 2 µg/ml or less and preferably 1 µg/ml or less.

PAE

Aminoglycoside antibiotics have a PAE for both staphylococci and gram-negative bacilli, meaning that suppression of bacterial growth persists despite concentrations of antibiotic below the MIC.[109,114,115] This permits longer intervals before another dose of aminoglycoside is given.

Postantibiotic leucocyte enhancement

Enhanced phagocytosis of aminoglycoside-exposed bacteria by host leukocytes has also been observed in vitro.[116] This phenomenon has been referred to as postantibiotic leukocyte enhancement (PALE). The absence of PALE may help explain the decreased efficacy of once-daily dosing that has been described in neutropenic animals as compared with nonneutropenic animals.[117]

The antibacterial effects of aminoglycosides can be impaired in a couple of settings. First, an acidic or an anaerobic environment is known to impair the activity of aminoglycosides.[118–120] Second, adaptive resistance refers to the phenomenon of transient reduction in rate of bacterial killing by an antibiotic following pre-exposure to that drug.[121] Adaptive resistance to aminoglycoside agents has been observed principally in P aeruginosa, but also in other gram-negative bacilli and more recently in staphylococci.[122,123] Once-daily dosing may circumvent the possibility of adaptive resistance through the provision of a drug-free interval.[109]

Toxicity

The major adverse effects of the aminoglycosides are nephrotoxicity and otovestibular toxicity. The aminoglycosides mediate toxic damage to the proximal convoluted tubules in the kidneys, and to the cochlear and vestibular bodies of the inner ear.[106,109] In addition, aminoglycosides can cause neuromuscular blockade due to interference of neurotransmission at neuromuscular junctions.[109] The uptake of aminoglycosides by renal cortical cells appears to be a saturable process.[106,109,124] Once proximal tubular cells are saturated with aminoglycoside, the higher peak serum concentrations seen with once-daily dosing should not cause greater intracellular accumulation of drug than is seen with multiple lower doses. In fact, renal cortical accumulation of gentamicin in rodents is lower following once-daily dosing regimens than after multiple daily doses, and greater increases in serum creatinine are seen with multiple-daily dosing regimens.[125]

Correlation of increased renal cortical accumulation of aminoglycosides with dosing frequency rather than with peak serum concentrations has been demonstrated in a cohort of human subjects undergoing nephrectomy for cancer.[124] There have been many clinical studies of nephrotoxicity of aminoglycosides. A recent review compiled a summary of the results of meta-analyses of once-daily dosing of aminoglycosides versus multiple-daily dosing.[113] Although some of these reported a decrease in nephrotoxicity with once-daily dosing, most of the meta-analyses demonstrated no significant decrease in nephrotoxicity.[126] However, once-daily administration of aminoglycoside was less likely to result in nephrotoxicity than twice-daily administration in the only randomized double-blind study of aminoglycoside use.[127]

Increased nephrotoxicity has been observed in the elderly; in patients who have elevated trough levels; with prolonged use; in patients who have diabetes mellitus; with concurrent use of vancomycin, loop diuretics, cyclosporine, and cisplatin; and when the drug is administered at time of rest as opposed to activity.[127–130]

Aminoglycoside therapy may result in both vestibular and cochlear toxicity.[131] In rats (but not in guinea pigs), gentamicin uptake into perilymph, endolymph, and inner ear tissues appears to be a saturable process, as in the kidney.[132] It is unknown whether gentamicin uptake is a saturable process in humans and it is unclear whether aminoglycoside accumulation in the inner ear predicts ototoxicity.[132]

Risk of ototoxicity has been associated with elevated trough levels of aminoglycoside, although some investigators have found no association between drug levels and ototoxicity after controlling for age.[133,134] Nonetheless, the suggestion that aminoglycoside uptake into inner ear fluids is saturable has raised the possibility that once-daily dosing of aminoglycosides may decrease ototoxicity. However, most published meta-analyses have reported no difference in ototoxicity between once- and multiple-daily dosing.[113]

Clinical Indications

The most common indication for aminoglycosides is combination therapy with other antimicrobial agents for serious gram-negative bacillary infections. In addition, the aminoglycosides are important drugs in the treatment of mycobacterial infections and in infections caused by less common pathogens, such as *Yersinia pestis*, *Brucella* spp, and *Francisella tularensis*.

The aminoglycosides are also used in combination with cell-wall–active antibiotics to provide synergistic bactericidal activity in treatment of serious gram-positive coccal infections such as staphylococcal, enterococcal, and streptococcal endocarditis.[84]

The major change in therapy with aminoglycosides has been the increasing use of single daily dosage for treatment of gram-negative bacillary infections versus divided daily doses. For example, the daily dose of gentamicin is usually 5 mg/kg. It can be given as 5 mg/kg in one single daily IV dose over 30 to 60 minutes or as 1.7 mg/kg IM or IV every 8 hours in gram-negative meningitis (FDA approved). Once-daily dosing should be performed in a manner that ensures a high C_{max}/MIC ratio for the pathogen being treated and ensures that trough levels are low enough to minimize toxicity and permit the loss of adaptive resistance. Maximizing concentrations of aminoglycosides by using single daily dosing optimizes the rate and extent of bactericidal activity and results in lower residual bacterial counts and longer intervals before significant regrowth occurs.

The potential for increased efficacy with once-daily aminoglycoside dosing has been evaluated in a multitude of randomized clinical trials. In general, these individual trials have lacked sufficient power to determine whether observed differences in efficacy between once-daily and multiple-daily dosage regimens were due to chance alone. Therefore, meta-analysis has been used to synthesize the data contained in these multiple studies. Most meta-analyses demonstrated an improvement (albeit small) in the clinical efficacy of once-daily aminoglycoside dosing.[113]

Overall, in vitro, animal, and existing clinical data suggest that once-daily administration of aminoglycosides may be more efficacious and less nephrotoxic, or at least not more nephrotoxic, than multiple-daily dosing. Giving the total 24-hour dose as a single dose, rather than in smaller divided doses, and using extended dosing intervals has now become the standard for use in gram-negative bacillary infections in many clinical settings.[113] This strategy may be especially appropriate for treatment of infections caused by borderline susceptible pathogens (eg, P aeruginosa), with MICs that are close to the breakpoint.[135]

The dosages of once-daily administration of gentamicin, netilmicin, and tobramycin have varied from 4–7 mg/kg/day in clinical trials.[135] A starting dose of 5 mg/kg has been suggested for adults 30 to 60 years of age with doses of 6 mg/kg for adults below 30 years and 4 mg/kg for those over 60.[113] Because of patient-to-patient variability, 4 mg/kg dosing does not always ensure sufficiently high peak concentrations to provide optimal activity against organisms such as P aeruginosa.[135] The use of 7 mg/kg dosing of gentamicin in 2148 adult inpatients was associated with only 27 incidents of nephrotoxicity and 3 of vestibulotoxicity; however, the median duration of therapy was only 3 days.[135] It has been suggested that the initial once-daily doses should be 7 mg/kg for gentamicin and tobramycin and 15 mg/kg for amikacin in the critically ill; the dose is then tapered to yield a C_{max}/MIC greater than or equal to 10.[109] Other investigators have suggested a dose of 5 mg/kg for gentamicin, which is more in line with the FDA-approved daily dosage.[106]

Two different approaches have been suggested to treat patients who have impaired renal function: reduction of daily drug dosage, and increase in dosing interval beyond 24 hours.[135,136] Intuitively, it seems most reasonable to give daily doses that will yield peak serum levels that result in an appropriate C_{max} and to stop administration as soon as feasible. Regardless of the approach used, vigilant monitoring of aminoglycoside serum levels is of utmost importance when renal function is decreased.

The doses of aminoglycosides used for synergistic bactericidal activity in the treatment of gram-positive coccal endocarditis have been lower than those used for serious gram-negative infections (target serum peak level of gentamicin 3 μg/mL). The most compelling data on the need for synergistic bactericidal activity requiring aminoglycosides concern enterococcal endocarditis. Although a significant PAE has been demonstrated against enterococci with aminoglycoside/beta-lactam combinations in vitro, no PAE was demonstrated in an animal model of enterococcal endocarditis.[137] Animal models of enterococcal endocarditis using single daily doses of aminoglycosides compared with 8-hour doses have yielded conflicting results.[84] The current recommendations from the American Heart Association state that until more data demonstrate that once-daily dosing of an aminoglycoside is as effective as multiple-daily dosing, gentamicin or streptomycin should be administered in multiple divided doses rather than a daily single dose to patients who have enterococcal endocarditis.[84]

Aminoglycoside antibiotics have been used in the treatment of pulmonary exacerbations in patients who have cystic fibrosis and P aeruginosa colonization.[138–141]

Antibiotic treatment of such exacerbations is typically prolonged, and often occurs in the home setting. Once-daily dosing for home therapy has obvious advantages. Evidence also suggests that inhaled tobramycin can reduce infective exacerbations and other health care costs in cystic fibrosis patients.[142–144] Debate continues, however, over whether aminoglycoside therapy significantly contributes to the long-term risk of nephrotoxicity in cystic fibrosis patients.[145]

Patients who have cystic fibrosis clear aminoglycosides at an increased rate.[146] Higher doses of aminoglycosides (eg, tobramycin at doses up to 15 mg/kg/d) once daily have been used successfully with little or no increase in nephrotoxicity,[147–152] although transient ototoxicity has been associated with these doses.[148]

Several different methods of monitoring once-daily aminoglycoside dosing have been suggested. Some investigators have suggested monitoring trough concentrations only, with dose adjustments for troughs greater than 2 μg/mL.[153,154] However, this approach does not allow clinicians to appreciate underdosage of drug, and trough levels of 2 μg/mL are too high and indicate reduced clearance with once-daily dosing.

Another proposed approach to monitoring of once-daily dosage is with a drug level taken 6 to14 hours after infusion and adjusting the doses according to a nomogram.[135,155,156] Suboptimal peaks are not recognized by this method. A third approach measures two levels (at 0.5–1 h and 6–14 h) and calculates the AUC.[157–159]

It has been proposed that aminoglycoside levels need not be measured with once-daily dosing in patients who have ClCr greater than 60 mL/min who receive fewer than 5 days of therapy.[135,160] However, levels should be checked in patients at increased risk for toxicity or clinical failure, such as the elderly, those receiving other nephrotoxic drugs, those with severe infections, or those expected to require longer than 5 days of treatment. In patients on long-term therapy, aminoglycoside levels should be measured weekly as long as the serum creatinine is stable.[135,160]

SUMMARY

This article reviews three classes of antibacterial agents that are uncommonly used in bacterial infections (other than mycobacterial infections) and therefore can be thought of as special-use agents. The polymyxins are reserved for gram-negative bacilli that are resistant to virtually all other classes of drugs. Rifampin is used therapeutically, mainly as a companion drug in treatment of refractory gram-positive coccal infections, especially involving foreign bodies. Rifaximin is a new rifamycin that is a strict enteric antibiotic approved for use for treatment of traveler's diarrhea and is showing promise as a possible agent for refractory *C difficile* infections. The aminoglycosides are used mainly as companion drugs for the therapy of resistant gram-negative bacillary infection and for gram-positive coccal endocarditis. The major change in use of aminoglycosides has been a shift to once-daily dosing in many situations.

REFERENCES

1. Hermsen ED, Sullivan CJ, Rotschafer JC. Polymyxins: pharmacology, pharmacokinetics, pharmacodynamics, and clinical applications. Infect Dis Clin North Am 2003;17(3):545–62.
2. Li J, Nation RL, Milne RW, et al. Evaluation of colistin as an agent against multiresistant gram-negative bacteria. Int J Antimicrob Agents 2005;25(1):11–25.
3. Kwa A, Kasiakou SK, Tam VH, et al. Polymyxin B: similarities to and differences from colistin (polymyxin E). Expert Rev Anti Infect Ther 2007;5(5):811–21.
4. Falagas ME, Kasiakou SK. Toxicity of polymyxins: a systematic review of the evidence from old and recent studies. Crit Care 2006;10(1):R27.

5. Zavascki AP, Goldani LZ, Li J, et al. Polymyxin B for the treatment of multidrug-resistant pathogens: a critical review. J Antimicrob Chemother 2007;60(6): 1206–15.

6. Michalopoulos AS, Karatza DC. Multidrug-resistant gram-negative infections: the use of colistin. Expert Rev Anti Infect Ther 2010;8(9):1009–17.

7. Tam VH, Chang KT, Abdelraouf K, et al. Prevalence, resistance mechanisms, and susceptibility of multidrug-resistant bloodstream isolates of pseudomonas aeruginosa. Antimicrob Agents Chemother 2010;54(3):1160–4.

8. Dixon RA, Chopra I. Leakage of periplasmic proteins from escherichia coli mediated by polymyxin b nonapeptide. Antimicrob Agents Chemother 1986;29(5): 781–8.

9. From AH, Fong JS, Good RA. Polymyxin B sulfate modification of bacterial endotoxin: effects on the development of endotoxin shock in dogs. Infect Immun 1979;23(3):660–4.

10. Gales AC, Reis AO, Jones RN. Contemporary assessment of antimicrobial susceptibility testing methods for polymyxin B and colistin: review of available interpretative criteria and quality control guidelines. J Clin Microbiol 2001; 39(1):183–90.

11. Clinical and Laboratory Standards Institute. Performance standards for antimicrobial susceptibility testing. Wayne (PA): Clinical and Laboratory Standards Institute (CLSI); 2008.

12. Marchaim D, Chopra T, Pogue JM, et al. Outbreak of colistin-resistant, carbapenem-resistant klebsiella pneumoniae in metropolitan detroit, michigan. Antimicrob Agents Chemother 2011;55(2):593–9.

13. Urban C, Tiruvury H, Mariano N, et al. Polymyxin-resistant clinical isolates of escherichia coli. Antimicrob Agents Chemother 2011;55(1):388–9.

14. Valencia R, Arroyo LA, Conde M, et al. Nosocomial outbreak of infection with pan-drug-resistant Acinetobacter baumannii in a tertiary care university hospital. Infect Control Hosp Epidemiol 2009;30(3):257–63.

15. Li J, Rayner CR, Nation RL, et al. Heteroresistance to colistin in multidrug-resistant acinetobacter baumannii. Antimicrob Agents Chemother 2006;50(9): 2946–50.

16. Hawley JS, Murray CK, Jorgensen JH. Colistin heteroresistance in acinetobacter and its association with previous colistin therapy. Antimicrob Agents Chemother 2008;52(1):351–2.

17. Falagas ME, Kasiakou SK. Colistin: the revival of polymyxins for the management of multidrug-resistant gram-negative bacterial infections. Clin Infect Dis 2005;40(9):1333–41.

18. Lim LM, Ly N, Anderson D, et al. Resurgence of colistin: a review of resistance, toxicity, pharmacodynamics, and dosing. Pharmacotherapy 2010;30(12):1279–91.

19. Muller C, Plesiat P, Jeannot K. A two-component regulatory system interconnects resistance to polymyxins, aminoglycosides, fluoroquinolones, and beta-lactams in Pseudomonas aeruginosa. Antimicrob Agents Chemother 2011;55(3):1211–21.

20. Livermore DM. Multiple mechanisms of antimicrobial resistance in Pseudomonas aeruginosa: our worst nightmare? Clin Infect Dis 2002;34(5):634–40.

21. Bengoechea JA, Skurnik M. Temperature-regulated efflux pump/potassium antiporter system mediates resistance to cationic antimicrobial peptides in Yersinia. Mol Microbiol 2000;37(1):67–80.

22. Li J, Nation RL, Turnidge JD, et al. Colistin: the re-emerging antibiotic for multidrug-resistant gram-negative bacterial infections. Lancet Infect Dis 2006;6(9): 589–601.

23. Zavascki AP, Goldani LZ, Cao G, et al. Pharmacokinetics of intravenous polymyxin B in critically ill patients. Clin Infect Dis 2008;47(10):1298–304.
24. Nation RL, Li J. Optimizing use of colistin and polymyxin B in the critically ill. Semin Respir Crit Care Med 2007;28(6):604–14.
25. Plachouras D, Karvanen M, Friberg LE, et al. Population pharmacokinetic analysis of colistin methanesulfonate and colistin after intravenous administration in critically ill patients with infections caused by gram-negative bacteria. Antimicrob Agents Chemother 2009;53(8):3430–6.
26. Reed MD, Stern RC, O'Riordan MA, et al. The pharmacokinetics of colistin in patients with cystic fibrosis. J Clin Pharmacol 2001;41(6):645–54.
27. Nation RL, Li J. Colistin in the 21st century. Curr Opin Infect Dis 2009;22(6): 535–43.
28. Markantonis SL, Markou N, Fousteri M, et al. Penetration of colistin into cerebrospinal fluid. Antimicrob Agents Chemother 2009;53(11):4907–10.
29. Jimenez-Mejias ME, Pichardo-Guerrero C, Marquez-Rivas FJ, et al. Cerebrospinal fluid penetration and pharmacokinetic/pharmacodynamic parameters of intravenously administered colistin in a case of multidrug-resistant *Acinetobacter baumannii* meningitis. Eur J Clin Microbiol Infect Dis 2002;21(3):212–4.
30. Ratjen F, Rietschel E, Kasel D, et al. Pharmacokinetics of inhaled colistin in patients with cystic fibrosis. J Antimicrob Chemother 2006;57(2):306–11.
31. Owen RJ, Li J, Nation RL, et al. In vitro pharmacodynamics of colistin against *Acinetobacter baumannii* clinical isolates. J Antimicrob Chemother 2007;59(3): 473–7.
32. Bergen PJ, Li J, Nation RL, et al. Comparison of once-, twice- and thrice-daily dosing of colistin on antibacterial effect and emergence of resistance: studies with *Pseudomonas aeruginosa* in an in vitro pharmacodynamic model. J Antimicrob Chemother 2008;61(3):636–42.
33. Gunderson BW, Ibrahim KH, Hovde LB, et al. Synergistic activity of colistin and ceftazidime against multiantibiotic-resistant *Pseudomonas aeruginosa* in an in vitro pharmacodynamic model. Antimicrob Agents Chemother 2003;47(3):905–9.
34. Giamarellos-Bourboulis EJ, Karnesis L, Giamarellou H. Synergy of colistin with rifampin and trimethoprim/sulfamethoxazole on multidrug-resistant *Stenotrophomonas maltophilia*. Diagn Microbiol Infect Dis 2002;44(3):259–63.
35. Rahal JJ. Novel antibiotic combinations against infections with almost completely resistant *Pseudomonas aeruginosa* and *Acinetobacter* species. Clin Infect Dis 2006;43(Suppl 2):S95–9.
36. Chitnis S, Chitnis V, Chitnis DS. In vitro synergistic activity of colistin with aminoglycosides, beta-lactams and rifampin against multidrug-resistant gram-negative bacteria. J Chemother 2007;19(2):226–9.
37. Petrosillo N, Ioannidou E, Falagas ME. Colistin monotherapy vs. combination therapy: evidence from microbiological, animal and clinical studies. Clin Microbiol Infect 2008;14(9):816–27.
38. Song JY, Lee J, Heo JY, et al. Colistin and rifampicin combination in the treatment of ventilator-associated pneumonia caused by carbapenem-resistant *Acinetobacter baumannii*. Int J Antimicrob Agents 2008;32(3):281–4.
39. Tascini C, Ferranti S, Messina F, et al. In vitro and in vivo synergistic activity of colistin, rifampin, and amikacin against a multiresistant *Pseudomonas aeruginosa* isolate. Clin Microbiol Infect 2000;6(12):690–1.
40. Principe L, D'Arezzo S, Capone A, et al. In vitro activity of tigecycline in combination with various antimicrobials against multidrug resistant acinetobacter baumannii. Ann Clin Microbiol Antimicrob 2009;8:18.

41. Hartzell JD, Neff R, Ake J, et al. Nephrotoxicity associated with intravenous colistin (colistimethate sodium) treatment at a tertiary care medical center. Clin Infect Dis 2009;48(12):1724–8.

42. Wallace SJ, Li J, Nation RL, et al. Subacute toxicity of colistin methanesulfonate in rats: comparison of various intravenous dosage regimens. Antimicrob Agents Chemother 2008;52(3):1159–61.

43. Bosso JA, Liptak CA, Seilheimer DK, et al. Toxicity of colistin in cystic fibrosis patients. DICP 1991;25(11):1168–70.

44. Garnacho-Montero J, Ortiz-Leyba C, Jimenez-Jimenez FJ, et al. Treatment of multidrug-resistant Acinetobacter baumannii ventilator-associated pneumonia (VAP) with intravenous colistin: a comparison with imipenem-susceptible VAP. Clin Infect Dis 2003;36(9):1111–8.

45. Rios FG, Luna CM, Maskin B, et al. Ventilator-associated pneumonia due to colistin susceptible-only microorganisms. Eur Respir J 2007;30(2):307–13.

46. Paul M, Bishara J, Levcovich A, et al. Effectiveness and safety of colistin: prospective comparative cohort study. J Antimicrob Chemother 2010;65(5): 1019–27.

47. Falagas ME, Bliziotis IA, Tam VH. Intraventricular or intrathecal use of polymyxins in patients with gram-negative meningitis: a systematic review of the available evidence. Int J Antimicrob Agents 2007;29(1):9–25.

48. Cascio A, Conti A, Sinardi L, et al. Post-neurosurgical multidrug-resistant acinetobacter baumannii meningitis successfully treated with intrathecal colistin. A new case and a systematic review of the literature. Int J Infect Dis 2010;14(7):e572–9.

49. Segal-Maurer S, Mariano N, Qavi A, et al. Successful treatment of ceftazidime-resistant Klebsiella pneumoniae ventriculitis with intravenous meropenem and intraventricular polymyxin B: case report and review. Clin Infect Dis 1999; 28(5):1134–8.

50. Gump WC, Walsh JW. Intrathecal colistin for treatment of highly resistant pseudomonas ventriculitis. Case report and review of the literature. J Neurosurg 2005;102(5):915–7.

51. Kofteridis DP, Alexopoulou C, Valachis A, et al. Aerosolized plus intravenous colistin versus intravenous colistin alone for the treatment of ventilator-associated pneumonia: a matched case-control study. Clin Infect Dis 2010;51(11): 1238–44.

52. Hartzell JD, Kim AS, Kortepeter MG, et al. Acinetobacter pneumonia: a review. MedGenMed 2007;9(3):4.

53. Tunkel AR, Hartman BJ, Kaplan SL, et al. Practice guidelines for the management of bacterial meningitis. Clin Infect Dis 2004;39(9):1267–84.

54. Beringer P. The clinical use of colistin in patients with cystic fibrosis. Curr Opin Pulm Med 2001;7(6):434–40.

55. Maragakis LL, Perl TM. Acinetobacter baumannii: epidemiology, antimicrobial resistance, and treatment options. Clin Infect Dis 2008;46(8):1254–63.

56. Matthaiou DK, Michalopoulos A, Rafailidis PI, et al. Risk factors associated with the isolation of colistin-resistant gram-negative bacteria: a matched case-control study. Crit Care Med 2008;36(3):807–11.

57. Huang DB, DuPont HL. Rifaximin–a novel antimicrobial for enteric infections. J Infect 2005;50(2):97–106.

58. Paramasivan CN, Sulochana S, Kubendiran G, et al. Bactericidal action of gatifloxacin, rifampin, and isoniazid on logarithmic- and stationary-phase cultures of Mycobacterium tuberculosis. Antimicrob Agents Chemother 2005;49(2): 627–31.

59. Cappelletty DM. Evaluation of an intracellular pharmacokinetic in vitro infection model as a tool to assess tuberculosis therapy. Int J Antimicrob Agents 2007; 29(2):212–6.

60. Wehrli W, Knusel F, Schmid K, et al. Interaction of rifamycin with bacterial RNA polymerase. Proc Natl Acad Sci U S A 1968;61(2):667–73.

61. Bundtzen RW, Gerber AU, Cohn DL, et al. Postantibiotic suppression of bacterial growth. Rev Infect Dis 1981;3(1):28–37.

62. Thornsberry C, Hill BC, Swenson JM, et al. Rifampin: spectrum of antibacterial activity. Rev Infect Dis 1983;5(Suppl 3):S412–7.

63. Pohlod DJ, Saravolatz LD, Somerville MM. In-vitro susceptibility of gram-positive cocci to LY146032 teicoplanin, sodium fusidate, vancomycin, and rifampicin. J Antimicrob Chemother 1987;20(2):197–202.

64. Klugman KP, Madhi SA. Emergence of drug resistance. Impact on bacterial meningitis. Infect Dis Clin North Am 1999;13(3):637–46, vii.

65. Watanakunakorn C, Tisone JC. Antagonism between nafcillin or oxacillin and rifampin against Staphylococcus aureus. Antimicrob Agents Chemother 1982; 22(5):920–2.

66. Zak O, Scheld WM, Sande MA. Rifampin in experimental endocarditis due to Staphylococcus aureus in rabbits. Rev Infect Dis 1983;5(Suppl 3):S481–90.

67. Kobasa WD, Kaye KL, Shapiro T, et al. Therapy for experimental endocarditis due to Staphylococcus epidermidis. Rev Infect Dis 1983;5(Suppl 3):S533–7.

68. Karchmer AW, Archer GL, Dismukes WE. Staphylococcus epidermidis causing prosthetic valve endocarditis: microbiologic and clinical observations as guides to therapy. Ann Intern Med 1983;98(4):447–55.

69. Friedland IR, Paris M, Ehrett S, et al. Evaluation of antimicrobial regimens for treatment of experimental penicillin- and cephalosporin-resistant pneumococcal meningitis. Antimicrob Agents Chemother 1993;37(8):1630–6.

70. Martinez-Lacasa J, Cabellos C, Martos A, et al. Experimental study of the efficacy of vancomycin, rifampicin and dexamethasone in the therapy of pneumococcal meningitis. J Antimicrob Chemother 2002;49(3):507–13.

71. Fitoussi F, Doit C, Geslin P, et al. Killing activities of trovafloxacin alone and in combination with beta-lactam agents, rifampin, or vancomycin against Streptococcus pneumoniae isolates with various susceptibilities to extended-spectrum cephalosporins at concentrations clinically achievable in cerebrospinal fluid. Antimicrob Agents Chemother 1999;43(10):2372–5.

72. Bassetti M, Repetto E, Righi E, et al. Colistin and rifampicin in the treatment of multidrug-resistant Acinetobacter baumannii infections. J Antimicrob Chemother 2008;61(2):417–20.

73. Baciewicz AM, Chrisman CR, Finch CK, et al. Update on rifampin and rifabutin drug interactions. Am J Med Sci 2008;335(2):126–36.

74. Mahatthanatrakul W, Nontaput T, Ridtitid W, et al. Rifampin, a cytochrome P450 3A inducer, decreases plasma concentrations of antipsychotic risperidone in healthy volunteers. J Clin Pharm Ther 2007;32(2):161–7.

75. Kwara A, Ramachandran G, Swaminathan S. Dose adjustment of the non-nucleoside reverse transcriptase inhibitors during concurrent rifampicin-containing tuberculosis therapy: one size does not fit all. Expert Opin Drug Metab Toxicol 2010;6(1):55–68.

76. Fraser A, Gafter-Gvili A, Paul M, et al. Antibiotics for preventing meningococcal infections. Cochrane Database Syst Rev 2006;4:CD004785.

77. Gardner P. Clinical practice. Prevention of meningococcal disease. N Engl J Med 2006;355(14):1466–73.

78. Rainbow J, Cebelinski E, Bartkus J, et al. Rifampin-resistant meningococcal disease. Emerg Infect Dis 2005;11(6):977–9.

79. Stefanelli P, Neri A, Carattoli A, et al. Detection of resistance to rifampicin and decreased susceptibility to penicillin in *Neisseria meningitidis* by real-time multiplex polymerase chain reaction assay. Diagn Microbiol Infect Dis 2007;58(2):241–4.

80. Cuevas LE, Kazembe P, Mughogho GK, et al. Eradication of nasopharyngeal carriage of *Neisseria meningitidis* in children and adults in rural Africa: a comparison of ciprofloxacin and rifampicin. J Infect Dis 1995;171(3):728–31.

81. Perlroth J, Kuo M, Tan J, et al. Adjunctive use of rifampin for the treatment of *Staphylococcus aureus* infections: a systematic review of the literature. Arch Intern Med 2008;168(8):805–19.

82. Morris AB, Brown RB, Sands M. Use of rifampin in nonstaphylococcal, nonmycobacterial disease. Antimicrob Agents Chemother 1993;37(1):1–7.

83. Bayston R, Nuradeen B, Ashraf W, et al. Antibiotics for the eradication of *Propionibacterium acnes* biofilms in surgical infection. J Antimicrob Chemother 2007; 60(6):1298–301.

84. Baddour LM, Wilson WR, Bayer AS, et al. Infective endocarditis: diagnosis, antimicrobial therapy, and management of complications: a statement for healthcare professionals from the Committee on Rheumatic Fever, Endocarditis, and Kawasaki Disease, Council on Cardiovascular Disease in the Young, and the Councils on Clinical Cardiology, Stroke, and Cardiovascular Surgery and Anesthesia, American Heart Association: endorsed by the Infectious Diseases Society of America. Circulation 2005;111(23):e394–434.

85. Norden CW. Experimental chronic staphylococcal osteomyelitis in rabbits: treatment with rifampin alone and in combination with other antimicrobial agents. Rev Infect Dis 1983;5(Suppl 3):S491–4.

86. Bliziotis IA, Ntziora F, Lawrence KR, et al. Rifampin as adjuvant treatment of gram-positive bacterial infections: a systematic review of comparative clinical trials. Eur J Clin Microbiol Infect Dis 2007;26(12):849–56.

87. Falagas ME, Bliziotis IA, Fragoulis KN. Oral rifampin for eradication of *Staphylococcus aureus* carriage from healthy and sick populations: a systematic review of the evidence from comparative trials. Am J Infect Control 2007; 35(2):106–14.

88. Simor AE, Phillips E, McGeer A, et al. Randomized controlled trial of chlorhexidine gluconate for washing, intranasal mupirocin, and rifampin and doxycycline versus no treatment for the eradication of methicillin-resistant *Staphylococcus aureus* colonization. Clin Infect Dis 2007;44(2):178–85.

89. Skalsky K, Yahav D, Bishara J, et al. Treatment of human brucellosis: systematic review and meta-analysis of randomised controlled trials. BMJ 2008;336(7646): 701–4.

90. Ranjbar M, Keramat F, Mamani M, et al. Comparison between doxycycline-rifampin-amikacin and doxycycline-rifampin regimens in the treatment of brucellosis. Int J Infect Dis 2007;11(2):152–6.

91. DuPont HL. Biologic properties and clinical uses of rifaximin. Expert Opin Pharmacother 2011;12(2):293–302.

92. Ripa S, Mignini F, Prenna M, et al. In vitro antibacterial activity of rifaximin against *Clostridium difficile*, *Campylobacter jejunii* and *Yersinia spp*. Drugs Exp Clin Res 1987;13(8):483–8.

93. DuPont HL, Jiang ZD. Influence of rifaximin treatment on the susceptibility of intestinal gram-negative flora and enterococci. Clin Microbiol Infect 2004; 10(11):1009–11.

94. Brigidi P, Swennen E, Rizzello F, et al. Effects of rifaximin administration on the intestinal microbiota in patients with ulcerative colitis. J Chemother 2002; 14(3):290–5.

95. Ouyang-Latimer J, Jafri S, VanTassel A, et al. In vitro antimicrobial susceptibility of bacterial enteropathogens isolated from international travelers to Mexico, Guatemala, and India from 2006 to 2008. Antimicrob Agents Chemother 2011; 55(2):874–8.

96. Valentin T, Leitner E, Rohn A, et al. Rifaximin intake leads to emergence of rifampin-resistant staphylococci. J Infect 2011;62(1):34–8.

97. DuPont HL, Jiang ZD, Ericsson CD, et al. Rifaximin versus ciprofloxacin for the treatment of traveler's diarrhea: a randomized, double-blind clinical trial. Clin Infect Dis 2001;33(11):1807–15.

98. Taylor DN, Bourgeois AL, Ericsson CD, et al. A randomized, double-blind, multicenter study of rifaximin compared with placebo and with ciprofloxacin in the treatment of travelers' diarrhea. Am J Trop Med Hyg 2006;74(6): 1060–6.

99. Steffen R, Sack DA, Riopel L, et al. Therapy of travelers' diarrhea with rifaximin on various continents. Am J Gastroenterol 2003;98(5):1073–8.

100. Pentikis HS, Connolly M, Trapnell CB, et al. The effect of multiple-dose, oral rifaximin on the pharmacokinetics of intravenous and oral midazolam in healthy volunteers. Pharmacotherapy 2007;27(10):1361–9.

101. Jiang ZD, DuPont HL, La Rocco M, et al. In vitro susceptibility of clostridium difficile to rifaximin and rifampin in 359 consecutive isolates at a university hospital in Houston, Texas. J Clin Pathol 2010;63(4):355–8.

102. McFarland LV. Emerging therapies for clostridium difficile infections. Expert Opin Emerg Drugs 2011. [Epub ahead of print].

103. Kokkotou E, Moss AC, Michos A, et al. Comparative efficacies of rifaximin and vancomycin for treatment of Clostridium difficile-associated diarrhea and prevention of disease recurrence in hamsters. Antimicrob Agents Chemother 2008;52(3):1121–6.

104. Berman AL. Efficacy of rifaximin and vancomycin combination therapy in a patient with refractory Clostridium difficile-associated diarrhea. J Clin Gastroenterol 2007;41(10):932–3.

105. Johnson S, Schriever C, Galang M, et al. Interruption of recurrent Clostridium difficile-associated diarrhea episodes by serial therapy with vancomycin and rifaximin. Clin Infect Dis 2007;44(6):846–8.

106. Drusano GL, Louie A. Optimization of aminoglycoside therapy. Antimicrob Agents Chemother 2011. [Epub ahead of print].

107. Falagas ME, Matthaiou DK, Bliziotis IA. The role of aminoglycosides in combination with a beta-lactam for the treatment of bacterial endocarditis: a meta-analysis of comparative trials. J Antimicrob Chemother 2006;57(4):639–47.

108. Lentino JR, Narita M, Yu VL. New antimicrobial agents as therapy for resistant gram-positive cocci. Eur J Clin Microbiol Infect Dis 2008;27(1):3–15.

109. Rea RS, Capitano B. Optimizing use of aminoglycosides in the critically ill. Semin Respir Crit Care Med 2007;28(6):596–603.

110. Cunha BA. New uses for older antibiotics: nitrofurantoin, amikacin, colistin, polymyxin B, doxycycline, and minocycline revisited. Med Clin North Am 2006;90(6): 1089–107.

111. Friedland I, Gallagher G, King T, et al. Antimicrobial susceptibility patterns in Pseudomonas aeruginosa: data from a multicenter Intensive Care Unit Surveillance Study (ISS) in the United States. J Chemother 2004;16(5):437–41.

112. Buijk SE, Mouton JW, Gyssens IC, et al. Experience with a once-daily dosing program of aminoglycosides in critically ill patients. Intensive Care Med 2002; 28(7):936–42.
113. Turnidge J. Pharmacodynamics and dosing of aminoglycosides. Infect Dis Clin North Am 2003;17(3):503–28, v.
114. McKenzie C. Antibiotic dosing in critical illness. J Antimicrob Chemother 2011; 66(Suppl 2):ii25–31.
115. Isaksson B, Nilsson L, Maller R, et al. Postantibiotic effect of aminoglycosides on gram-negative bacteria evaluated by a new method. J Antimicrob Chemother 1988;22(1):23–33.
116. Craig W. Pharmacodynamics of antimicrobial agents as a basis for determining dosage regimens. Eur J Clin Microbiol Infect Dis 1993;12(Suppl 1):S6–8.
117. Kapusnik JE, Hackbarth CJ, Chambers HF, et al. Single, large, daily dosing versus intermittent dosing of tobramycin for treating experimental pseudomonas pneumonia. J Infect Dis 1988;158(1):7–12.
118. Baudoux P, Bles N, Lemaire S, et al. Combined effect of pH and concentration on the activities of gentamicin and oxacillin against Staphylococcus aureus in pharmacodynamic models of extracellular and intracellular infections. J Antimicrob Chemother 2007;59(2):246–53.
119. Simmen HP, Battaglia H, Kossmann T, et al. Effect of peritoneal fluid pH on outcome of aminoglycoside treatment of intraabdominal infections. World J Surg 1993;17(3):393–7.
120. Harrell LJ, Evans JB. Anaerobic resistance of clinical isolates of Staphylococcus aureus to aminoglycosides. Antimicrob Agents Chemother 1978;14(6): 927–9.
121. Barclay ML, Begg EJ. Aminoglycoside adaptive resistance: importance for effective dosage regimens. Drugs 2001;61(6):713–21.
122. Skiada A, Markogiannakis A, Plachouras D, et al. Adaptive resistance to cationic compounds in Pseudomonas aeruginosa. Int J Antimicrob Agents 2011;37(3): 187–93.
123. Chandrakanth RK, Raju S, Patil SA. Aminoglycoside-resistance mechanisms in multidrug-resistant Staphylococcus aureus clinical isolates. Curr Microbiol 2008;56(6):558–62.
124. Verpooten GA, Giuliano RA, Verbist L, et al. Once-daily dosing decreases renal accumulation of gentamicin and netilmicin. Clin Pharmacol Ther 1989;45(1):22–7.
125. Bennett WM, Plamp CE, Gilbert DN, et al. The influence of dosage regimen on experimental gentamicin nephrotoxicity: dissociation of peak serum levels from renal failure. J Infect Dis 1979;140(4):576–80.
126. Mavros MN, Polyzos KA, Rafailidis PI, et al. Once versus multiple daily dosing of aminoglycosides for patients with febrile neutropenia: a systematic review and meta-analysis. J Antimicrob Chemother 2011;66(2):251–9.
127. Rybak MJ, Abate BJ, Kang SL, et al. Prospective evaluation of the effect of an aminoglycoside dosing regimen on rates of observed nephrotoxicity and ototoxicity. Antimicrob Agents Chemother 1999;43(7):1549–55.
128. Barbieri CD, Oliveira GM, Zanetta DM, et al. Prevalence and risk factors for aminoglycoside nephrotoxicity in intensive care units. Antimicrob Agents Chemother 2009;53(7):2887–91.
129. Baciewicz AM, Sokos DR, Cowan RI. Aminoglycoside-associated nephrotoxicity in the elderly. Ann Pharmacother 2003;37(2):182–6.
130. Rougier F, Claude D, Maurin M, et al. Aminoglycoside nephrotoxicity. Curr Drug Targets Infect Disord 2004;4(2):153–62.

131. Rybak LP, Ramkumar V. Ototoxicity. Kidney Int 2007;72(8):931–5.
132. Tran Ba Huy P, Bernard P, Schacht J. Kinetics of gentamicin uptake and release in the rat. Comparison of inner ear tissues and fluids with other organs. J Clin Invest 1986;77(5):1492–500.
133. Gatell JM, Ferran F, Araujo V, et al. Univariate and multivariate analyses of risk factors predisposing to auditory toxicity in patients receiving aminoglycosides. Antimicrob Agents Chemother 1987;31(9):1383–7.
134. Ariano RE, Zelenitsky SA, Kassum DA. Aminoglycoside-induced vestibular injury: maintaining a sense of balance. Ann Pharmacother 2008;42(9): 1282–9.
135. Nicolau DP, Freeman CD, Belliveau PP, et al. Experience with a once-daily aminoglycoside program administered to 2,184 adult patients. Antimicrob Agents Chemother 1995;39(3):650–5.
136. Prins JM, Weverling GJ, de Blok K, et al. Validation and nephrotoxicity of a simplified once-daily aminoglycoside dosing schedule and guidelines for monitoring therapy. Antimicrob Agents Chemother 1996;40(11):2494–9.
137. Graham JC, Gould FK. Role of aminoglycosides in the treatment of bacterial endocarditis. J Antimicrob Chemother 2002;49(3):437–44.
138. Smyth AR, Tan KH. Once-daily versus multiple-daily dosing with intravenous aminoglycosides for cystic fibrosis. Cochrane Database Syst Rev 2006;3: CD002009.
139. Ratjen F. Treatment of early *Pseudomonas aeruginosa* infection in patients with cystic fibrosis. Curr Opin Pulm Med 2006;12(6):428–32.
140. Wood DM, Smyth AR. Antibiotic strategies for eradicating *Pseudomonas aeruginosa* in people with cystic fibrosis. Cochrane Database Syst Rev 2006;1: CD004197.
141. Smyth A, Tan KH, Hyman-Taylor P, et al. Once versus three-times daily regimens of tobramycin treatment for pulmonary exacerbations of cystic fibrosis–the TOPIC study: a randomised controlled trial. Lancet 2005;365(9459):573–8.
142. Weiner JR, Toy EL, Sacco P, et al. Costs, quality of life and treatment compliance associated with antibiotic therapies in patients with cystic fibrosis: a review of the literature. Expert Opin Pharmacother 2008;9(5):751–66.
143. Dopfer R, Brand P, Mullinger B, et al. Inhalation of tobramycin in patients with cystic fibrosis: comparison of two methods. J Physiol Pharmacol 2007; 58(Suppl 5 Pt 1):141–54.
144. Lenoir G, Antypkin YG, Miano A, et al. Efficacy, safety, and local pharmacokinetics of highly concentrated nebulized tobramycin in patients with cystic fibrosis colonized with *Pseudomonas aeruginosa*. Paediatr Drugs 2007; 9(Suppl 1):11–20.
145. Goss CH. Should we stop using intravenous gentamicin in patients with cystic fibrosis? Thorax 2008;63(6):479–80.
146. de Groot R, Smith AL. Antibiotic pharmacokinetics in cystic fibrosis. Differences and clinical significance. Clin Pharmacokinet 1987;13(4):228–53.
147. Vic P, Ategbo S, Turck D, et al. Efficacy, tolerance, and pharmacokinetics of once daily tobramycin for pseudomonas exacerbations in cystic fibrosis. Arch Dis Child 1998;78(6):536–9.
148. Bragonier R, Brown NM. The pharmacokinetics and toxicity of once-daily tobramycin therapy in children with cystic fibrosis. J Antimicrob Chemother 1998; 42(1):103–6.
149. Banerjee D, Stableforth D. The treatment of respiratory pseudomonas infection in cystic fibrosis: what drug and which way? Drugs 2000;60(5):1053–64.

150. Beringer PM, Vinks AA, Jelliffe RW, et al. Pharmacokinetics of tobramycin in adults with cystic fibrosis: implications for once-daily administration. Antimicrob Agents Chemother 2000;44(4):809–13.

151. Byl B, Baran D, Jacobs F, et al. Serum pharmacokinetics and sputum penetration of amikacin 30 mg/kg once daily and of ceftazidime 200 mg/kg/day as a continuous infusion in cystic fibrosis patients. J Antimicrob Chemother 2001; 48(2):325–7.

152. Touw DJ, Knox AJ, Smyth A. Population pharmacokinetics of tobramycin administered thrice daily and once daily in children and adults with cystic fibrosis. J Cyst Fibros 2007;6(5):327–33.

153. Al-Lanqawi Y, Capps P, Abdel-hamid M, et al. Therapeutic drug monitoring of gentamicin: evaluation of five nomograms for initial dosing at Al-Amiri hospital in Kuwait. Med Princ Pract 2007;16(5):348–54.

154. Barclay ML, Kirkpatrick CM, Begg EJ. Once daily aminoglycoside therapy. Is it less toxic than multiple daily doses and how should it be monitored? Clin Pharmacokinet 1999;36(2):89–98.

155. Bailey TC, Little JR, Littenberg B, et al. A meta-analysis of extended-interval dosing versus multiple daily dosing of aminoglycosides. Clin Infect Dis 1997; 24(5):786–95.

156. Tod MM, Padoin C, Petitjean O. Individualising aminoglycoside dosage regimens after therapeutic drug monitoring: simple or complex pharmacokinetic methods? Clin Pharmacokinet 2001;40(11):803–14.

157. Barclay ML, Duffull SB, Begg EJ, et al. Experience of once-daily aminoglycoside dosing using a target area under the concentration-time curve. Aust N Z J Med 1995;25(3):230–5.

158. Paterson DL, Robson JM, Wagener MM, et al. Monitoring of serum aminoglycoside levels with once-daily dosing. Pathology 1998;30(3):289–94.

159. Bartal C, Danon A, Schlaeffer F, et al. Pharmacokinetic dosing of aminoglycosides: a controlled trial. Am J Med 2003;114(3):194–8.

160. Urban AW, Craig WA. Daily dosage of aminoglycosides. Curr Clin Top Infect Dis 1997;17:236–55.

Index

Note: Page numbers of article titles are in **boldface** type.

A

Achilles tendon rupture, in fluoroquinolone therapy, 804–805
Acinetobacter, resistance in, 660–661
Active efflux, as resistance mechanism, 649
Alcohols, for hand hygiene, 709
Amikacin, dosing of, in renal failure, 681–682, 690
Aminoglycosides, 828–833
    activity of, 828–829
    clinical indications for, 831–833
    dosing of, in renal failure, 681–682
    inactivating enzymes of, 649
    mechanism of action of, 828–829
    pharmacokinetics of, 829–830
    resistance to, 829
        in *Acinetobacter,* 660–661
        in enterococci, 650–651
    serum levels of, in renal failure, 691–692
    toxicity of, 830–831
Amoxicillin, dosing of, in renal failure, 688
AmpC gene, in Gram-negative rods, 659–660
Ampicillin
    dosing of, in renal failure, 688
    resistance to, 663
Anthrax, fluoroquinolones for, 808, 811
Antibacterial agents. *See also specific agents and types of agents.*
    fluoroquinolones. *See* Fluoroquinolones.
    for Gram-positive bacterial infections, **723–742**
    glycylcyclines, **761–791**
    in renal failure, **677–702**
    ketolids, **761–791**
    macrolides, **761–791**
    new beta-lactam type, **743–760**
    new uses for, **819–842**
    resistance to. *See* Resistance.
    topical, **703–721**
Antiseptics, 703–706
Arrhythmias, in fluoroquinolone therapy, 805
Arteriovenous hemodialysis, continuous, antibacterial agent dosing with, 694
Arteriovenous hemofiltration, continuous, antibacterial agent dosing with, 694
Arthropathy, in fluoroquinolone therapy, 804–805
Azelaic acid, 705

Med Clin N Am 95 (2011) 843–854
doi:10.1016/S0025-7125(11)00051-4
0025-7125/11/$ – see front matter © 2011 Elsevier Inc. All rights reserved.

medical.theclinics.com

Moving?

Make sure your subscription moves with you!

To notify us of your new address, find your **Clinics Account Number** (located on your mailing label above your name), and contact customer service at:

Email: journalscustomerservice-usa@elsevier.com

800-654-2452 (subscribers in the U.S. & Canada)
314-447-8871 (subscribers outside of the U.S. & Canada)

Fax number: 314-447-8029

Elsevier Health Sciences Division
Subscription Customer Service
3251 Riverport Lane
Maryland Heights, MO 63043

*To ensure uninterrupted delivery of your subscription, please notify us at least 4 weeks in advance of move.